THE EXPANDING ROLE
OF FOLATES AND
FLUOROPYRIMIDINES IN
CANCER CHEMOTHERAPY

ADVANCES IN EXPERIMENTAL MEDICINE AND BIOLOGY

Recent Volumes in this Series

THE EXPANDING ROLE OF FOLATES AND FLUOROPYRIMIDINES IN CANCER CHEMOTHERAPY

Edited by

Youcef Rustum and
John J. McGuire

Roswell Park Memorial Institute
Buffalo, New York

PLENUM PRESS • NEW YORK AND LONDON

Library of Congress Cataloging in Publication Data

International Symposium on the Expanding Role of Folates and Fluoropyrimidines in
Cancer Chemotherapy (1988: Buffalo, N.Y.)
   The expanding role of folates and fluoropyrimidines in cancer chemotherapy /
edited by Youcef Rustum and John J. McGuire.
      p.   cm. — (Advances in experimental medicine and biology; v. 244)
   "Proceedings of an International Symposium on the Expanding Role of Folates and
Fluoropyrimidines in Cancer Chemotherapy, held April 28-29, 1988, in Buffalo, New
York" — T.p. verso.
   Includes bibliographies and index.
   ISBN 0-306-43100-9
   1. Fluoropyrimidines — Therapeutic use — Testing — Congresses. 2. Folinic acid —
Therapeutic use — Testing — Congresses. 3. Fluorouracil — Therapeutic use — Testing —
Congresses. 4. Cancer — Chemotherapy — Congresses. I. Rustum, Youcef M. II.
McGuire, John J. III. Title. IV. Series.
   [DNLM: 1. Fluorouracil — therapeutic use — congresses. 2. Folic Acid — therapeutic
use — congresses. 3. Neoplasms — drug therapy — congresses. QZ 267 16175e 1988]
RC271.F55I59 1988
616.99′4061 — dc19
DNLM/DLC   88-38105
for Library of Congress   CIP

Proceedings of an International Symposium on the Expanding Role of
Folates and Fluoropyrimidines in Cancer Chemotherapy,
held April 28-29, 1988, in Buffalo, New York

© 1988 Plenum Press, New York
A Division of Plenum Publishing Corporation
233 Spring Street, New York, N.Y. 10013

Printed in the United States of America

PREFACE

Although 5-fluorouracil (FUra) is the drug of choice for the treatment of patients with advanced colorectal cancer, this agent has limited effectiveness with a reported response rate of 10-20% and a duration of response of only 6-9 months. The large percentage of treatment failures with this agent has spurred a continuing effort to delineate the mechanism(s) of resistance to FUra and to evaluate approaches that would selectively modulate the therapeutic efficacy of this agent.

The therapeutic efficacy of FUra has been attributed to its selective incorporation into RNA and to its inhibition of thymidylate synthase, leading to potent inhibition of DNA synthesis. Studies of cell lines in vitro and model systems in vivo have demonstrated that although mechanisms of sensitivity and resistance to FUra are multifactorial, in the presence of citrovorum factor (CF, 5-formyltetrahydrofolate) the site of action of FUra becomes predominantly the pronounced and prolonged inhibition of thymidylate synthase. This action is the result of stabilization of the covalent ternary complex between FdUMP, an active metabolite of FUra, 5,10-methylenetetrahydrofolates, and thymidylate synthase. This effect of CF is thus an example of the concept of metabolic modulation.

CF is commercially available as a racemic mixture of diastereoisomers (6R and 6S). The 6R isomer is considered to be biologically inactive; the 6S isomer is the biologically active form that is metabolized intracellularly to form the various folate cofactor pools including 5,10-methylenetetrahydrofolates. Although the extent of metabolism of folates in normal and tumor tissues has not been clearly delineated, it is possible that in some tumor tissues the formation of folylpolyglutamates is a function of both the dose and schedule of CF administration. Thus, it appears that for optimal modulation of FUra activity several factors must be considered simultaneously. These include the dose and schedule of administration of CF, the intracellular concentrations of the various folylpolyglutamate forms, the level of thymidylate synthase, and the degree and duration of inhibition of thymidylate synthase. The latter is also influenced by the absolute and relative intracellular concentrations of FdUMP and the competing metabolite, dUMP.

This symposium had four goals:

1) To discuss the biochemical, pharmacological and molecular determinants of response to FUra in combination with CF (FUra/CF).

2) To identify conditions for optimal modulation of FUra activity.

3) To update and review the response rate and duration of response of patients treated with this combination.

4) To define the future direction for this combination in patients with advanced malignancies.

On day one of this symposium, studies related to the first two goals were discussed. Identification and evaluation of determinants of response to FUra in combination with CF were emphasized. The role of the 6R and 6S diastereomers of CF, and the effects of the schedule and route of administration of CF in FUra modulation were points of focus.

On the second day of this symposium, a review and update of the clinical results with FUra/CF in patients with various malignancies were discussed. Since various doses and schedules of FUra and CF have been employed clinically, it was hoped that knowledge would be gained as to the optimal conditions for FUra modulation. The question of whether CF is selectively modulating the therapeutic efficacy of FUra was addressed by a number of the participants. It was clear that the clinical pattern of host tissue toxicity of FUra had been altered by CF, with mucositis and gastrointestinal toxicities predominating.

The results of these various clinical trials, based on strong rationales derived from in vitro and in vivo laboratory studies, reinforces the need for further laboratory investigations aimed at optimization of conditions and parameters responsible for selective modulation of FUra by CF. It is clearly evident from the results of clinical trials conducted to date that a better understanding of the role of dose, schedule and route of administration of CF in the selective modulation of fluoropyrimidines is required.

On behalf of the organizing committee (Drs. Rustum, Creaven, McGuire, Mihich and Mittelman), we would like to take this opportunity to thank the speakers, discussants and attendees for their valuable contributions to this symposium. The success of this symposium should be credited to the tireless efforts of Ms. Gayle Bersani and Ms. Geri Wagner to whom we are indebted. We would like also to thank Ms. Cheryl Melancon and Ms. Mae Brown for their help in typing manuscripts, transcribing the discussions, and preparing correspondence.

Major support of this symposium was generously provided by Burroughs Wellcome, the Lederle Division of American Cyanamid, Kyowa Hakko Kogyo, Co., and the Food and Drug Administration. Without their generous financial support this 2 day symposium would not have been possible. Additional support was provided by Hoffman-LaRoche, Bristol Myers, Upjohn, and Marine Midland Bank.

This symposium was held to honor Maire T. Hakala, Ph.D. for her outstanding contributions to the field of cancer research. Recently, Maire retired from active scientific duties following 31 years of productive research at Roswell Park Memorial Institute. It is her research on mechanisms of action of fluoropyrimidines alone and in combination with CF that provided the scientific basis for the development of clinical trials at Roswell Park Memorial Institute and elsewhere. We all shall miss her and wish her the best in all future endeavors.

Youcef M. Rustum   John J. McGuire
Co-Editor   Co-Editor

CONTENTS

OVERVIEW: RATIONAL BASIS FOR DEVELOPMENT OF

FLUOROPYRIMIDINE/5-FORMYLTETRAHYDROFOLATE COMBINATION CHEMOTHERAPY[*]

F.M. Huennekens, Y.D. Montejano and K.S. Vitols

Division of Biochemistry
Department of Basic and Clinical Research
Research Institute of Scripps Clinic
La Jolla, California 92037

SUMMARY

Fluorodeoxyuridylate (FdUMP) and thymidylate synthase (TS) are one of the better understood systems of drug-target interaction in cancer chemotherapy. Isolation and characterization of TS (initially from *Lactobacillus casei* and later from a variety of other sources), cloning and sequencing of the gene, determination of the 3-D structure of the enzyme by X-ray diffraction, and elucidation of the structure of both the catalytic intermediate and the enzyme-inhibitor complex have revealed critical parameters of the target at the molecular level. Potentiation of FdUMP binding by 5,10-methylenetetrahydrofolate (CH_2-FH_4), discovered at the enzymatic level, has been exploited to increase the clinical effectiveness of fluoropyrimidines. CH_2-FH_4 can be generated from folate, 5-methyltetrahydrofolate, or 5-formyltetrahydrofolate (citrovorum factor, CF); the latter is the compound of choice for therapeutic regimens. Transformation of CF to CH_2-FH_4 can occur via two pathways: (a) CF —> 5,10-methenyltetrahydrofolate —> CH_2-FH_4; or (b) CF —> tetrahydrofolate —> CH_2-FH_4. The relative importance of these pathways in various cells is not yet clear. The role of CH_2-FH_4 in FdUMP toxicity, and its central position in folate coenzyme-dependent C_1 metabolism, emphasize the need for development of methods to quantitate intracellular levels of this compound.

EMPIRICAL AND RATIONAL APPROACHES TO DRUG DEVELOPMENT: SEPARATE ROADS TO A COMMON OBJECTIVE

Cancer chemotherapy continues to improve, although still too slowly, by optimizing the regimens of existing drugs and by the development of new drugs. The latter is accomplished either by an empirical approach in which large numbers of compounds (naturally-occurring or synthetic) are screened for anti-tumor activity or by a rational approach in which smaller numbers of specific compounds are synthesized with some *a priori* target or strategy in mind. Each approach has its merits; each has

---

[*] This is publication 5359-BCR from the Research Institute of Scripps Clinic. Experimental work was supported by Grant CA-39836 (Outstanding Investigator Award) from the National Cancer Institute and Grant CH-31 from the American Cancer Society.

1

produced useful drugs. Acivicin, for example, was encountered in a survey
of fermentation broths, and maytansine was found in the extract of an
exotic plant. Tiazofurin and N-(phosphonacetyl)-aspartate (PALA),
alternatively, were synthesized for specific purposes, viz., to inhibit
IMP dehydrogenase and aspartate transcarbamoylase.

Despite these and other clear accomplishments, there still lurks the
belief that "rational" is a complimentary term, while "empirical" is one
of opprobrium. More balanced views, fortunately, have placed this matter
in proper perspective. Hitchings (1), for example, has commented that
"One has heard a great deal about the need for, and the possibility of, a
rational chemotherapy. In the minds of some, chemotherapy would be
rational only when new agents could be produced on demand, fully formed,
like the heroes who arose from the dragon's teeth of Jason. Perhaps this
rational chemotherapy will arrive in one glorious stroke of genius. It
seems more likely, however, that it will arrive by small increments of
progress and for this reason unheralded". And, similarly, Friedkin (2)
advised that "Insight alone, although seemingly superior to the empirical
approach, is not enough. Our knowledge is too fragmentary. We may be in
the position to make a good guess about potential efficacy but we cannot
predict toxicity. After we are all through inhibiting our favorite
enzymes, we simply cannot be certain that our treated patient will still
have a clear mind, good circulation, a steady heart, clear skin, toes that
don't tingle, kidney and liver in good shape, and unblemished
chromosomes".

Acceptance of fluoropyrimidines as important agents in the
chemotherapeutic arsenal has resulted from the work of a number of
investigators, travelling on both empirical and rational roads. The use
of 5-formyltetrahydrofolate (folinate; citrovorum factor) to potentiate
the cytotoxicity of fluoropyrimidines stands as an excellent example of a
rational approach based upon an understanding of the target enzyme
(thymidylate synthase) and of the pathways for interconversion of folate
coenzymes. These subjects are reviewed briefly in the following sections.

FLUOROPYRIMIDINES IN CANCER CHEMOTHERAPY

The chemical synthesis of 5-fluorouracil (FUra)[1] by Heidelberger and
colleagues in 1957, and the subsequent demonstration of its cytotoxicity
toward several animal tumors (3), stimulated research in many
laboratories. The close structural relationship of FUra to uracil, and
reversal of its cytotoxicity by thymine, suggested that the drug
interfered in some manner with the conversion of uracil to thymine.
Subsequent work proceeded in two general directions: (a) identification
of the fluoropyrimidine species responsible for the cytotoxicity; and (b)
delineation of the target enzyme.

Fluorouracil is metabolized by two different pathways (Fig. 1).
Reaction with deoxyribose-1-P yields the deoxynucleoside (FdUrd), which
becomes phosphorylated to 5-fluorodeoxyuridylate (FdUMP). Alternatively,

---

1. Abbreviations: FUra, 5-fluorouracil; FdUrd, fluorodeoxyuridine; FUrd,
fluorouridine; FdUMP, fluorodeoxyuridylate; TS, thymidylate synthase; F,
folate; FH_2, dihydrofolate; FH_4, tetrahydrofolate; 5-CHO-FH_4 (also CF), 10-
CHO-FH_4, 5,10-CH-FH_4 (or CH-FH_4), 5,10-CH_2-FH_4 (or CH_2-FH_4) and 5-CH_3-FH_4,
5-formyl-, 10-formyl-, 5,10-methenyl-, 5,10-methylene-, and 5-methyl-
tetrahydrofolate.

2

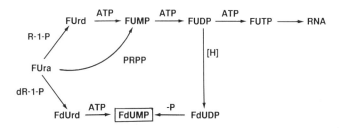

Fig. 1. Metabolism of 5-fluorouracil. For abbreviations, see footnote 1.

reaction of the base with PRPP produces 5-fluorouridine (FUrd) which, after conversion to the nucleoside triphosphate, can be incorporated into RNA. Although interference with RNA function is important, the primary basis for cytotoxicity of FUra is believed to be the inhibition of thymidylate synthase by FdUMP. Discovery of this target/drug combination was made independently by the laboratories of Cohen (4) and Heidelberger (5).

THYMIDYLATE SYNTHASE

Recognition of TS as the enzyme responsible for the conversion of dUMP to dTMP began with the work of Friedkin and Kornberg (6), who demonstrated that, in extracts of *Escherichia coli*, the reaction required serine (as the C_1 source) and FH_4. Further studies by Humphreys and Greenberg (7), using extracts of rat thymus, implicated 5,10-methylene-tetrahydrofolate (CH_2-FH_4) as the co-substrate with dUMP, and the lack of requirement for any additional oxido-reduction components led these investigators to conclude that the tetrahydrofolate moiety supplied the reducing power for the methylene —> methyl conversion. The overall stoichiometry for dTMP synthesis was thus established:

$$CH_2\text{-}FH_4 + dUMP \xrightarrow{\text{TS}} FH_2 + dTMP \qquad (1)$$

It was soon recognized, however, that the *continuous* synthesis of dTMP required regeneration of CH_2-FH_4 via a cyclic process (Fig. 2) involving TS, dihydrofolate reductase and serine hydroxymethyltransferase. Since TS

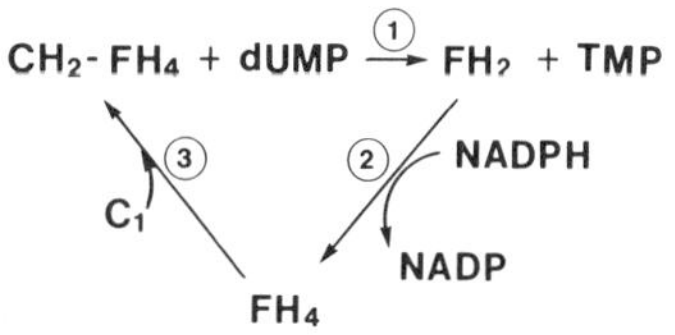

Fig. 2. Thymidylate synthesis cycle. 1, thymidylate synthase; 2, dihydrofolate reductase; 3, serine hydroxymethyltransferase.

was the target for FUra (as FdUMP) and dihydrofolate reductase had been identified previously as the target for Methotrexate (8), this cycle became the focus of attention for investigators in both the antifolate and fluoropyrimidine fields.

Initial studies with TS were conducted with partially purified preparations from different sources (reviewed in (9)). The enzyme was then purified to homogeneity and crystallized from Methotrexate-resistant strains of L. casei (10,11). Although it was not known at the time, the elevated levels of TS (up to several hundred-fold), and also of dihydro-folate reductase, were the result of drug-induced gene amplification in these mutants. For a number of years the L. casei enzyme served as the prototype TS. Key properties common to various thymidylate synthases (e.g., dimeric structure consisting of two 35 kDa peptides, and the presence of one critical -SH group among the total of four in the dimer) were first encountered in the bacterial enzyme.

In subsequent studies, TS was isolated from other sources (reviewed in (12)) and amino acid and gene sequences are being determined (reviewed in (13,14)). The three-dimensional structure of the L. casei enzyme has been determined recently by X-ray diffraction (15). The kinetics and mechanism of the enzyme-catalyzed reaction (eq. 1) and its inhibition by FdUMP have been investigated extensively (reviewed in (12)). Some salient findings are: (a) Polyglutamates of CH_2-FH_4 show significantly lower K_m values than the monoglutamate (16). (b) The dimeric enzyme displays a curious half-of-active-sites behavior with respect to the binding of dUMP and FdUMP. Depending upon the conditions used (e.g., presence or absence of CH_2-FH_4), one or two molecules of these nucleotides are bound to the complex of identical subunits (reviewed in (12)). (c) In both the enzyme-catalyzed reaction (eq. 1) and the aborted reaction in the presence of -FdUMP, the first step involves the critical -SH group (see above), identified as Cys-198 in the L. casei enzyme (17), reacting with the 5,6-double bond in dUMP to form an enzyme-substrate complex. This activates C-5, allowing it to react with the 5-iminium cation form of CH_2-FH_4. The resulting intermediate (whose structure was first proposed by Friedkin (18)), has the -CH_2 group bridged between N-5 of tetrahydrofolate and C-5 of the pyrimidine. Ejection of the proton from C-5, and attack by a hydride ion emanating from C-6 of tetrahydrofolate, cleaves the linkage to N-5 to yield dTMP and dihydrofolate. A similar sequence (reviewed in (12) and (19)) occurs when FdUMP is present at the pyrimidine binding site, but the inability to release fluorine from C-5 produces a stable enzyme-substrate-inhibitor complex (Fig. 3).

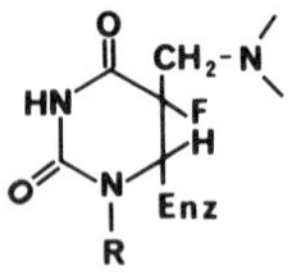

Fig. 3.   Complex of TS with substrate (CH_2-FH_4) and inhibitor (FdUMP). -CH_2-N$\langle$ denotes N-5 of tetrahydrofolate and the bridging methylene group (linked covalently to C-5 of the pyrimidine). Enz denotes enzyme whose -SH group is linked covalently to C-6 of the pyrimidine.

POTENTIATION OF THE BINDING OF 5-FLUORODEOXYURIDYLATE TO THYMIDYLATE SYNTHASE

Studies on the interaction of TS with FdUMP demonstrated that drug binding is enhanced in the presence of CH_2-FH_4 (reviewed in (12)). Although in enzyme catalysis, binding of one substrate often induces conformational changes in the protein that enhance binding of the second substrate, the situation is more complicated with TS. Both the normal and inhibited reaction proceed via an ordered sequence in which the pyrimidine nucleotide interacts first (20), and subsequent binding of CH_2-FH_4 produces a ternary complex in which the substrates are fused covalently and one of them (dUMP or FdUMP) is also linked covalently to the enzyme (see above).

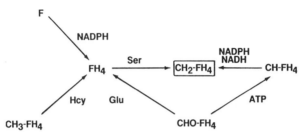

Fig. 4.   Pathways for generation of 5,10-methylenetetrahydrofolate.

From these considerations, it seemed possible that the cytotoxicity of fluoropyrimidines could be maximized if high intracellular levels of CH_2-FH_4 were attained. The latter compound, however, is ordinarily present at relatively low concentrations in cells (see below), and co-administration of CH_2-FH_4, even in cell culture experiments, is not feasible because of its lability. Inspection of the network of reactions linking various C_1-FH_4 adducts (Fig. 4) suggests that the desired build-up of the 5,10-methylene derivative can be achieved by several routes: (a) from F, via the NADPH-dependent reduction to FH_4, followed by addition of the CH_2 group from serine; (b) from CH_3-FH_4, via the B_{12}-dependent methionine synthetase, to yield FH_4 (and hence, CH_2-FH_4); and (c) from CHO-FH_4, via two possible pathways (conversion to FH_4 or CH-FH_4). Processing of CH-FH_4 would then involve reduction by the NADPH- or NADH-dependent CH_2-FH_4 dehydrogenase. 5-Formyltetrahydrofolate is the agent of choice, because it is more stable than the methyl derivative and more readily transported into cells than folate. Translating theory into practice, several groups (21-23) reported that incubation of tumor cells with high levels of CHO-FH_4 increased their sensitivity to FUra. Representative results, from the work of Dr. Maire Hakala and her colleagues illustrating the effectiveness of the CHO-FH_4/FUra combination against S-180 and Hep-2 cells, are summarized in Table I. It is thus fitting that the present Symposium, which includes the extension of this therapeutic regimen to cancer patients, honors Maire for her fundamental contributions in this field.

Table I. Potentiation of FUra Toxicity by CF*

Cells	Drug	IC_{50}
		μM
Hep-2	FUra	430
	FUra + CF (300 μM)	170
S-180	FUra	7.2
	FUra + CF (300 μM)	1.7

* Data have been calculated from Chart 2 in reference (23).

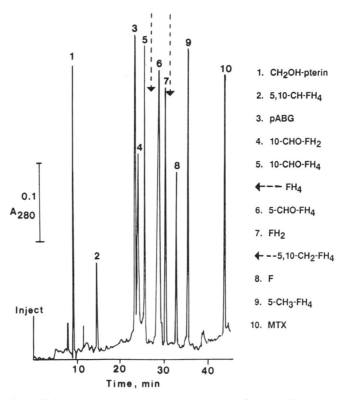

1. CH_2OH-pterin
2. 5,10-CH-FH_4
3. pABG
4. 10-CHO-FH_2
5. 10-CHO-FH_4
   ← -- FH_4
6. 5-CHO-FH_4
7. FH_2
   ← --5,10-CH_2-FH_4
8. F
9. 5-CH_3-FH_4
10. MTX

Fig. 5. HPLC of folate compounds. Experimental details as in (28) except that the gradient was changed to: 100% A for 4 min; 40% B for 1 min; linear gradient to 100% B for 60 min; 100% A for 20 min (the latter at 1.5 ml/min). Elution position of CH_2-FH_4 and FH_4 are indicated by arrows.

6

INTRACELLULAR LEVELS OF 5,10-METHYLENETETRAHYDROFOLATE

The ability of CH_2-FH_4 to potentiate the cytotoxicity of fluoropyrimidines, as well as its central role in folate-dependent C_1-metabolism, has made it desirable to be able to determine intracellular levels of this compound. This is difficult, however, because the levels are low (ca. 1 pmol/10^6 cells) and the compound dissociates into HCHO and FH_4 (24). Thus, Moran et al. (25) and Fujii et al. (26), using chromatography on DEAE-cellulose and Sephadex G-25 to separate and quantitate the various intracellular folates, reported composite values for FH_4 plus CH_2-FH_4. More recently, reversed-phase HPLC has improved the resolution of intracellular folates; a representative profile of folate standards, using a solvent system similar to that of Duch et al. (27), is

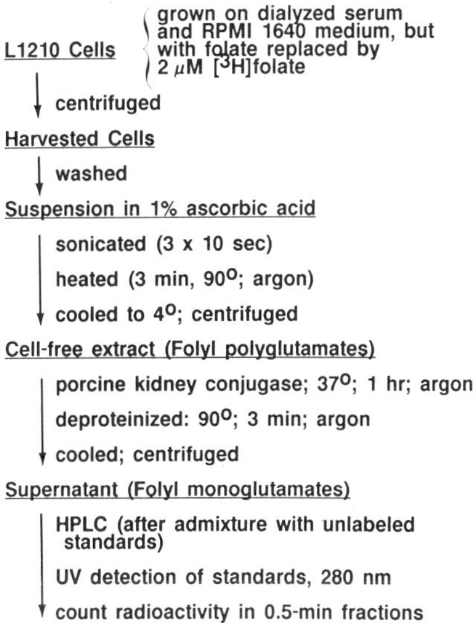

L1210 Cells — grown on dialyzed serum and RPMI 1640 medium, but with folate replaced by 2 μM [^{3}H]folate

↓ centrifuged

Harvested Cells

↓ washed

Suspension in 1% ascorbic acid

| sonicated (3 x 10 sec)

| heated (3 min, 90°; argon)

↓ cooled to 4°; centrifuged

Cell-free extract (Folyl polyglutamates)

| porcine kidney conjugase; 37°; 1 hr; argon

| deproteinized: 90°; 3 min; argon

↓ cooled; centrifuged

Supernatant (Folyl monoglutamates)

| HPLC (after admixture with unlabeled standards)

| UV detection of standards, 280 nm

↓ count radioactivity in 0.5-min fractions

Fig. 6.   Processing of intracellular folates for HPLC analysis. Experimental details as in (28).

illustrated in Fig. 5. The elution position of CH_2-FH_4 between FH_2 and F was determined by working at neutral pH and removing excess HCHO (which perturbs the HPLC solvent system) from the preparation. However, when intracellular folates are measured, the lability of CH_2-FH_4 is difficult to circumvent. In these procedures, cells are grown on [^{14}C]folate and the lysate is processed as shown in Fig. 6. Folates are released from proteins by heat-denaturation and excess glutamates are removed by treatment of the folylpolyglutamates with conjugase. Lowering of the pH by the presence of ascorbic acid (added to protect the reduced folates and to optimize conjugase activity) and the elevated temperature accelerate the dissociation of CH_2-FH_4.

At present, an enzymatic trapping method developed by Priest (29) appears to be most suitable for quantitating intracellular CH_2-FH_4. This involves treating the cell lysate immediately with [^{3}H]FdUMP and *L. casei* TS. The CH_2-FH_4 polyglutamates bind to the enzyme, along with an equivalent amount of the labeled fluoropyrimidine. All proteins are then precipitated, and the amount of radioactivity is determined. A method being developed in this laboratory, which would allow CH_2-FH_4 to be determined via the HPLC procedure, treats the cell lysate, prior to the conjugase step, with NADPH-dependent CH_2-FH_4 reductase to generate 5-CH_3-FH_4 from the labile CH_2-FH_4. The latter is then quantitated via the increased amount of 5-CH_3-FH_4 over the untreated control.

CONVERSION OF 5-FORMYLTETRAHYDROFOLATE TO 5,10-METHYLENETETRAHYDROFOLATE

Exposure of cells to CHO-FH_4 increases the intracellular level of various folate compounds including CH_2-FH_4, but the details of this process are not entirely clear. As described above (cf. Fig. 4), two pathways are possible: one initiated by the ATP-dependent isomerization of CHO-FH_4 to the methenyl derivative, and the other by the glutamate-dependent transformylation of CHO-FH_4. Enzymes catalyzing the isomerization reaction have been isolated from *L. casei* (30) and rabbit liver (31) and the transformylase has been obtained from pig liver (32). The occurrence of these two enzymes, and their relative contributions toward the mobilization of CHO-FH_4, have not yet been investigated in various cells. High levels of these enzymes in tumor cells (relative to normal cells) would facilitate a selective effect of CHO-FH_4 in potentiating the cytotoxicity of fluoropyrimidines. Similar considerations are involved in evaluating the "rescue" of Methotrexate-treated cells by CHO-FH_4, except that the reverse situation (higher levels of the mobilizing enzyme(s) in normal cells) is desirable.

5-Formyltetrahydrofolate is an enigma among the C_1-tetrahydrofolate complexes. It can be synthesized chemically by heating 10-CHO-FH_4 in basic solution (33) or by the carbodiimide-promoted formylation of FH_4 (34). Knowledge of the former reaction has engendered the suspicion that part of the 5-CHO-FH_4, isolated from natural sources (e.g., (35)) or appearing in HPLC profiles, may have arisen as an artifact from endogenous 10-CHO-FH_4. If so, reported levels of 5-CHO-FH_4 may be erroneously high. The existence of two enzymes capable of directing 5-CHO-FH_4 into the C_1-FH_4 pool, however, argues that the compound is naturally-occurring and that it serves as a stable storage form of reduced folate.

ACKNOWLEDGMENT

The authors are indebted to Ms. Susan Burke for typing and editorial assistance in the preparation of this manuscript.

REFERENCES

1. G. H. Hitchings, *Trans*. N.Y. *Acad*. *Sci*. 23:700 (1961).
2. M. Friedkin, E. J. Crawford, and L. T. Plante, *Ann*. N.Y. *Acad*. *Sci*. 186:209 (1971).
3. C. Heidelberger, N. K. Chaudhuri, P. Danenberg, D. Mooren, L. Griesbach, R. Duschinsky, R. J. Schnitzer, E. Pleven, and J. Scheiner, *Nature* 179:663 (1957).
4. S. S. Cohen, J. G. Flaks, H. D. Barner, M.R. Loeb, and J. Lichensteiner, *Proc*. *Natl*. *Acad*. *Sci*. U.S.A. 44:1004 (1958).

5. P. V. Danenberg, B. J. Montag, and C. Heidelberger, <u>Cancer</u> <u>Res</u>. 18:335 (1958).

6. M. Friedkin and A. Kornberg, <u>in</u>: "The Chemical Basis of Heredity", W. D. McElroy and B. Glass, eds., Johns Hopkins Press, Baltimore, pp. 609-614 (1957).

7. G. K. Humphreys and D. M. Greenberg, <u>Arch</u>. <u>Biochem</u>. <u>Biophys</u>. 78:275 (1958).

8. M. J. Osborn, M. Freeman, and F. M. Huennekens, <u>Proc</u>. <u>Soc</u>. <u>Exp</u>. <u>Biol</u>. <u>Med</u>. 97:429 (1958).

9. R. L. Blakley, "Biochemistry of Folic Acid and Related Pteridines", North-Holland, Amsterdam, p. 236 (1969).

10. T. C. Crusberg, R. Leary, and R. L. Kisliuk, <u>J</u>. <u>Biol</u>. <u>Chem</u>. 245:5292 (1970).

11. R. B. Dunlap, N. G. L. Harding, and F. M. Huennekens, <u>Biochemistry</u> 10:88 (1971).

12. D. V. Santi and P. V. Danenberg <u>in</u>: "Folates and Pterins", Vol. 1, R. L. Blakley and S. J. Benkovic, eds., John Wiley, New York, pp. 345-398 (1984).

13. F. Maley, M. Belfort, and G. Maley, <u>Adv</u>. <u>Enzyme</u> <u>Regul</u>. 22:413 (1983).

14. F. Maley, F. K. Chu, D. K. West, and G. F. Maley <u>in</u>: "Chemistry and Biology of Pteridines", B. A. Cooper and V. M. Whitehead, eds., Walter de Gruyter, Berlin, pp. 613-629 (1986).

15. L. W. Hardy, J. S. Finer-Moore, W. R. Montfort, M. O. Jones, D. V. Santi, and R. M. Stroud, <u>Science</u> 235:448 (1987).

16. R. L. Kisliuk, Y. Gaumont, E. Lafer, C.M. Baugh, and J. A. Montgomery, <u>Biochemistry</u> 20:929 (1981).

17. R. L. Bellisario, G. F. Maley, D. V. Guarino, and F. Maley, <u>J</u>. <u>Biol</u>. <u>Chem</u>. 254:1296 (1979).

18. M. Friedkin, <u>Fed</u>. <u>Proc</u>. <u>Fed</u>. <u>Am</u>. <u>Soc</u>. <u>Exp</u>. <u>Biol</u>. 18:230 (1959).

19. M.A. Moore, F. Ahmed, and R. B. Dunlap, <u>J</u>. <u>Biol</u>. <u>Chem</u>. 261:12745 (1986).

20. A. Lockshin and P. V. Danenberg, <u>Biochem</u>. <u>Pharm</u>. 30:127 (1981).

21. S. Waxman, H. Bruckner, A. Wagle, and C. Schreiber, <u>Proc</u>. <u>Am</u>. <u>Assoc</u>. <u>Cancer</u> <u>Res</u>. 19:149 (1978).

22. B. Ullman, M. Lee, D. W. Martin, and D. V. Santi, <u>Proc</u>. <u>Natl</u>. <u>Acad</u>. <u>Sci</u>. <u>U.S.A</u>. 75:980 (1978).

23. R. M. Evans, J. D. Laskin, and M. T. Hakala, <u>Cancer</u> <u>Res</u>. 41:3288 (1981).

24. M. J. Osborn, P. T. Talbert, and F. M. Huennekens, <u>J</u>. <u>Am</u>. <u>Chem</u>. <u>Soc</u>., 82:4921 (1960).

25. R. G. Moran, W. C. Werkheiser, and S. F. Zakrzewski, <u>J</u>. <u>Biol</u> <u>Chem</u>. 251:3569 (1976).

26. K. Fujii, T. Nagasaki, and F. M. Huennekens, <u>J</u>. <u>Biol</u>. <u>Chem</u>. 257:2144 (1982).

27. D. S. Duch, S. W. Bowers and C. A. Nichol, <u>Anal</u>. <u>Biochem</u>. 130:385 (1983).

28. K. S. Vitols, Y. Montejano, T. Duffy, L. Pope, G. Grundler, and F. M. Huennekens, <u>Adv</u>. <u>Enzyme</u> <u>Regul</u>. 26:17 (1987).

29. V. Kesavan, P. Sur, M. T. Doig, K. J. Scanlon, and D. G Priest, <u>Cancer</u> <u>Lett</u>. 30:55 (1986).

30. C. E. Grimshaw, G. B. Henderson, G. G. Soppe, G. Hansen, E. J. Mathur, and F. M. Huennekens, <u>J</u>. <u>Biol</u>. <u>Chem</u>. 259:2728 (1984).

31. S. Hopkins and V. Schirch, <u>J</u>. <u>Biol</u>. <u>Chem</u>. 259:5618 (1984).

32. M. Silverman, J. C. Keresztesy, G. J. Koval, and R. C. Gardiner, <u>J</u>. <u>Biol</u>. <u>Chem</u>. 226:83 (1957).

33. B. Roth, M. E. Hultquist, M. J. Fahrenbach, D. B. Cosulich, H. P. Broquist, J. A. Brockman, J. M. Smith, R. P. Parker, E. L. R. Stokstad, and T. H. Jukes, <u>J</u>. <u>Am</u>. <u>Chem</u>. <u>Soc</u>. 74:3274 (1952).

34. R. G. Moran and P. D. Colman, <u>Anal</u>. <u>Biochem</u>. 112:70 (1982).

35. H. E. Sauberlich and C. A. Baumann, <u>J</u>. <u>Biol</u>. <u>Chem</u>. 176:165 (1948).

DISCUSSION OF DR. HUENNEKENS' PRESENTATION

Dr. Mihich: Resistance to fluoropyrimidines could be associated with
a change in affinity for the inhibitor of the target enzyme
thymidylate synthase. This was the first example of this mechanism
of resistance. Now that we have advanced in studies of the control
of enzyme synthesis and function through advances of molecular
biology, has that observation been followed up at the genetic level
and what is known about the mechanism through which this affinity
change in the ternary complex occurs?

Dr. Huennekens: I can't speak to any work in the genetic field. It is
true I think, that the problem of resistance to fluoropyrimidines in
some ways is parallel to what we see in resistance to MTX. In the
latter case there are a number of different mechanisms which have
been identified both in cellular systems and, in some cases, in
patients. We know we have gene amplification where there's an
elevated level of dihydrofolate reductase, we have reductase with
defective MTX binding, we have defective transport, defective polyglutamylation. I guess (except polyglutamylation) similar events
have been found in fluorouracil resistant cells, that is transport
deficient cells, cells that are unable to make FdUMP, and enzyme with
reduced affinity. Certainly gene amplification has been seen because
in the original work with the L.casei thymidylate synthase, we and
Roy Kisliuk were very fortunate we had a methotrexate resistant subline of L.casei which had an elevated level not only of dihydrofolate
reductase but of the synthase as well. Bruce Dunlap has recently
shown that those 2 genes are very close together in the bacterial
system. One can say there are certain prototype mechanisms of
resistance which you see with antimetabolites and one is not surprised to see them with fluorouracil as well.

Dr. Mihich: The isoenzyme part has not been followed up yet?

Dr. Huennekens: I would have to defer to people who are currently
working with TS from various sources on that. Does anyone have a
comment on that?

Dr. Bertino: There are several examples of altered enzymes of
thymidylate synthase as a mechanism of resistance. I don't think the
exact site of mutation has been mapped yet for those enzymes.

Dr. Spears: The Silverman pathway for transformylation of glutamate,
giving the one-step activation of CF to tetrahydrofolate, is not for
certain to my knowledge. Is there more evidence for it using purified enzyme and second, do you know of a cheap source, other than
Rick Moran's method of synthesis, of [^{14}C] formyltetrahydrofolate?

Dr. Huennekens: No, I don't of any other sources. The synthetic
procedures are described and are reasonably straight forward. In
answer to your first question, the work of Silverman was followed up
by Tabor and Rabinowitz and Wyngaarden working on the same enzyme.
Although that work is 3 decades old, I think it's quite substantial
and was done very extensively. The enzyme was purified from several
different sources and characterized as only Jesse Rabinowitz would do
with 14 or 15 tables and figures. To the best of my knowledge no one
recently has done much with this, although it would seem to be a
fairly important factor.

Dr. McGuire: I think that Bob MacKenzie of McGill looked at the formiminotranferase reaction and showed that the formylglutamate transferase seemed to be in his homogeneous preparation of that enzyme; it seemed to be a side reaction carried on at a very low rate relative to the formiminotransferase reaction.

Dr. Huennekens: It has also been suggested that you might somehow go from formimino directly to formyl, but to the best of my knowledge that doesn't occur. When you transfer a formimino group off of 5-formiminotetrahydrofolate (which you get in histidine breakdown), it goes to methenyl; you lose the ammonia and cyclize at the same time yielding the methenyl derivative. I think the loss of an (-NH) would be chemically rather unlikely.

Dr. Hakala: It is not always true that thymidylate synthase and dihydrofolate reductase are regulated together. We observed 20 years ago that in MTX-resistant sublines of S-180, developed in the presence of thymidine, the level of TS was very low while the DHFR was quite high. The pathways were uncoupled.

Dr. Huennekens: I shouldn't have implied that that is an inevitable consequence of gene amplification. There are many cases where only one is amplified. We were fortunate though in the L.casei instance that both were amplified and so that subline became a very rich source of both enzymes. As I mentioned, Bruce Dunlap's recent work has shown that the 2 genes are adjacent in the bacterium. I'm sure it could be otherwise in other cells.

Dr. Bertino: Considering that methylenetetrahydrofolate is subject to many interconversons, are you surprised that we can increase the levels of that co-factor in cells and that it is not under tight regulation?

Dr. Huennekens: Yes, I am surprised but the fact is, I guess you can.

Dr. Bertino: Are there data that suggest what the limits of this elevation are by perturbation with extracellular leucovorin?

Dr. Huennekens: My impression is that you can get perhaps a 5-fold expansion of the pool. I think the levels are about 1 pmol/10^6 cells, at least in Ll210. The expansion of course has to come at the expense of something, presumably of the input folates. To come back to your earlier comment though, it is true that when you have something with 4 different pathways going in and out, it would be nice to block the pathways that lead out because that would perhaps be another way of helping to raise the level of methylenetetrahydrofolate. Another question I think, is whether the methylenetetrahydrofolate is free or is bound to one or more enzymes. An analogy would be methionine synthase which has the B_{12} co-enzyme on it. In its catalytic mechanism the B_{12} goes through a cycle where the methyl group comes from methyltetrahydrofolate and converts the co-enzyme to methyl B_{12}. Then it loses the methyl group and becomes B_{12S} which is the very highly labile Co^{+1} and that is so reactive, even with water, that it is not surprising that all the B_{12} is bound with the methionine synthetase and very carefully protected. Its conceivable that the methylenetetrahydrofolate because of its lability might be similarly bound, if so that might be a limitation as to the upper level that you could accumulate in a cell.

THE NATURAL AND UNNATURAL DIASTEREOMERS OF LEUCOVORIN:
ASPECTS OF THEIR CELLULAR PHARMACOLOGY

Richard Bertrand and Jacques Jolivet

Institut du Cancer de Montréal
1560 Sherbrooke st. east
Montréal, Québec, Canada

INTRODUCTION

A mixture of the natural ((6S)-LV) and unnatural ((6R)-LV) diastereomers of leucovorin (LV, (6RS)-LV) is administered clinically in combination with 5-fluorouracil (FUra) to overcome drug resistance due to insufficient intracellular folate concentrations (1). Initially described as a growth factor for *Pediococcus cerevesiae*, LV has a S chirality at the 6 carbon of the tetrahydropterine ring (2). Following intravenous administration of a mixture of the (6S) and (6R) isomers of leucovorin to patients, plasmatic (6S)-LV disappears rapidly with a $T_{0.5}$ of 30 min. while (6R)-LV has a slower clearance ($T_{0.5}$ of 7.5 hours) (1,3). The natural isomer is readily transported into cells where it has no known folate cofactor activity. Greenberg was the first to show that LV was converted to another folate involved in purine biosynthesis (4). The first enzymatic step involved was later found to be methenyltetrahydrofolate synthetase (5-formyltetrahydrofolate cyclodehydrase, EC 6.3.3.2) which catalyzes the irreversible and stereospecific ATP and Mg^{2+}-dependent transformation of (6S)-LV to N^{5-10}-methenyltetrahydrofolate. Sheep liver enzyme activity was first partially purified (5) and the enzyme was more recently highly purified and characterized from *Lactobacillus casei* (6) and rabbit liver (7). We have recently obtained and characterized highly purified human liver methenyltetrahydrofolate synthetase (8) and will describe in the following paper its purification and characteristics. We next took advantage of the enzyme characteristics to prepare stereochemically pure (6R)-LV (9) and will present its transport characteristics and biological activity in human leukemic CCRF-CEM cells.

MATERIALS AND METHODS

Chemicals. Folic acid ($PteGlu_{1 or 5}$) and (6RS)-LV were purchased from B. Schircks Laboratories (Jona, Switzerland). Methotrexate (MTX) was obtained from the National Cancer

Institute (Bethesda MD) and MTX-Glu$_5$ provided by Dr. C.M. Baugh (Department of Biochemistry, University of South Alabama, Mobile, AL) and Dr. C.J. Allegra (National Cancer Institute, Bethesda MD). [3',5',7,9 -^{3}H] folic acid (20 mCi/µmole) and [3',5',7,9 -^{3}H] methotrexate (20 mCi/µmole) were purchased from Moraveck Biochemicals Inc. (Brea, Cal.). [^{3}H]-labelled and unlabelled (6S)-LV were prepared as described previously by Moran and Colman (10) and [^{3}H]-(6S)-N^5-CH$_3$-H$_4$-PteGlu and unlabelled (6S)-N^5-CH$_3$-H$_4$PteGlu made as described by Chanarin and Perry (11). N$^{5-10}$-CH$^+$-H$_4$PteGlu and N^{10}-HCOH$_4$-PteGlu were synthesized as per Rabinowitz (12) and the potassium salt of (6RS)-LV made from the calcium salt by exposure to potassium oxalate and removal of the calcium oxalate formed by centrifugation. H$_2$PteGlu$_{1 or 5}$ and (6S)-H$_4$PteGlu$_{1 or 5}$ were prepared as follows: PteGlu$_n$ was first reduced to H$_2$-PteGlu$_n$ by sodium hydrosulfite (13) following which H$_2$PteGlu$_n$ was further reduced to (6S)-H$_4$PteGlu$_n$ with partially purified *Lactobacillus casei* DHFR obtained from the New England Enzyme Center (Boston, MA). All folates were purified by reverse phase HPLC as described by Sirotnak et al (14) with peak purity recontrolled as per Allegra et al (15). Amino-hexyl-Sepharose-4B, Blue Sepharose CL-6B, Sephadex G-25 and G-200 were obtained from Pharmacia Fine Chemicals (Uppsala, Sweden). All other chemicals were of reagent grade and purchased from Boehringer-Mannheim (Penzberg, F.R.G.), Sigma (St-Louis MO) or Fisher Scientific Co. (Fair Lawn, NJ).

5-HCO-H$_4$PteGlu-aminohexyl-Sepharose. The affinity column was prepared as follows: (6RS)-LV (50 mg) was dissolved in 20 ml of distilled deionized water and added to a suspension of activated (pH 4.5) AH-Sepharose-4B (5 g). The mixture was stirred for 30 min at 25°C before adding 1-ethyl-3-(3-dimethyl-aminopropyl)carbodiimide (250 mg) and the pH was adjusted to 6.0. The final mixture was washed and stored at 4°C in 50 mM Pipes, 50mM β-mercaptoethanol (pH 6.0).

Assay system. Methenyltetrahydrofolate synthetase activity was measured by monitoring the increase in absorbance at 360 nm due to the formation of N$^{5-10}$-CH$^+$-H$_4$PteGlu (ϵ_{360} = 25.1 x 10^3 M^{-1} cm^{-1}) (16). Reactions were carried out in quartz cuvettes of either 1 or 10 cm optical path-lengh and the temperature was maintained at 30°C using a water-jacketed sample compartment. The assay mixture contained 50 mM 2-(N-Morpholino)-ehanesulfonic acid (Mes), 10 mM β-mercaptoethanol, 10 mM magnesium acetate, 0.5 mM ATP and 0.2 mM LV.

Purification of methenyltetrahydrofolate synthetase. Human liver was obtained at autopsy and kept at -80°C. Approximately 40 g was homogenized in 100 ml of 20 mM 1,4-Piperazinediethanesulfonic acid (PIPES), 20 mM β-mercaptoethanol, 10 mM magnesium acetate at pH 7.0 (PMM buffer) and the homogenate was centrifuged at 12 000 x g for 30 min. The supernatant was saturated at 70% with solid (NH$_4$)$_2$SO$_4$ and the mixture was stirred for 30 min. After centrifugation (12000 x g, 30 min) the precipitate was resuspended in a minimal volume of PMM buffer (pH 7.0) and desalted by centrifugation (5000 x g, 10 min) through a 3 X 8 cm column of Sephadex G-25. All steps were performed at 4°C. The fraction containing protein was then applied to a Blue Sepharose column (1.6 X 100 cm) which had been equilibrated at 4°C with PMM buffer at pH 7.0. The column was then washed with 4 liters of PMM

buffer containing 0.1% (v/v) Tween 20 (PMMT buffer), and
0.35M KCl at pH 7.0. Enzyme activity was eluted with 500 ml
PMMT buffer in 0.35 M KCl containing 0.1 mM (6RS)-LV (calcium
salt). Fractions containing activity were dialyzed twice
against 24 liters of PMMT buffer containing 24 g acid-washed
activated charcoal. KCl 0.15 M was added to the dialyzed
solution and the pH adjusted to 6.5. The solution was applied
to the affinity column (1 X 30 cm) equilibrated with PMMT
buffer containing 0.15 M KCl at pH 6.5. The column was then
washed with 1 liter of the same buffer and elution of the
enzyme was accomplished by applying 1mM (6RS)-LV (potassium
salt). The enzyme was dialyzed against charcoal as described
above prior to kinetic analysis. One unit of enzyme activity
corresponds to 1 μmole of product/min, and specific activity
is expressed as units/mg of protein.

Synthesis of (6R)-N⁵-HCO-H₄PteGlu. (6R,S)-LV (0.2 mM)
was incubated at 30°C overnight with 0.1 unit of purified methenyltetrahydrofolate synthetase in a reaction mixture of 50
ml containing 50mM MES, 10 mM β-mercaptoethanol, 10 mM Mg
acetate and 1.0 mM ATP at pH 6.0. The reaction was followed
spectrophotometrically by monitoring the increase in absorbance at 360 nm due to the formation of N^{5-10}-CH⁺-H₄PteGlu.
After the reaction was completed, the mixture was lyophilized
and purified by reverse-phase HPLC (14). Fractions containing
(6R)-LV were pooled, lyophilized and peak purity recontrolled
as described (15). Stereochemical purity was monitored by
chiral HPLC (17). Tritium-labelled (6R)-LV was obtained similarly from [³H]-(6R,S)-LV which had been prepared by the
carbodiimide-induced formylation of [³H]-(6R,S)-H₄PteGlu (10)
synthesized chemically by the borohydrate reduction of [³H]-
PteGlu (18).

Cell culture. The human lymphoid cell line CCRF-CEM was
obtained from Dr. George P. Browman (Hamilton, Ont) and grown
in RPMI medium 1640 (Gibco, Grand Island, NY) supplemented
with 10% heat-deactivated fetal bovine serum (Gibco), 3.6 mM
(L)-glutamine, penicillin (100 units/ml) and streptomycin
(100 μg/ml) (Gibco). The cells were folate-depleted in
folate-free RPMI medium 1640 supplemented with 10% charcoal-
treated fetal bovine serum, 50 μM hypoxanthine, 10 μM
thymidine, 3.6 mM L-glutamine, 100 units/ml penicillin and
100 μg/ml streptomycin.

Transport experiments. Transport assays were performed
as described by Henderson et al (19) both in an anion-free
buffer (20 mM 4-(2-Hydroxyethyl)-1-piperazinethanesulfonic
acid (HEPES), 225 mM sucrose adjusted to pH 7.4 with MgO) and
in an anionic buffer (20 mM HEPES, 140 mM NaCl, 10 mM KCl, 2
mM MgCl₂, adjusted to pH 7.4 with NaOH) at 37°C. Time-
dependent uptake was measured for up to 120 minutes in the
presence of 5 μM [³H]-(6R)-LV (225 μCi/μmole) and
concentration-dependent influx experiments were performed
using 5 minute exposures from 0 to 20 μM [³H]-(6R)-LV (225
μCi/μmole). Non-specific cell membrane binding was determined
by parallel experiments done at 4°C. Inhibition experiments
were performed using 5 minute exposures to varying concentrations of (6R)-LV in the presence of four fixed concentrations of labelled substrates (MTX (255 μCi/μmole), PteGlu
(238 μCi/μmole), (6S)-LV (208 μCi/μmole) and (6S)-N⁵-CH₃-
H₄PteGlu (170 μCi/μmole)). At selected intervals, cells were

washed three times in ice-cold phosphate buffered saline at pH 7.4 (PBS). The washed pellets were lysed in distilled water, sonicated and part of the sonicate was assayed for radioactivity while a Bradford protein determination was performed on the rest of the sample (20).

RESULTS

Purification and properties of the enzyme

Methenyltetrahydrofolate synthetase was purified 49,000-fold from human liver obtained at autopsy. A summary of the purification protocol is shown in Table I. The enzyme is extremely labile at 4°C but can be well stabilized with a non-ionic detergent, Tween 20. At the final purification step, the specific activity at 30°C and pH 6.0 was 37 µmoles min^{-1} mg^{-1}, wich corresponds to a turnover number of 1000 min^{-1}. The enzyme has a single-size subunit with a molecular weight of 27,000 according to SDS-polyacrylamide gel elec-trophoresis. The molecular weight of the native enzyme was also determined to be 27,000 by gel filtration on Sephadex G-200. The isoelectric point was estimated to be at pH 7.0 by isoelectric focusing under denaturing conditions. The K_m values of (6RS)-LV, (6S)-LV, (6S)-LV pentaglutamate and ATP were found to be 4.4 µM, 2.0 µM, 0.6 µM and 20 µM res-pectively. The enzyme is stereospecific for (6S)-LV and binds substrates in a sequential as opposed to a ping-pong mecha-nism. The ability of various folate analogues to inhibit the activity of the synthetase was determined by varying the con-centration of LV in the presence of different fixed concen-trations of inhibitors. Results are summarized in Table II.

(6R)-N^5-HCO-H$_4$PteGlu synthesis

(6R,S)-LV was incubated with methenyltetrahydrofolate synthetase until no N$^{5-10}$-CH$^+$-H$_4$PteGlu formation could be de-tected spectrophotometrically. Following purification, a com-pound with a U.V. absorption spectra (OD$_{max}$ 285 nm) and a re-tention time on HPLC identical to authentic (6S)-LV was iden-tified. Polarimetric analysis of the compound showed an oppo-site circular dichroic spectra to (6S)-LV. The isolated substance was not a substrate for purified human liver

TABLE I

PURIFICATION OF HUMAN METHENYLTETRAHYDROFOLATE SYNTHETASE

	Volume (ml)	Protein (mg)	Units	Spec.Act.	Purification (-fold)	
Supernatant	110	1910	1.45	7.6x10^{-4}	1	(100%)
70% (NH$_4$)$_2$SO$_4$	22	1430	1.11	7.8x10^{-4}	1	(77%)
Blue Sepharose	330	0.39	0.93	2.4	3160	(64%)
LV-Sepharose	18	0.02	0.74	37	48680	(51%)

TABLE II

KINETIC CONSTANTS AND INHIBITION CONSTANTS FOR HUMAN LIVER METHENYLTETRAHYDROFOLATE SYNTHETASE

Substrate	Inhibitor	K_m [a] (μM)	K_i [b] (μM)
(6RS)-5-HCO-H_4PteGlu$_1$	-----	4.4	---
(6S)-5 HCO-H_4PteGlu$_1$	-----	2.0	---
(6S)-5-HCO-H_4PteGlu$_5$	-----	0.6	---
(6RS)-5-HCO-H_4PteGlu$_1$	PteGlu$_1$	---	55
(6RS)-5-HCO-H_4PteGlu$_1$	PteGlu$_5$	---	3.5
(6RS)-5-HCO-H_4PteGlu$_1$	H_2PteGlu$_1$	---	50
(6RS)-5-HCO-H_4PteGlu$_1$	H_2PteGlu$_5$	---	3.8
(6RS)-5-HCO-H_4PteGlu$_1$	H_4PteGlu$_1$	---	>400
(6RS)-5-HCO-H_4PteGlu$_1$	5-CH_3-H_4PteGlu$_1$	---	18
(6RS)-5-HCO-H_4PteGlu$_1$	MTX-Glu$_1$	---	>350
(6RS)-5-HCO-H_4PteGlu$_1$	MTX-Glu$_5$	---	15
(6S)-5-HCO-H_4PteGlu$_5$	MTX-Glu$_5$	---	16

[a] K_m values were determined by double reciprocal (1/V vs. 1/[S]) plots using three different fixed concentrations of ATP at 34 μM, 17 μM and 8.5 μM. All points represent averages of five measurements.
[b] K_i values were estimated from replots of data (K_m/V_{max} vs [I]) taken from double reciprocal (1/V vs. 1/[S]) plots using three different fixed concentrations of inhibitors. Each point represents an average of three measurements.

methenyltetrahydrofolate synthetase in a standard assay mixture. Further evidence that the product was N^5-HCO-H_4PteGlu was obtained by acidifying the preparation to pH 1.5 and detecting the spontaneous formation of N^{5-10}-CH^+-H_4PteGlu (OD_{max} 355nm) (11). Stereochemical purity was monitored by chiral HPLC (17). Variable contamination by (6S)-LV was detected and only preparations with no detectable (6S)-LV were used for all experiments. Overall yields of 60% to 70% of the (6R)-LV and 24% to 36% of the [^{3}H]-(6R)-LV initially present in the diastereomer mixture were recovered after column purification and lyophilisation.

Transport characteristics

Time-dependent uptake and concentration-dependent influx experiments illustrated in fig.1 revealed that (6R)-LV was poorly transported into CCRF-CEM cells with K_{Ts} of 10 μM compared to 0.3 μM for (6S)-LV in an anion-free buffer and 45 μM compared to 1.0 μM for the natural isomer in the anionic buffer. Inhibition studies indicated that (6R)-LV was a competitive inhibitor of MTX, PteGlu, (6S)-LV and (6S)-N^5-CH_3-H_4-PteGlu influx. Results are summarized in Table III.

TABLE III Influx and inhibition constants for various folates versus (6R)-N5-HCO-H4PteGlu.

Substrate	Anion-free Buffer			Anionic Buffer		
	K_t	V_{Max}	K_i	K_t	V_{Max}	K_i
(6R)-N5-HCO-H4PteGlu	10	4.0	---	45	4.0	--
(6S)-N5-HCO-H4PteGlu	.3	4.0	1.9	1.0	4.3	30
(6S)-N5-CH3-H4PteGlu	.2	3.9	1.6	1.2	4.6	25
PteGlu	16	4.3	3.0	56	4.7	45
MTX	.7	4.0	2.2	4.4	4.5	28

K_t and K_i values are expressed in μM and V_{max} values in pmoles/mg/min. They were respectively determined from Lineweaver-Burke and Dixon plots. All values represent the mean result of duplicate experiments. Composition of the anion-free and anionic buffers are described in Methods.

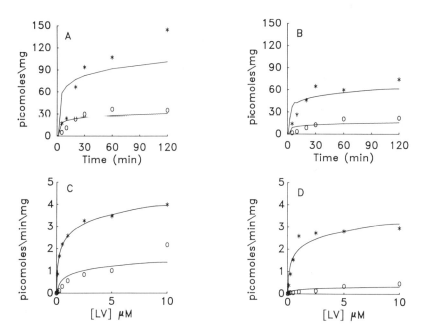

Fig.1 Time-dependent and concentration-dependent uptake of (6R)-N5-HCO-H4PteGlu by CCRF-CEM cells. CCRF-CEM cells were exposed to 5μM [3H]-(6R)-LV (O) or 5μM [3H]-(6S)-LV (*) for up to 120 minutes in an anion-free (Panel A) or an anionic buffer (Panel B) or for 5 minutes at various [3H]-(6R)-LV (O) or [3H]-(6S)-LV (*) concentrations in either an anion-free (Panel C) or anionic buffer (Panel D). Uptake was measured as described in Methods and represents determinations made at 37°C minus non-specific binding determined at 4°C. Results represent the mean of duplicate experiments.

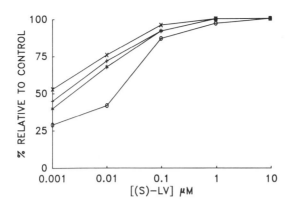

**Fig.2 Growth response curves of folate-depleted CCRF-CEM
cells.** CCRF-CEM cells (2 x 10^5/ml) were folate-depleted as
described in Methods and transferred to folate-free RPMI-1640
and 10% charcoal-treated fetal bovine serum simultaneously
containing different concentrations of (6S)-LV and (6R)-LV.
The (6S)-LV concentrations used are plotted on the abscissa.
Percent cell growth relative to control cells grown in 10 μM
folic acid is illustrated by line graphs: the (X) line
represents cells grown with no (6R)-LV added to the (6S)-LV,
(+) with 1μM (6R)-LV, (*) 10μM and (O) 100μM. Cell counts
were determined visually using an hemacytometer after three
cell doublings. Results represent the mean of duplicate experiments.

Biological activity

(6R)-LV failed to promote the growth of folate-depleted
CCRF-CEM cells at 10 μM while the same concentration of
either (6S)-LV or (6RS)-LV supported cell growth equal to
that seen in control cells exposed to 10 μM folic acid. When
cells were grown in folate-free media simultaneously
containing (6S)-LV and (6R)-LV (Fig 2), growth rates
diminished by 50% when the (6S)-LV/(6R)-LV concentration
ratio was 1:100,000, by 35% at 1:10,000, 11% at 1:1000 and
4.6% at 1:100 compared to control cells exposed to (6S)-LV
only.

DISCUSSION

LV is given clinically as a mixture of its natural and
unnatural diastereomers either in combination with FUra to
enhance its antitumor activity or in association with MTX as
a rescue agent. This reduced folate is probably a physiological component of the intracellular folate pools as it
is found in mammalian cells exposed to folic acid as the only
source of folates (15). Its mode of intracellular synthesis
or physiological role remain unknown however (21) and it has
no known folate cofactor activity per se. LV is the specific
substrate for methenyltetrahydrofolate synthetase (MTHFS), an
enzyme which irreversibly transforms it to 5-10 methenyltetrahydrofolate. Again, the physiological function of this

reaction is unknown although possible hypotheses include: a) LV as a folate storage form anabolized into the active folate pools by MTHFS; b) LV as a toxic byproduct of intra-cellular folate metabolism with MTHFS as a detoxifying enzyme. Further knowledge of the cellular pharmacology of both diastereomers of LV and the enzyme MTHFS has become important in view of the folate's increasing clinical use. We have thus recently purified human MTHFS to homogeneity and determined its kinetics and affinity for polyglutamate substrates. (6S)-LV pentaglutamate was found to have increased affinity for the enzyme compared to the monoglutamate although the lower K_m value observed was not accompanied by any significant change in the apparent V_{max} suggesting that the polyglutamate chain increases substrate binding to the enzyme but does not modify the active site (22). Folate and antifolate polyglutamates are also known to be better inhibitors of certain folate-dependent enzymes than their monoglutamate forms. This was again shown for MTHFS as PteGlu$_5$ (K_i =3.5 µM), H_2PteGlu$_5$ (K_i =3.8 µM) and MTX-Glu$_5$ (K_i =15 µM) were much more potent inhibitors of the enzyme than folic acid (K_i =55 µM), H_2PteGlu (K_i =50 µM) or MTX (K_i >350 µM). The K_m values for (6RS)-LV and (6S)-LV were found to be 4.4 µM and 2.0 µM respectively, suggesting that the unnatural isomer is not a substrate or an inhibitor of the synthetase. We next took advantage of this characteristic and prepared (6R)-LV by incubating a stereoisomer mixture of LV with MTHFS which eventually metabolized all the (6S)-LV, leaving stereochemically pure (6R)-LV as assayed by a recently described chiral chromatography assay (17).

Since folate and antifolate transport in eucaryotic cells is mediated by a specific membrane-associated transport protein (19,23,24), we next examined (6R)-LV transport characteristics to determine its specific uptake and membrane interactions with other folates and the antifolate MTX. (6R)-LV was poorly transported into CCRF-CEM cells, 45-fold less than (6S)-LV in a physiological-like anionic buffer and 33-fold less in an anion-free buffer (which optimizes transport conditions) but the unnatural diastereomer was a potent inhibitor of the uptake of various folates. V_{max} values for all folates and MTX influx in the presence of (6R)-LV were identical to those reported previously by Henderson et al (19) using the same assay system indicating specific binding of the unnatural isomer to the folate transport protein. K_t and K_i values increased in the anionic physiological-like buffer suggesting that the presence of extracellular anions reduced the binding efficiency of (6R)-LV to the transport protein, an observation already made for other folates and MTX (19).

Cell culture experiments indicated that 10µM (6R)-LV could not support the growth of folate-depleted human leukemic CCRF-CEM cells. This can be explained partly because of (6R)-LV's poor cellular influx and partly because it is not a substrate for MTHFS. When CCRF-CEM cells were exposed simultaneously to varying concentrations of (6R)-LV and (6S)-LV, the unnatural diastereomer could, at very large concentration ratios relative to the natural diastereomer, decrease the cell growth response of the folate-depleted cells to the latter. This observation probably reflects (6R)-LV's weak ability to compete with (6S)-LV's influx in physiological buffers.

The clinical significance of the transport inhibition of folates by (6R)-LV is as yet unknown altough prolonged high plasma levels of the unnatural isomer are regularly obtained following i.v. administration of high-doses of the racemic mixture (1). Such observations suggest the possible interference with influx of different folates which can possibly influence treatment outcome when (6R)-LV is given in association with FUra.

ACKNOWLEDGEMENTS

We thank Dr. K.E. Choi and R.L. Schilsky for performing the chiral HPLC assays. This work was supported by grants from the Medical Research Council of Canada and the National Cancer Institute of Canada. Studentship support was from the Cancer Research Society of Montreal and the National Cancer Institute of Canada.

REFERENCES

(1) MACHOVER D, GOLDSCHMIDT E, CHOLLET P, METZGER G, ZITTOUN J,MARQUET J, VANDENBULCKE JM, MISSET JL, SCHWARZENBERG L,FOURTILLAN JB, GAGET H, MATHE G., Treatment of advanced colorectal and gastric adenocarcinomas with 5-fluorouracil and high-dose folinic acid, J. Clin. Oncol., 4: 685-696, 1986.
(2) COSULICH DB, SMITH JM, BROQUIST HP., Diastereomer of leucovorin, J. Amer. Chem. Soc., 74: 4215-16, 1952.
(3) STRAW JA, SZAPARY D, WYNN WT., Pharmacokinetics of the diastereomer of leucovorin after intravenous and oral administration to normal subjects, Cancer Res., 44: 3114-3119, 1984.
(4) GREENBERG GR., A formylation factor, J. Am. Chem. Soc., 76: 1458-1459, 1954
(5) GREENBERG DM, WYNSTON LK, NAGABHUSHANAM A., Further studies on N^5-formyltetrahydrofolic acid cyclodehydrase, Biochemistry 4: 1872-1878, 1965
(6) GRIMSHAW CE, HENDERSON GB, SOPPE GG, HANSWEN G, MATHUR EJ, HUENNEKENS FM.,Purification and properties of 5,10-methenyltetrahydrofolate synthetase from Lactobacillus casei, J. Biol. Chem., 259: 2728-2733, 1984.
(7) HOPKINS S, SCHIRCH V., 5,10-Methenyltetrahydrofolate synthetase. Purification and properties of the enzyme from rabbit liver, J. Biol. Chem., 259: 5618-5622, 1984.
(8) BERTRAND R, MACKENZIE RE, JOLIVET J., Human liver methenyltetrahydrofolate synthetase: improved purification and increased affinity for folates polyglutamate substrates,Biochim. Biophys. Acta, 911: 154-161, 1987.
(9) BERTRAND R, JOLIVET J., Synthesis, transport characteristics and biological activity of the unnatural diastereomer of leucovorin, in preparation.
(10) MORAN RG, COLMAN PD. A simple procedure for the synthesis of high specific activity tritiated (6S)-5-formyltetrahydrofolate, Anal. Biochem., 122: 70-78, 1982.
(11) CHANARIN I, PERRY J., A simple method for the preparation of 5-methyltetrahydropteroylglutamic acid, Biochem. J., 105: 633- 635, 1967.

(12) RABINOWITZ JC.   Preparation and properties of 5,10-me-
     thenyltetrahydrofolic acid and 10-formyltetrahydrofolic
     acid, Meth.in Enzymol., 814-815, 1963.
(13) COWARD JK, PARAMESWARAN KN, CASHMORE AR, BERTINO JR.,
     7,8-Dihydropteroyl oligo-τ-l-glutamates: Synthesis and
     kinetic studies with purified dihydrofolate reductase
     from mammalian sources, Biochemistry, 13: 3899-3903,
     1974
(14) SIROTNAK FM, GOUTAS LJ, JACOBSEN DM, MINES LS,BARRUECO
     JR, GAUMONT Y, KISLIUK RL., Carrier-mediated transport
     of folate compound in L1210 cells, Biochem. Pharmacol.,
     36, 10: 1659-1667, 1987.
(15) ALLEGRA CJ, FINE RL, DRAKE JC, CHABNER BA., The effect
     of methotrexate on intracellular folate pools in human
     MCF-7 breast cancer cells, J. Biol. Chem., 261: 6478-
     6485, 1986.
(16) RABINOWITZ JC., in The Enzymes (Boyer P.D., Lardy H. and
     Myrback K., eds.), Vol 2: 185-252, Academic Press, New-
     York, 1960.
(17) CHOI KE, SCHILSKY RL., Resolution of the stereoisomers
     of leucovorin and 5-methyltetrahydrofolate by chiral
     HPLC, Anal. Biochem., 168: 398-404, 1988.
(18) BLAIR JA, SAUNDERS KJ., A convenient method for the pre-
     paration of 5-methyltetrahydrofolic acid, Anal.
     Biochem., 34: 376, 1970.
(19) HENDERSON GB, TSUJI JM, KUMAR HP., Characterization of
     the individual transport routes that mediate the influx
     and efflux of methotrexate in CCRF-CEM human
     lymphoblastic cells, Cancer Res., 46: 1633-1638, 1986.
(20) BRADFORD M., A rapid and sensitive method for the quan-
     titation of μg of protein utilizing the principle of
     protein dye binding, Anal. Biochem., 72: 248, 1976.
(21) McKENZIE RE.,Biogenesis and interconversion of substi-
     tuted tetrahydrofolates, in Folates and Pterins, R.L.
     Blakley and S.J. Benkovik eds., New-York, 293-296, 1984.
(22) McGUIRE JJ, BERTINO JR., Enzymatic synthesis and func-
     tion of folylpolyglutamates, Mol. Cell. Biochem., 39:
     19-48, 1981.
(23) NAHAS A, NIXON PF,BERTINO JR., Uptake and metabolism of
     5-formyltetrahydrofolate by L1210 leukemia cells, Cancer
     Res., 32: 1416-1421, 1972.
(24) HUENNEKENS FM, VITOLS KS, HENDERSON GB., Transport of
     folate compounds in bacterial and mammalian cells,
     Adv.Enzymol., 47: 313-346, 1978.

DISCUSSION OF DR. JOLIVET'S PRESENTATION

Dr. Bertino: In view of the fact that CF is so rapidly converted to $5\text{-}CH_3\text{-}H_4\text{PteGlu}$ you probably want to consider using that in these experiments, as well as CF.

Dr. Jolivet: There is a problem with stability there; it is reasonably stable, but in these experiments which last a few days, I'm quite sure that it is broken down to a large extent. So we have continued using CF because we're sure what is in the culture medium with CF and we're not sure with $5\text{-}CH_3\text{-}H_4\text{PteGlu}$.

Dr. Schilsky: I just wanted to make a couple of comments. We've looked at the cellular pharmacology of the isomers in human colon cancer cells, HT29 cells, and we are at about the same level of accomplishment as you are with the CEM cells. The data look very similar. We found that the transport of the 6R isomer is about 30-fold less than the 6S isomer in colon cancer cells. The 6R isomer does support the growth of folate depleted colon cancer cells but it's about 400-fold less potent in doing so. We've not been able to see any inhibition of uptake of 6S by 6R but we've only looked at concentration ratios as high as a 1000:1 and it may be that at those concentration ratios there is not any inhibition.

Dr. McGuire: I'm trying to figure out which pathway is the most important for CF activation. Did you say that the formiminotransferase is only present in liver, in terms of tissue distribution?

Dr. Jolivet: It has been found mostly in liver and kidney, but not in all the tissues which have been looked at. I think it is a tissue specific enzyme. It's not a ubiquitous enzyme like 5,10-methenyl-tetrahydrofolate synthetase which has been found in all the tissues in which we've looked. Of course the K_m for CF for the formimino-transferase is 10-fold higher also. Both these facts suggest that it's probably a secondary pathway.

Dr. McGuire: So your feeling is that the primary pathway is the 5,10-methenyltetrahydrofolate synthetase.

Dr. Jolivet: Yes. We've looked at many cell cultures, many human tissues from autopsy including liver, and we find it in most tissues. Indeed it can be found all the way to L.casei. It's an enzyme which is highly conserved. This has caused us problems. We've been trying to generate antibodies to the pure protein but have been unable to generate any antibodies, throughout many species. I'm wondering if that is because it is well conserved throughout evolution. That is interesting since nobody knows what its role is.

Dr. Rustum: I noticed in your uptake experiment with the R versus S, the highest R-isomer concentration was around 10 μM. Yet for the inhibition assays you went to a much higher concentration. As you know, the plasma concentration in patients is on the order of 80-100 μM. Have you looked at the transport of R-isomer at a concentration around 100 μM or so?

Dr. Jolivet: No we haven't, because of the expense. Practically, we've only been able to generate concentrations up to 10 μM in tissue culture experiments.

Dr. Rustum: The higher concentrations might be important for interference with the further metabolism of S-CF in the cells.

Dr. Jolivet: As you noticed in the cell culture experiments we did go up to 100 μM non-radioactive R-CF which is easier and less expensive to make. Certainly for the range of concentrations we used in the transport experiments, we could clearly generate K_i values which gives you an idea of the inhibitory potential of these compounds. In tissue culture you have to go to 100 μM which is above our estimated K_i in physiological buffers (30 μM) for the transport of R versus S. There you start seeing effects on cell growth but only at those very high concentrations and very high ratios of R to S. That is why I have a feeling this interaction is mostly operative at the later time points of the elimination of R and S isomers, where you see this large ratio.

Dr. Rustum: I know you use HPLC to separate the R and S. Can you give us an estimation of the purity of your R-isomer?

Dr. Jolivet: These samples were analyzed by Richard Schilsky. Not all of our samples are pure and in some preparations, probably depending on enzyme stability, there is some remaining S-isomer; we didn't, of course, use these preparations for experiments. In some preparations we could not identify any S-isomer by the chiral HPLC assay.

Dr. Rustum: We are pursuing similar lines of investigation and we've isolated the R-isomer from urine of patients treated with high dose CF. We used the HPLC for separation of this but the best we can do at the present time is about 98% pure. We are not satisfied with that since if you have 2% contamination of the S-isomer it can give you problems.

Dr. Jolivet: Another way to look at that is to use L.casei and see what the growth promoting potential of the preparation is. We get around 1500-fold less growth with R than with S, meaning that there is probably still some contamination but it is at a very, very low level. It's probably impossible to get completely pure.

DISTRIBUTION AND METABOLISM OF CALCIUM LEUCOVORIN IN NORMAL AND TUMOR TISSUE

Robert J. Mullin, Barry R. Keith and David S. Duch

Department of Medicinal Biochemistry
Wellcome Research Laboratories
Research Triangle Park, NC 27709

INTRODUCTION

Thymidylate synthase catalyzes the formation of thymidylate from deoxyuridine monophosphate in a reaction which employs the folate cofactor CH_2-H_4PteGlu both as methyl donor and reductant. The TS inhibitor FUra has been widely used clinically for the treatment of solid tumors, particularly colorectal carcinomas. Inhibition of TS by FUra occurs following its metabolism to FdUMP and formation of a ternary complex involving TS, FdUMP and CH_2-H_4PteGlu (1-3). An increased interest in the use of FUra stems from the observations in tissue culture (4,5) and in extracts of human colon adenocarcinoma xenographs (6) that the antitumor effects of FUra can be potentiated by the administration of exogenous folates in the form of calcium leucovorin. The results of these studies indicated that the response of many tumors to FUra is limited by the intracellular concentration of CH_2-H_4PteGlu and that the metabolism of 5-CHO-H_4PteGlu to CH_2-H_4PteGlu following cellular uptake expands this cofactor pool. With increased intracellular levels of CH_2-H_4PteGlu, the half-life of the ternary complex is increased, resulting in increased cytoxicity. In support of this model, enlargement of the CH_2-H_4PteGlu pool following administration of 5-CHO-H_4PteGlu has been demonstrated in tissue culture (7).

Clinically FUra as a single agent has been the primary treatment for colorectal carcinoma. However responses to FUra alone are of short duration and occur in only 15-20 percent of the patients treated (8,9). The pioneering clinical studies of Machover et al. (10), based on the preclinical studies described above, led to a large number of clinical studies which showed an improved response rate in patients with colorectal carcinoma following therapy using FUra combined with calcium leucovorin (11). The clinical studies were designed to achieve plasma folate concentrations of 10 uM, the concentration which resulted in maximum potentiation of FUra cytotoxicity in tissue culture (5). However in these clinical studies there was no evidence that these levels were achieved in tissues. An animal model suitable for examining questions concerning the effects of scheduling, routes of administration and intracellular folate pools on the potentiation of FUra by calcium leucovorin has not been demonstrated. Studies using L1210 in vivo (12) could not demonstrate potentiation of FUra by concurrent calcium leucovorin infusion and studies in our laboratory (unpublished) employing colon 38 adenocarcinoma in vivo were also unsuccessful. In order to determine whether the lack of potentiation of FUra by calcium leucovorin in rodent tumors was related to the folate cofactor levels attained in tumor tissue, the folate pools of both normal (liver) and neoplastic (colon 38 adenocarcinoma) tissues following administration of calcium leucovorin were determined. These tissues were also assayed for 5,10-methenyltetrahydrofolate synthetase (EC 6.3.3.2), the enzyme responsible for entry of 5-CHO-H_4PteGlu into the folate interconversion process. The results of these studies indicate differences between liver and tumor concerning the metabolism of 5-CHO-H_4PteGlu following uptake into tissues.

MATERIALS AND METHODS

Folate standards were prepared as previously described (14) with the exception of H_4PteGlu which was prepared by the enzymatic reduction of H_2PteGlu (14). Calcium leucovorin (5-CHO-H_4PteGlu) was from Burroughs Wellcome Co. Dowex 50 was purchased from Bio-Rad Laboratories. The colon 38 adenocarcinoma (obtained from Southern Research Institute, Birmingham, Alabama) was maintained in C57BL/6 mice as subcutaneous axillary implants. Passage time was 21-28 days.

Tissue folate analysis was performed using modifications of published methods (13). Following extraction of folates from tissues, the samples were digested for three hours at 37° with rat plasma conjugase (15) with a 4:1 ratio of sample to plasma. Digestion was stopped and plasma proteins were precipitated by incubating for 5 min at 95°. Samples were clarified by centrifugation at 30,000 x g for 5 min and adjusted to pH 4.5 with 1 $\underline{M}$ acetic acid. Samples were then quickly passed over 0.5 X 2.5-cm columns of Dowex 50 X-4, 200-400 mesh, $NH4^+$ form (13). The Dowex eluate was concentrated and further purified by use of a C18 Bond Elute cartridge (Analytichem International). Prior to application of the sample, cartridges were rinsed with 5 ml methanol, 10 ml of water, 1 ml of 10 $\underline{mM}$ PicA, 5 ml of water and 5 ml of 0.1% sodium ascorbate containing 0.1% mercaptoethanol. Following application of the sample, the cartridges were washed with 10 ml of 0.1% sodium ascorbate containing 0.1% mercaptoethanol. Samples were eluted with 1 ml of methanol and dried under nitrogen. Recovery of standard folates was similar to values previously reported (13). Following reconstitution in 0.1% sodium ascorbate containing 0.1% mercaptoethanol samples were analyzed by HPLC (13) with detection by UV absorbance. Data was collected and analyzed with a DS-80 microcomputer. Plasma samples were prepared by centrifuging heparinized blood collected from the vena cava for 10 min at 1000 x g. A volume of the plasma was removed and mixed with an equal volume of 1% ascorbate containing 1% mercaptoethanol at 95°. The mixture was then kept at 95° for 5 min, and following cooling, was centrifuged for 30 min at 12,500 x g. The clear supernatant was then analyzed directly by HPLC (13). When necessary, samples were flushed with N_2 and stored at -70°.

Tissue and plasma folates were quantitated by comparison with folate standards and the tissue results are adjusted for the standards carried through the above process. In these studies, cofactor pools refer to the sum of levels of $10\text{-}CHO\text{-}H_4PteGlu$, $H_4PteGlu$, $H_2PteGlu$, and $5\text{-}CH_3\text{-}H_4PteGlu$, while total folate pools refers to the sum of the levels of the cofactor pool plus the $5\text{-}CHO\text{-}H_4PteGlu$ pool.

Liver and colon 38 tumor tissue were assayed for 5,10-methenyltetrahydrofolate synthetase activity as described by Bertrand et al. (16). Protein concentrations were determined by the BCA method described by Smith et al. (17).

RESULTS

In studies in our laboratory, C57Bl/6 mice carrying the 1,2-
dimethylhydrazine dihydrochloride-induced colon 38 adenocarcinoma
subcutaneously have proven to be refractory to potentiation of the
antitumor effects of FUra by calcium leucovorin. In an attempt to
determine the basis of this response, plasma, liver, and tumor folate
levels were monitored for a 24 hour period following i.p.
administration of 400 mg/kg of calcium leucovorin.

Total Folate Levels. Plasma, liver and tumor all demonstrated
elevated total folate levels in response to the leucovorin dose
administered (Table 1). Plasma demonstrated the greatest relative
increase, nearly 130-fold, reaching concentrations of 1 mM 5 min
following administration. The tumor also reached maximal levels at
5 min, increasing 24-fold to 71.7 nmol/g tissue. At the 5 min time
point the liver and tumor have equal levels of total folates. The
liver reached maximal levels of 170.9 nmol/g tissue at 30 min,
increasing 5.5-fold over control levels. Relative to the tumor the
liver showed the greater absolute change in folate content. In spite
of 10-fold higher initial folate levels, the liver accumulated more
folate per gram of tissue (140 nmol/g) than did the tumor (69 nmol/g).
The liver and tumor tissues also differed in that the total folate
content of the liver continued to increase at a time when the tumor
folate content began to decline. At the 2 hour time point, the liver
remained at nearly 90 percent of its maximally-achieved levels while
the tumor had fallen to below 45 percent of its maximum content. The
plasma showed an even greater decline, dropping to 6 percent of its
maximum after 2 hours. Folate levels in all tissues had returned to
control levels within 24 hours after leucovorin administration.

Folate Pool Analysis. The analysis of the folates in mouse
plasma following leucovorin administration revealed that for the most
part plasma folates were present as 5-CHO-H_4PteGlu. 5-CH_3-H_4PteGlu
appeared to be present but was nearly undetectable by these methods
except for the 30 min and 2 hr time points. At these points, 5-CH_3-
H_4PteGlu was present at concentrations of 5 and and 13 uM
respectively, which represents 1 and 21 per cent of the total plasma

Table 1. Total Folate Levels in Plasma, Liver and Colon 38 Tumor
Following a 400 mg/kg i.p. Dose of Calcium Leucovorin.

Time (min)	Plasma[1]	Liver[2]	Tumor[2]
0	7.8 ± 3.2	30.7 ± 5.2	3.0 ± 0.8
5	1033.1 ± 52.2	72.1 ± 31	71.7 ± 65.7
30	443.1 ± 76.6	170.9 ± 19.7	65.3 ± 15.8
120	263.3 *	151.1 ± 43.8	31.8 ± 10.8
360	7.5 ± 0.5	56.1 ± 4.6	26.2 *
1380	3.1 ± 2.2	38.9 ± 4.7	3.5 ± 0.4

[1] $u\underline{M}$. These results are from a single experiment with duplicate analysis.
[2] nmol/g tissue. The results are the mean of duplicate experiments with standard deviations.
In each experiment tissues from multiple animals were pooled prior to analysis.
* Due to loss of sample these results represent single determinations.

folates at these times. Preliminary studies with oral administration of leucovorin indicated that following either 50 or 400 mg/kg doses of leucovorin, 5-CHO-H_4PteGlu was seen as the principal plasma folate, and was present at concentrations of 4 and 140 uM thirty minutes after administration of the respective doses.

Changes in the folate pools in liver over the 24 hours following leucovorin administration are summarized in Figure 1. Several points can be drawn from this data. The response at the earliest time points indicates that the folate being taken up is 5-CHO-H_4PteGlu rather than 5-CH$_3$-H_4PteGlu. If 5-CH$_3$-H_4PteGlu were being taken up, some degree of accumulation would be expected. This, however, does not occur. A comparison of the 5 min and 2 hour time points indicates that 5-CHO-H_4PteGlu appears to undergo metabolism in the liver since the 5-CHO-H_4PteGlu levels did not change whereas the total folate level has more

than doubled (Fig. 1 and Table 1). At 6 hours, the folate pools had
declined substantially but were still nearly two-fold higher than
control levels. Folate pools returned to baseline levels with regard
to both total folate levels and cofactor distribution within 24 hours.
Over the 24 hour time course the 5-CH$_3$-H$_4$PteGlu pool showed relatively
little change.

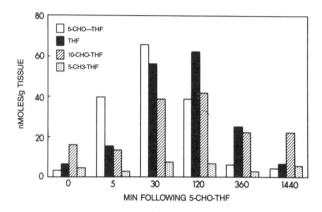

Figure 1. Liver folate levels following a 400 mg/kg dose of calcium
leucovorin.

Two pools, both capable of acting as enzymatic cofactors, that
show the greatest increase are 10-CHO-H$_4$PteGlu and H$_4$PteGlu. The
H$_4$PteGlu pool represents a summation of both H$_4$PteGlu and CH$_2$-
H$_4$PteGlu, since the latter folate congener is converted to H$_4$PteGlu by
this as well as most reported methods of direct cofactor analysis. At
the 5 min time point the major change in the liver folate pools,
excluding the expansion of the 5-CHO-H$_4$PteGlu pool, is the expansion
of the H$_4$PteGlu pool. At subsequent time points both the H$_4$PteGlu and
10-CHO-H$_4$PteGlu pools show considerable expansion, reaching their
maximum levels of just over 40 and 60 nmol/g tissue respectively at 2
hours. This represents an increase of 2.6-fold for 10-CHO-H$_4$PteGlu
and nearly 10-fold for H$_4$PteGlu. The CH$_2$-H$_4$PteGlu pool is thought to
expand to a similar extent as the H$_4$PteGlu pool, and low levels of
this congener were detectable after leucovorin treatment, having
remained intact through sample preparation and analysis.

The analysis of the folate pools in the colon 38 tumor is summarized in Figures 2 and 3. The most striking result of this study can clearly be seen in Figure 2. This tumor exibits a marked and substantial uptake of 5-CHO-H_4PteGlu but is unable to metabolize it to enlarge the cofactor pools in a manner comparable to that seen in the liver. On a relative scale, considering that the baseline levels of folates in tumor are some ten-fold lower than in the liver (Table 1) the tumor is as proficient at metabolizing 5-CHO-H_4PteGlu to other cofactors forms as is the liver, raising the total cofactor pool some five-fold at the 2 hour time point. However in light of the size of the available 5-CHO-H_4PteGlu pool the tumor appears incapable of significantly metabolizing this pool to the other cofactor forms.

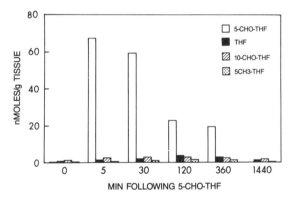

Figure 2. Total reduced folate levels in colon 38 adenocarcinoma following an i.p. dose of 400 mg/kg calcium leucovorin.

The nature of folate metabolism in the tumor can be seen in Fig. 3. The folate distribution in tumors from untreated animals is similar to that seen in liver with 10-CHO-H_4PteGlu representing the largest fraction followed by H_4PteGlu and then 5-CH_3-H_4PteGlu. Following administration of 5-CHO-H_4PteGlu, the tumor differs from the liver in that the 10-CHO-H_4PteGlu pool remains the largest cofactor pool for at least 30 min. At the 2 hour time point H_4PteGlu was the largest cofactor pool. In the liver H_4PteGlu was the major folate cofactor as early as the 5 min time point. The tumor also showed a four-fold increase in 5-CH_3-H_4PteGlu at the 2 hour time point.

The increase in 5-CH₃-H₄PteGlu appears to mirror its appearance in the plasma and may reflect direct uptake of this compound rather than the intracellular metabolism of 5-CHO-H₄PteGlu. In a fashion similar to the liver, folate levels in the tumor returned to baseline levels within 24 hours of the leucovorin dose. However, in contrast to the plasma and liver, total folates and cofactor pool in tumor were still substantially elevated at the 6 hour time point (Table 1, Fig. 3).

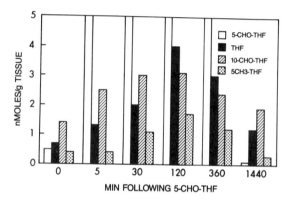

Figure 3. Reduced folate cofactor levels in colon 38 adenocarcinoma following an i.p. dose of 400 mg/kg calcium leucovorin.

The enzyme 5,10-methenyltetrahydrofolate synthetase catalyzes the conversion of 5-CHO-H₄PteGlu to 5,10-CH⁺-H₄PteGlu and serves as the entry point for 5-CHO-H₄PteGlu into the intracellular cofactor pool. The differences in the ability of liver and tumor to utilize 5-CHO-H₄PteGlu to elevate cofactor pools could be due to differences in the activity of this enzyme in the two tissues. As might be expected from the results presented above, the liver contains substantial amounts of this enzyme whereas the activity in the tumor is at the lower limits of detection for this method.

DISCUSSION

In an attempt to explain the inability of leucovorin to potentiate the antitumor effect of FUra in the colon 38 adenocarcinoma we have measured the changes in folate pools in liver, tumor and plasma of mice bearing this tumor following administration of calcium leucovorin. Following uptake of exogenous $5\text{-}CHO\text{-}H_4PteGlu$, the liver and tumor demonstrate noticeable differences in the metabolism of this compound. Extensive metabolism occurs in the liver as reflected by the expansion of the cofactor pool. The changes observed in the cofactor levels suggest that metabolism is through $CH_2\text{-}H_4PteGlu$ dehydrogenase (EC 1.5.1.5) with $H_4PteGlu$, the major observable metabolite, representing a summation of both the $H_4PteGlu$ and the $CH_2\text{-}H_4PteGlu$ pools. The liver fails to maintain elevated folate pools in the absence of elevated plasma folate levels. This is evident from the return to near normal folate levels seen within six hours after leucovorin administration (Fig. 1). This decline in liver closely parallels the decline seen in plasma and indicates that continuous administration or multiple frequent dosing of calcium leucovorin would be required to maintain elevated folate levels in tissues.

The response of the folate pools in tumor to exogenous leucovorin is rather different from that of liver in these studies. The major difference is the near inability of the tumor to metabolize $5\text{-}CHO\text{-}H_4PteGlu$ (Fig. 2 and 3). The basis for the inability of the tumor to greatly expand its folate cofactor pool in light of the available $5\text{-}CHO\text{-}H_4PteGlu$ appears to be due to the low levels of $CH^+\text{-}H_4PteGlu$ synthetase, the enzyme responsible for this metabolic step. Presently the role of this enzyme in therapies involving leucovorin, as has been discussed by Bertrand et al. (16), is being explored in our laboratory. There is also the possibility that tumor metabolism may occur through $5\text{-}CH_3\text{-}H_4PteGlu$ since its levels also increase in the tumor following its appearance in the plasma. However, cofactor pool expansion at 5 min precedes the expansion of the $5\text{-}CH_3H_4PteGlu$ pool (Fig. 3).

The nature of the metabolism that does occur in the tumor also differs from that seen in the liver. At the 5 min time point, the greatest absolute change in the tumor is the expansion of the 10-CHO-H_4PteGlu pool (Fig. 2). This may be a reflection of the presence of the NAD-dependent CH_2-H_4PteGlu dehydrogenase, an enzyme present primarily in transformed mammalian cells (18). The total folate content and individual cofactor pools in tumor returned to baseline levels within 24 hours, again indicating that additional administration of calcium leucovorin would be required to maintain elevated tissue folate pools. Interestingly, if one compares the relative expansion of the total cofactor pools normalized to baseline folate levels in the respective tissues the two tissues appear similar, both increasing approximately four-fold at the two hour time point. This may reflect a facet of the poorly understood mechanism of folate homeostasis.

The distribution of plasma folates following administration of calcium leucovorin raises an important question concerning the validity of employing mouse models to examine metabolism of exogenous leucovorin. With the lack of metabolism of 5-CHO-H_4PteGlu to 5-CH_3-H_4PteGlu seen in this study and elsewhere (19), this system fails to accurately mimic that in humans where there is considerable metabolism of (1)-5-CHO-H_4PteGlu to 5-CH_3-H_4PteGlu (20,21). While methotrexate uptake studies indicate that the transport of 5-CHO-H_4PteGlu and 5-CH_3-H_4PteGlu are comparable (22,23) the metabolism of each of these cofactors following uptake into cells is rather different. The entry of 5-CH_3-H_4PteGlu into the folate intercoversion pathway is tied to methionine biosynthesis since the only route of 5-CH_3-H_4PteGlu metabolism is conversion to H_4PteGlu while acting as a cofactor for methionine synthetase. The entry of 5-CHO-H_4PteGlu into the interconversion process is regulated by CH^+-H_4PteGlu synthetase. The balance of these two enzymes is apt to be crucial in the potentiation of FUra cytotoxicity as pharmacokinetic studies indicate that tissues are presented with both 5-CHO-H_4PteGlu and 5-CH_3-H_4PteGlu following leucovorin administration.

In conclusion, examination of liver and colon 38 folate pools has indicated differences in both the degree of metabolism of 5-CHO-H_4PteGlu and in the nature of this metabolism. Analysis of the plasma folates has raised questions concerning the employment of murine models for leucovorin administration, considering the lack of metabolism of 5-CHO-H_4PteGlu to 5-CH_3-H_4PteGlu.

REFERENCES

1. D.V. Santi, and C.S. McHenry, 5-Fluoro-2'-Deoxyuridylate: Covalent Complex with Thymidylate Synthetase, Proc. Natl. Acad. Sci. 69:1855 (1972).

2. R.J. Langenbach, P.V. Danenberg, and C. Heidelberger, Thymidylate Synthetase: Mechanism of Inhibition by 5-Fluoro-2'-Deoxyuridylate, Biochem. Biophys. Res. Comm. 48:1565 (1972).

3. D.V. Santi, C.S. McHenry, and H. Sommer, Mechanism of Interaction of Thymidylate Synthetase with 5-Fluorodeoxyuridylate. Biochem. 13:471 (1974).

4. B. Ullman, M. Lee, D.W. Martin, and D.V. Santi, Cytotoxicity of 5-Fluoro-2'-Deoxyuridine: Requirement for Reduced Folate Cofactors and Antagonism by Methotrexate. Proc. Natl. Acad. Sci. 75:980 (1978).

5. R.M. Evans, J.D. Laskin, M.T. Hakala, Effects of Excess Folates and Deoxyinosine on the Activity of and Site of Action of 5-Fluorouracil, Cancer Res. 41:3288 (1981).

6. J.A. Houghton, S.J. Maroda, J.O. Phillips, and P.J. Houghton, Biochemical Determinants of Responsiveness to 5-Fluorouracil and its Derivatives in Xenografts of Human Colorectal Adenocarcinomas in Mice, Cancer Res. 41:144 (1981).

7. D.G. Priest, M.T. Doig, and M. Mangum, Response of Mouse Hepatoma Cell Methylenetetrahydrofolate Polyglutamates to Folate Deprivation, Biochim. Biophys. Acta 756:253 (1983).

8. R.B. Livingston, and S. Carter, Single Agents in Cancer Chemotherapy. Plenum, New York, 1970, pp. 195-256.

9. H.L. Davis, Chemotherapy of Large Bowel Cancer. Cancer 50:2638 (1982).

10. D. Machover, L. Schwarzenberg, E. Goldschmidt, J.M. Tourane, B. Michalski, M. Hatat, T. Dorval, J.L. Misset, C. Jasmin, R. Maral, and G. Mathe', Treatment of Advanced Colorectal and Gastric Adenocarcinomas with 5-Fluorouracil Combined with High-Dose Folinic Acid: A Pilot Study. Cancer Treatment Rep. 66:1803 (1982).

11. J.C. Grem, D.F. Hoth, J.M. Hamilton, S.A. King, and B. Leyland-Jones, Overview of Current Status and Future Direction of Clinical Trials with 5-Fluorouracil in Combination with Folinic Acid, Cancer Treatment Rep. 71:1241 (1987).

12. P. Klubes, I. Cerna, and M.A. Meldon, Effect of Concurrent Calcium Leucovorin Infusion on 5-Fluorouracil Cytotoxicity Against Murine L1210 Leukemia, Cancer Chemother. Pharmacol. 6:121 (1981).

13. D.S. Duch, S.W. Bowers, and C.A. Nichol, Analysis of Cofactor Levels in Tissues Using High Performance Liquid Chromatography, Anal. Biochem. 130:385 (1983).

14. C.K. Mathews, and F.M. Huennekens, Enzymatic Preparation of the (1)-Diastereoisomers of Tetrahydrofolic Acid, J. Biol. Chem. 235:3304 (1960).

15. D.W. Horne, C.L. Krumdieck, and C. Wagner, Properties of Folic Acid Gamma-Glutamyl Hyrolase (Conjugase) in Rat Bile and Plasma. J. Nutr. 111: 442 (1981).

16. R. Bertrand, R.E. MacKenzie, and J. Jolivet, Human Liver Methenyltetrahydrofolate Synthetase: Improved Purification and Increased Affinity for Folate Polyglutamate Substrates, Biochem. Biophys. Acta. 911:154 (1987).

17. P.K. Smith, R.I. Krohn, G.T. Hermanson, A.K. Mallia, F.H. Gartner, E.K. Provenzano, E.K. Fujimoto, N.M. Goeke, B.J. Olson, and D.C. Klenk, Measurement of Protein Using Bicinchoninic Acid. Anal. Biochem. 150:76 (1985).

18. N.R. Meija, and R.E. MacKenzie, NAD-Dependent Methylenetetrahydrofolate Dehydrogenase Is Expressed by Immortal Cells, J. Biol. Chem. 260:14616 (1985).

19. M. Trotz, C. Wegner, and H. Nau, Valproic Acid-Induced Neural Tube Defects: Reduction by Folinic Acid in the Mouse, Life Sci. 41:103 (1987).

20. J.A. Straw, D. Szapary, and W.T. Wynn, Pharmacokinetics of the Diastereoisomers of Leucovorin after Intravenous and Oral Administration to Normal Subjects, Cancer Res. 44:3114 (1984).

21. B. McGuire, L. Sia, P. Leese, M. Gutierrez, and E.L.R. Stokstad, Pharmacokinetics of Leucovorin Calcium Given Intravenously, Intramuscularly, and Orally to Human Subjects, In NCI Monograph "Development of Folates and Folic Acid Antagonists in Cancer Chemotherapy", p.47, (1987).

22. F.M. Sirotnak, P.L. Chello, D.M. Moccio, R.L. Kisluk, G. Combepine, Y. Gaumont, and J.A. Montgomery, Stereospecificity at Carbon 6 of Formyltetrahydrofolate as a Competitive Inhibitor of Transport and Cytotoxicity of Methotrexate in vitro, Biochem. Pharmacol. 28:2993 (1979).

23. P.L. Chello, F.M. Sirotnak, E. Wong, R.L. Kisliuk, Y. Gaumont, and G. Combepine, Further Studies of Stereospecificity at Carbon 6 for Membrane Transport of Tetrahydrofolates, Biochem. Pharmacol. 31:1527 (1982).

DISCUSSION OF DR. DUCH'S PRESENTATION

Dr. Hines: Have you looked at similar doses of methyltetrahydrofolate, because in man at least, the majority of the CF is converted to methyl. At the high dose levels there may be a different pathway or mechanism and the methylene may be affected more.

Dr. Duch: Possibly, yes. No, we haven't done that yet.

Dr. Bertino: Your data would indicate that the level of the methionine synthase enzyme is also low in the tumor because presumably the mouse also converts leucovorin to 5-methyltetrahydrofolate rapidly. Have you measured the methionine synthase?

Dr. Duch: No we haven't. Even in some of the other studies where people have looked at levels of methionine synthase in the methionine requiring cells, there seems to be a fairly high level in those cells that have methionine requirements, so it may not be methionine synthase itself, but something else.

Dr. Peters: Your results on the folate pools actually demonstrate that you should not give CF 16 hours before FUra. We did some experiments in the colon 38 tumor model in which we gave CF 1 hour before FUra. We demonstrated that CF could potentiate the anti-tumor activity of FUra not only in this tumor model but also some other tumor models. How this relates to the reduced folate pools is not yet clear because we didn't measure the folate pools, we only measured the anti-tumor activity. But we also saw that you should give CF several times probably to keep the pools high (at least that is our idea). Based on your results, our idea is indeed a good one.

Dr. Duch: Yes, it is. We know now the probable reason we didn't see potentiation is because of the schedule of CF used. The data indicate that giving it 1 hour before FUra will put you right in the range where you are achieving maximum tissue levels of reduced folates.

Dr. Peters: It also demonstrates that the schedule used by groups in the L1210 model was the wrong one. They used very low leucovorin concentrations not 400 but 200 mg/kg.

Dr. Duch: Yes.

Dr. Houghton: Two points. One, you said on your last slide that at 120 min you still had about a 50-50 distribution of 6R and 6S in the plasma and yet there seems to be a very marked depression. That seems to be strange because 6S-CF is cleared much more rapidly.

Dr. Duch: Yes, that surprised us also. One thing that we did find was that there wasn't a lot of conversion of 5-formyl in the mouse; we didn't see large increases in plasma levels of 5-methyl and that bothered us. However, there was a study awhile back that also showed that you don't get a lot of 5-methyl formed in mice. It may be a function of the dose that we are giving; that we are saturating the conversion system for one thing. We are going to do a dose response and see what we get at different doses to see whether that holds up or whether the percentage of 5-methyl increases. I think Joe Rustum would say that we probably will see changes.

Dr. Houghton: You see a decrease in the tissue folates which parallels loss of folates in plasma. Have you looked to see whether you're forming folylpolyglutamates in these tissues?

Dr. Duch: Not yet, no.

Dr. Schilsky: It appears that CF is not very efficiently metabolized in the colon 38 model. Do you know, if in fact, that the cytotoxicity of FUra can be potentiated by CF in that model system?

Dr. Duch: No, we don't; we haven't gone back and done those studies yet. So we don't know the answer.

Dr. Rustum: Have you looked at other schedules and routes of administration, for example, ip., p.o. or by i.v. injection.

Dr. Duch: We looked crudely at oral treatment and just looked at a comparison of plasma levels. We haven't done anything in tissues yet and that is one of things that we're trying to do also; but orally, the levels in plasma are lower than we see by giving it i.p., that's about the only thing we can say at this point.

Dr. Rustum: You have not given multiple i.p. doses.

Dr. Duch: Not yet, no.

Dr. Greco: Would you have any data or would you know people that would have data on the effects of FUra and/or metabolites on the pharmaco-kinetics of 6R or 6S-CF and/or metabolites.

Dr. Duch: No.

Dr. Greco: Would you speculate on what you think one might have and how important it might be to look for such a thing?

Dr. Duch: No, we don't have any data on that because we haven't looked at the combinations yet of the 2 drugs; we've been concentrating on leucovorin. I don't know whether one would effect the metabolism of the other, I really have no idea.

Dr. McGuire: You're looking only at the monoglutamate pool in these experiments or you're looking at everything inside the cell after you've gone through some procedure.

Dr. Duch: These go through conjugase treatment and an isolation. So we're looking at total folates. It's not only monoglutamates.

Dr. McGuire: You wouldn't lose selectively one of those polyglutamate pools going through extractions and conjugase treatment.

Dr. Duch: No, we did recoveries on each one so that's all taken care of.

ROLE OF DOSE, SCHEDULE AND ROUTE OF ADMINISTRATION OF 5-FORMYLTETRA-

HYDROFOLATE: PRECLINICAL AND CLINICAL INVESTIGATIONS

Y.M. Rustum, L. Liu, and Z. Zhang

Grace Cancer Drug Center and Experimental Therapeutics
Roswell Park Memorial Institute
Buffalo, NY 14263

INTRODUCTION

During the last 30 years, 5-fluorouracil (FUra)* has been the drug
of choice for treatment of patients with adenocarcinoma of the colon.
This agent is also active against breast carcinoma and has significant
activity in carcinoma of the head and neck. In all cases, but especially
in colon carcinoma, the response rate is low and the duration of response is relatively short, on the order of 6 to 9 months.

Although determinants of response to FUra are multifactorial, in
vitro cytotoxicity has been attributed to its incorporation into
cellular RNA (1-5) and DNA (6-8) and to its potent inhibition of thymidylate synthase (9-16). Under in vivo conditions, however, factors such
as drug delivery to the target tissue may be affected by the pharmacokinetic properties of FUra and also by the dose and mode of its administration. Once the drug is delivered to the target tissue in sufficient
concentrations, factors such as cellular transport, activation to the
level of FdUMP and FUTP, retention of FdUMP, incorporation into cellular
RNA and DNA, levels of thymidylate synthase and cellular folate cofactor
pools, alone and/or in combination may play an important role in determining the therapeutic selectivity of FUra. The importance of one or
combinations of these factors may vary among cells of different types
and between tumor and normal cells.

Additional factors which influence the activity of FUra include:
circulating and cellular concentrations of normal metabolites such as
deoxyinosine, uridine and thymidine; the intracellular concentrations of
the competing metabolite, dUMP; and the circulating and endogenous concentrations of reduced folates. In vitro and in vivo studies revealed

---

*Abbreviations used are: FUra, 5-fluorouracil; FdUMP: 5-fluorodeoxy-
uridine monophosphate; TS, thymidylate synthase; dLCF, folinic acid,
(leucovorin, 5-formyltetrahydrofolic acid); $5-CH_3FH_4$, 5-methyltetra-
hydrofolic acid; $5,10-CH_2FH_4$, 5,10-methylenetetrahydrofolic acid;
$T_{1/2}$, elimination half-life; SSc: steady-state concentration; FUTP,
FUra triphosphate; AUC, area under the concentration time curve.

that regardless of the mechanism of action of FUra, in the presence of
excess 5-formyltetrahydrofolate the critical site of action of FUra
becomes thymidylate synthase, yielding potent and prolonged inhibition
of DNA synthesis. Furthermore, potentiation of the cytotoxic action of
FUra was highly dependent on the dose and duration of exposure to 5-
formyltetrahydrofolate.

Clinically, FUra and 5-formyltetrahydrofolate are being used at different doses and schedules and routes of administration. The aim of
this investigation is to evaluate the role of dose, schedule and route
of administration of 5-formyltetrahydrofolate in the therapeutic efficacy of FUra. Although investigations were carried out primarily in
rats bearing colon carcinoma, clinical pharmacological results will also
be discussed. Clinical experiences will be reported elsewhere in this
Symposium by Dr. Petrelli in colon cancer and by Dr. Arbuck in gastric
and other diseases.

METHODS

Clinical Protocols

Pharmacokinetic parameters of i.v. dLCF were evaluated in patients
with advanced colorectal cancer and oral and i.v. dLCF in patients with
lung carcinoma. Three clinical protocols were utilized and are outlined
in Table 1.

Specimens

Multiple blood specimens were obtained during the 2 h, 5 days continuous infusion and oral administration of dLCF and at various times
thereafter. Specimens were collected in heparinized tubes containing
sodium ascorbate (1 mg/ml). Tumor tissue specimens obtained during, and
in selected cases after termination of, dLCF + FUra treatment were frozen quickly on dry ice and stored in liquid nitrogen. Small specimens
were used for histopathology.

Table 1. Clinical Protocols for FUra Modulation by dLCF

Agent	Dose (mg/m^2)	Route	Schedule
dLCF	500	i.v.	2 h infusion
FUra	500-600	i.v.	push at 1 h after the start of dLCF infusion
dLCF	500	i.v.	5 days infusion
FUra	600	i.v.	5 days infusion
dLCF	125	p.o.	Q 1 h X4
FUra	450-600	i.v.	push at 4 h

Sample Processing

Quantitation of dLCF, 5-CH$_3$FH$_4$ and FUra were carried out by HPLC
as previously described by Trave et al. (17). The biologically active
isomer, 6S-CF was quantitated by microbiological assay with Pediococcus

40

cerevisiae. Intracellular $5,10\text{-}CH_2FH_4$ pools were quantitated using _Lactobacillus_ _casei_ TS and ^3H-FdUMP. Thymidylate synthase inhibition assays were carried out as described by Moran et al. (18).

Pharmacokinetic Studies in Rats

Pharmacokinetic studies of dLCF were carried out in normal rats and rats bearing transplantable colon carcinomas. Following cannulation of the rat's jugular vein, blood samples (0.1-0.2 ml/point) were collected in sodium ascorbate, centrifuged, extracted and processed for HPLC analysis. Up to 12 samples from each rat were obtained within 48 h.

Antitumor Activity

Antitumor activity of FUra alone and in combination with dLCF was carried out as follows: for leukemia cells, 10^6 cells were transplanted i.p. to DBA2/J mice and treatments were initiated 24 h later. For solid tumors, 0.1 gm of tumor pieces were transplanted s.c. and 7-10 days later when tumor sizes were approximately 0.5 to 1.0 gm, treatments were initiated.

Continuous i.v. Infusion

Continuous i.v. infusion of FUra alone and in combination with dLCF were carried out as described previously by Danhauser and Rustum (19).

Pharmacokinetic Evaluation

The elimination half-lives ($T_{1/2}$) were evaluated by 0.693/k where k is the apparent first-order elimination rate constant (slope of the linear regressed terminal portion of the log concentration vs. time curve). Areas under the concentration vs. time curve (AUC) were calculated by the trapezoidal rule; the area from the last data point detected to infinity was estimated by first order extrapolation according to C_z/k, where C_z was the last concentration detected.

For the 5 days continuous infusion schedule, parameters evaluated were: steady-state plasma concentration (SSc) and AUC; AUC from time zero to 120 h were calculated by the trapezoidal rule; AUC from 120 h to infinity were evaluated by first-order extrapolation using the mean elimination rate constant from patients treated with the 2 h infusion schedule.

RESULTS

Modulation of FUra Cytotoxicity by dL-CF

The role of dLCF dose and duration of exposure in the potentiation of FUra cytotoxicity against mouse cell line S-180 were investigated _in vitro_ and the data are summarized in Table 2.

It was initially determined by Hakala and her coworkers (15,16), that 20 μM dLCF (10 μM 6S-CF) and exposure for 24 h were the optimal conditions for modulation of FUra cytotoxicity. The data in Table 2 are an extension of those studies and demonstrate further that not only the dose was important but the duration of exposure was also critical. For example, incubation with 5 μM dLCF for 120 h produced similar cytotoxicity potentiation of FUra as obtained with 20 μM and exposure for 2 h. In the design of optimal regimens for FUra modulation by folate, the dose and duration of infusions should be taken into consideration.

Table 2. Modulation of Fluoropyridine Cytotoxicity by dLCF against
S-180 Cells: Role of Dose and Schedule

Duration of Exposure to dLCF (H)	IC_{50} (μM) of FUra at dLCF Concentrations of			
	1	5	10	20 μM
2	4.7	3.2	1.6	1.3
24	3.5	2.3	1.1	0.7
120	2.8	1.4	0.8	0.5

Pharmacokinetic Parameters of dLCF and Its Metabolites in Patients

Pharmacokinetic data of dLCF, LCF and $5-CH_5CH_4$ in colon carcinoma patients treated by the 2 h and by 5 d continuous i.v. infusion
of dLCF and in patients with lung carcinoma receiving the oral CF are
summarized in Table 3.

Table 3. Pharmacokinetic Properties of Reduced Folates in Plasma of
Patients with Advanced Colorectal Cancer. dLCF was Infused
as $500/mg/m^2/2$ hr or by 5 Days Continuous Infusion, or as
125 $mg/m^2/1h$ x4 Orally.

dLCF Schedule (mg/m^2)	dLCF		6S-LCF		$5-CH_3FH_4$	
	Peak[+]/S.S.[++]	AUC*	Peak[+]/S.S.[++]	AUC*	Peak[+]/S.S.[++]	AUC*
2H 500	96±38	71±22	24±6	2.7±1.5	17±8	14±5
5D 500	76±28	480±113	1.2±0.5	6±3.9	12±5	83±38
p.o. 125x4	4.6±1.9	375±89	0.5±1.0	–	4.3±2.1	43±21

[+]peak plasma concentration of folates (μM).
[++]plasma steady state (S.S.) concentration of folates (μM).
*Area under the concentration time curve (mM.min).

The data in Table 2 indicate that the AUC for dLCF and $5-CH_3FH_4$
were the highest when dLCF was administered by the 5 d infusion or p.o.
The peak plasma concentration of 6S-CF for the 2 h, 5 d and p.o. were
24±6, 1.2±5 and less than 0.5 μM, respectively. An example of the
plasma pharmacokinetic profile of dLCF and its metabolites following a 2
h, 5 d continuous i.v. infusion, and oral administration of dLCF (500
mg/m^2) are shown in Fig. 1. The data in Table 3 and Fig. 1 indicate
that the $t_{1/2}$ for dCF, LCF and $5-CH_3$ following an i.v. administration of dLCF were 8, 0.8 and 7 hr, respectively and greater than 6 h for
LCF following an oral administration of dLCF. The data in Table 3 also
indicate that while the peak plasma concentrations of LCF following the
2 h infusion of dLCF were over 20-fold higher than the achieved steady
state concentration, the AUC's for LCF were about 2-fold higher following a continuous infusion of dLCF. The plasma clearance of dLCF, how-

ever, were similar following an i.v. administration of dLCF (22±8 vs 20±7 ml/min), LCF clearance was significantly higher during the 5 d infusion than after the 2 h infusion (176±803 vs 398±241).

Relationship between Plasma LCF, Cellular 5,10,CH_2 and Inhibition of TS

The data in Table 4 indicate that with higher peak plasma concentration of LCF (24±6 μM) by the 2 h schedule, a greater increase in the cellular concentration of 5,10-CH_2FH_4 and correspondingly greater inhibition of TS were observed.

Data not shown here indicate while there was no significant differences on the pharmacokinetic properties of dLCF and its metabolites between previously treated and untreated patients, the lack of significant perturbation of cellular folate pools under conditions of continuous infusion of dLCF may be due to differences in the nature of the disease previously treated vs previous untreated patients and/or to a difference in the transport and activation of folate which may be influenced by the schedule of drug administration. Previously treated patients may require higher steady state plasma concentrations than 1 M LCG in order to modify sufficiently cellular folate. This hypothesis is now under investigation in our laboratory.

Table 4. Relationship between Plasma AUC of LCF, Intracellular Concentrations of 5,10 Methylenetetrahydrofolates (5,10-CH_2FH_4) and inhibition of Thymidylate Synthase (TS) in Previously Untreated and Treated Patients with Advanced Colorectal Carcinoma Following Treatment with FUra (500-600 mg/m[2] i.v. Push) and dLCF (500 mg/m[2]) by either 2 h or Daily for Five Days Continuous Infusion.

Schedule	N	Stage	LCF Peak[C]	LCF AUC[C]	5,10,CH_2FH_4 [D] Pre	5,10,CH_2FH_4 [D] Post/During	TS[E] Pre	TS[E] Post/During
2h	8	A	24±6	3.1±1.8	41±4	160±33	55±38	8±6
5d	5	B	1.2±5	6.0±3.9	38±39	75±32	38±46	23±6

A = Previously untreated patients
B = Previously treated patients
C = Area under the concentration time curve (mM.min), peak and steady state are expressed in μM

D = Expressed as pmol/mg protein
E = Expressed as fmol/mg protein

Pharmacokinetic Parameters of dLCF Administered at Different Doses, Schedules and Routes to Normal Rats

The area under the concentration time curve for CF and 5-CH_3FH_4 are summarized in Table 5. These data indicate that at 400 mg/kg dose, the AUC for dLCF and 5-CH_3FH_4 varied according to the mode of administration of dLCF. The AUC values for 5-CH_3FH_4 were in the order of 2h > 2d inf.> i.v. push>p.o. The dLCF to CH_3FH_4 ratios indicate greater metabolism to 5-CH_3FH_4 when dLCF was administered by infusion or by the oral route. Similar results were obtained at dLCF doses of 50,100, and 200 mg/kg. Greater than 10 μM-LCF was detected in rats' plasma following an i.v. administration of 100 mg/kg dLCF. In man, administration of 500 mg/m[2] dLCF by 2 h or 5 day continuous i.v. infusions, yielded 5.1 and 5.7 CF/5CH_3FH_4 ratios, respectively.

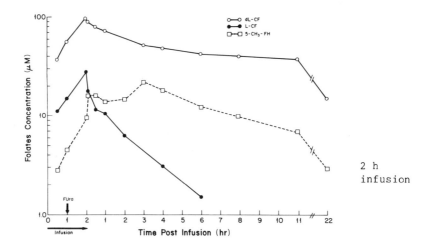

2 h
infusion

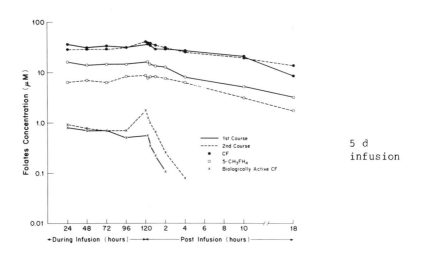

5 d
infusion

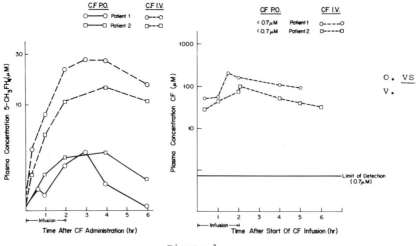

O. VS
V.

Figure 1

Table 5. Plasma AUC values and the AUC Ratios of CF to $5\text{-}CH_3FH_4$ Following i.v. and Oral Administration of 400 mg/kg CF.

| Schedule | AUC (μM/hr) | | CF/$5\text{-}CH_3FH_4$ Ratio |
	CF	$5\text{-}CH_3FH_4$	
i.v. push (400 mg/kg)	498.1±7.4	19.3±17.4	26.2
2 hr infusion (400 mg/kg)	734.3±96.6	119.6±96.6	6.1
2 days infusion (400 mg/kg/d)	253.4	114.9	2.2
p.o. q1hr x4 (100 mg/kg/hr)	10.4±2.9	4.1±0.4	2.5

Modulation of the Antitumor Activity of FUra Against Transplantable Mouse Tumors

The antitumor activity of FUra alone and in combination with dLCF against mice and rats bearing transplantable tumors was investigated and the results are summarized in Table 6. The effects of dLCF administration on the modulation of TS-folate cofactor pools were also evaluated.

The administration of dLCF at the 400 mg/kg by 2 h i.v. infusion in combination with FUra and yielding a peak plasma concentration of LCF on the order of 50 μM, did not modify significantly the antitumor activity against L1210, P-1798, C-26 and C-38. Except for the mouse colon tumors and B-16 melanoma, the pre-existing TS folate cofactor pools were relatively high. Treatment with dLCF did not alter significantly tumor tissue folates nor their response to FUra combination. In contrast, treatment of mice bearing B-16 melanoma and rats with colon tumor with dLCF modified the antitumor activity of FUra. These preliminary results indicate that the effect of dLCF treatment is tumor specific and the basis for these differences need to be investigated.

Table 6. Folate Cofactor Pools and In Vivo Antitumor Activity of FUra (100 mg/kg, i.v. push) Alone and in Combination with 2h i.v. Infusion of dLCF (400 mg/kg).

| Tumor | Type | TS-Folate Cofactor (pmol/mg protein) | | ILS (%) | |
		-dLCF	+dLCF	-dLCF	+dLCF
L1210	Leukemia	142	220	60	70
P1798	Lymphosarcoma	130	195	300	290
C-26	Colon	48	ND[+]	10	15
C-38	Colon	33	ND	20	10
B-16	Melanoma	9	122	5	80
-	Colon, rats	98	ND	150	280

[+]Not done.

CONCLUDING REMARKS AND FUTURE DIRECTION

Studies conducted in man and rats utilizing dLCF administered by different routes (i.v. and p.o.) and different schedules short vs continuous i.v. infusion, once a week and daily for 5 days demonstrated that the pharmacokinetic properties of CF and its metabolites are influenced by these factors. Furthermore, while alteration of the intracellular TS-folate cofactor pools seem to be a function of the dose and duration of exposure to dLCF, delivery of sufficient concentration of CF to the target cells may be a function of the peak or higher steady state plasma concentrations of LCF.

Administration of dLCF by short infusion did not modify the therapeutic efficacy of FUra in all of the tumors tested. Lack of such modulation seems to correlate with the inability to modulate equally the intracellular concentration of $5,10$-CH$_2$FH$_4$ in the tumors tested (Table 6). These data suggested the need to evaluate other schedules and routes of administration of dLCF in order to optimize conditions for achieving maximum therapeutic selectivity of FUra.

Future investigations should include: 1) extent and differential cellular metabolism of CF in normal vs tumor tissues following an administration of dLCF at different routes, schedules and routes of administration; 2) influence of dCF on the transport and metabolism of LCF by tumor and normal tissues under different ratios of dLCF to LCF; 3) refinement and development of new methodologies for the measurement of the kinetics of inhibition and recovery of thymidylate synthase as well as various intracellular folates and metabolites. Difficulties associated with these measurements from clinical materials have been encountered and limits the identification of critical determinants of response to FUra in combination with dLCF.

References

1. D.S. Martin, R.L. Stolfi, R.C. Sawyer, and C.W. Young. The application of biochemical modulation with a therapeutically inactive modulating agent in clinical trials of cancer chemotherapy. Cancer Treat. Rep., 69:421-423 (1985).
2. D.S. Martin, R.L. Stolfi, and S. Spiegelman, Striking augmentation of the in vivo anticancer activity of 5-fluorouracil by combination with pyrimidine nucleosides: an RNA effect, Proc. Am. Assoc. Cancer Res. 19:221 (1978).
3. R. Nayak, D.S. Martin, R.L. Stolfi, J. Furth, and S. Spiegelman. Pyrimidine nucleosides enhance the anticancer activity of 5-fluorouracil and augment its incorporation into nuclear RNA, Proc. Am. Assoc. Cancer Res. 19:1963 (1978).
4. D.S. Martin, R.L. Stolfi, R.C. Sawyer, R. Nayak, S. Spiegelman, C.W. Young, and T. Woodcock. An overview of thymidine, Cancer 45:1117-1128 (1980).
5. R.I. Glazer and K.D. Hartman. The effect of 5-fluorouracil on the synthesis and methylation of low molelcular weight nuclear RNA in L1210 cells, Mol. Pharmacol., 17:245-249 (1979).
6. D.W. Kufe, P.P. Major, E.M. Egan, and E. Loh. 5-Fluoro-2'-Deoxyuridine incorporation into L1210 DNA. J. Biol. Chem., 256:8885-8888 (1981).
7. P.V. Danenberg, C. Heidelberger, M. Mulkins, and A.R. Peterson. the incorporation of 5-fluoro-2'-deoxyuridine into dNA of mammalian tumor cells. Biochem. Biophys. Res. Commun. 102:654-558 (1981).
8. J.D. Schuetz, H.J. Wallace, and R.B. Diasio. 5-Fluorouracil incorporation into DNA of CF-1 mouse bone marrow cells as a possible mechanism of toxicity, Cancer Res. 44:1358-1363 (1984).
9. D.V. Santi, C.S. McHenry, and H. Sommer. Mechanism of interaction of thymidylate synthetase with 5-fluorodeoxyuridylate. Biochemistry, 13:471-480 (1974).

10. P.V. Danenberg. The role of reduced folates in the enhanced binding of FdUMP to dTMP synthetase. In: The Current Status of 5-Fluorouracil Leucovorin Calcium Combination, Bruckner, H.W. and Rustum, Y.M. eds., p. 5-11, Park Row Publishers, New York (1984).

11. J.A. Houghton and P.J. Houghton. On the mechanism of cytotoxicity of fluorinated pyrimidines in four human colon adenocarcinoma xenografts maintained in immune-deprived mice, Cancer, 45:1159-1167 (1980).

12. J.A. Houghton, S.J. Maroda, J.O. Philips, and P.J. Houghton. Biochemical determinants of responsiveness to 5-fluorouracil and its derivatives in xenografts of human colorectal adenocarcinomas in mice. Cancer Res., 41:144-149 (1981).

13. J.A. Houghton, C. Schmidt and P.J. Houghton. The effect of derivatives of folic acid on the fluorodeoxyuridylate-thymidylate synthetase covalent complex in human colon xenografts. Eur. J. Cancer Clin. Oncol., 18:347-354 (1982).

14. J.A. Houghton and P.J. Houghton. Basis for the interaction of 5-Fluorouracil and leucovorin in colon adenocarcinoma. In: The Current Status of 5-Fluorouracil-Leucovorin Calcium Combination, Bruckner, H.W. and Rustum, Y.M., eds., p. 23-32, Park Row Publishers, New York (1984).

15. R.M. Evans, J.D. Laskin and M.T. Hakala. Effect of excess folates and deoxyinosine on the activity and site of action of 5-fluorouracil. Cancer Res., 41:3288-3295 (1981).

16. M-B. Yin, S.F. Zakrzewski and M.T. Hakala. Relationship of cellular folate cofactor pools to activity of 5-fluorouracil. Mol. Pharmacol. 23:190-197 (1983).

17. F. Trave, Y.M. Rustum, N. Petrelli, L. Herrera, A. Mittelman, C. Frank and P.J. Creaven, Plasmic tumor tissue pharmacology of high dose intravenous 5-formyltetrahydrofolate in combination with 5-fluorouracil in patients with advanced colorectal carcinoma, J. Clinical Oncology 6:1184 (1988).

18. R.J. Moran, C.P. Spears and C. Heidelberger, Biochemical determinants of tumor sensitivity to the fluorouracil: Ultrasensitive method for the determination of 5-fluorodeoxyuridine monophosphate and thymidylate synthase, Proc. Natl. Acad. Sci. USA 76:1456 (1969).

19. L. Danhauser and Y.M. Rustum, A method for continuous drug infusion in unrestarained rats: Its application in the evaluation of the toxicity of 5-fluorouracil/thymidine combination, J. Lab. Clin. Med. 92:1047 (1979).

DISCUSSION OF DR. RUSTUM'S PRESENTATION

Dr. Santi: Does anyone know the effect of CF on FUra incorporation into RNA?

Dr. Rustum: Dr. Hakala did such studies in culture and found that CF has no significant effect on that parameter. We have done a few studies, using radiolabel in the rat tumor, and we also saw no significant effect on the incorporation of FUra into total RNA.

Dr. Hines: Joe, as you know we've looked at only 6 patients prospectively using a 500 mg oral loading dose of CF 12 hr pre-operatively at the time of the de novo removal of tumor (all colon cancer patients). Interestingly, at 12 hr when the tissues are frozen, the total reduced folate pools are ranging between 0.9 and as high as 4 μM. Not surprisingly these are mostly polyglutamate folates.

Dr. Bertino: How do they relate to pretreatment pools?

Dr. Rustum: We've got some of the specimen from Dr. Hines. We haven't had a chance to do the analysis as of yet.

Dr. Mihich: Do you know whether uptake of CF is different in the tumors in which you cannot observe an increase in ILS and which have relatively low pools to start?

Dr. Rustum: We have identified tumors with differential sensitivity to FUra modulation. Now we know we have given enough CF so delivery to the tumor is no longer an obstacle. As far as the intracellular modulation of reduced folates, we have not done these studies as of yet.

Dr. Mittelman: In the oral study, there were 13 patients, and in only 3 or 4 could you measure a plasma levels of 6S-CF, but you could see the other 5 formyl metabolite. What is that telling us?

Dr. Rustum: I think that probably could tell us several things. One is we know that 6S-CF is preferentially absorbed by the GI mucosa but not 6R-CF so it may have been taken up by tissues, metabolized, and not released into circulation. There is also degradation in the stomach because of the acid pH, etc. So there are many factors involved with this and I think the issue right now is to look at the polyglutamates, the extent of metabolism of CF by the oral route versus i.v. route by different schedule to see whether we really have differential metabolism between normal and tumor tissues. But this is telling us something, we don't know what, and I think it opens a lot of avenues for future investigations.

Dr. Bertino: A simple explanation is that 6S-CF which is absorbed goes to the liver first and is converted to 5-methyltetrahydrofolate. So you don't see very much of a blood level of the CF unless you use higher doses.

Dr. Rustum: It's possible, yes. There is extremely high first pass metabolism and unless you saturate that you get very small quantities of the 6S-isomer on board.

Dr. Straw: When you give oral dosing, the tumor and most tissues never see L-5-formyl, they're going to see 5-methyl. Is this a problem with oral dosing? One interpretation of my pharmacokinetic analysis is that in humans given very large doses of CF, there is an intra-cellular pool of folates which is in equilibrium with plasma 5-methyl but doesn't appear to be in equilibrium with 5-formyl. So one might argue from that that it's the plasma levels of 5-methyl which are important and not the plasma levels of 5-formyl.

Dr. Rustum: In the rat model, a comparison of the pharmacokinetics of 6S-CF by the i.v. route versus the oral route shows there is no detectable 6S-CF by the oral route and there is around 20-30 μM of 6S-CF from the i.v. The potentiation of the antitumor activity is almost identical. So I think we have to be very careful how much emphasis we place on plasma levels of reduced folates. I think what's important is tissue concentrations and metabolism.

Dr. Spears: Does CF perhaps have some other mechanism because you don't see the potentiation of ILS in mice so much. I think one has to be really cautious because TdR levels in mouse plasma may be 10 μM and no amount of CF would increase TS mechanism under those circumstances.

Dr. Rustum: Let me comment first. The concentrations of thymidine in mouse plasma is below the 1 μM level.

Dr. Spears: Ann Jackman says in her review it is 10 M and anyway Dr. Bertino has found that 0.1 μM TdR can rescue CCRF-CEM cells in vitro. So below 1 μM does not rule out a thymidine rescue autologous effect or perhaps dietary effects. Have you looked at transport in-hibitors that would perhaps decrease salvage mechanisms like benzyl-acyclouridine or dietary thymidine effects or dipyridamole that might bring out a TS mechanism?

Dr. Rustum: We have not done those experiments.

Dr. Schilsky: I want to make a comment about our experience with oral CF administration. We've been using oral CF in a regimen for patients with head and neck cancer and we give 100 mg orally every 4 hours continuously for over a period of 5 days. When one looks at the plasma concentrations, on the average, you see total reduced folate concentrations of about 7 μM. This is comprised primarily of total CF which is about 3 micromolar (of which about 10% is 6S-CF, the remainder being 6R-CF) and the remaining reduced folate is 5-methyltetrahydrofolate. I agree with you that when you give it orally, you get very little 6S-CF probably because of this first pass effect and rapid metabolism to 5-methyltetrahydrofolate.

Dr. Rustum: The 5-methyl may also be very important. Dr. Hakala and others have demonstrated that one can get modulation with the 5-methyl, at least in tissue culture cell lines, although sometimes you need a little higher concentration. We should not overlook the potential contribution of 5-methyl to the modulation of FUra.

Dr. Schilsky: Also, if the relative concentrations of 6R-CF to L-reduced folates are important, one may see a more favorable concentration ratio following oral administration than following intravenous administration.

Dr. Houghton: Given your data with oral CF showing that one may generate 5-methyl, which may be active, and Dave Duch's data which suggested that in the liver you got very high metabolism to 5-CH$_3$, has anybody looked at a primary model of hepatoma with FUra. It could be that if you have a moderately differentiated hepatoma it is going to have the same kind of characteristics as we see in liver. I think that maybe a very good model to look at this interaction in.

Dr. Rustum: I agree. We haven't looked at that, but we did look at the toxicity. When we give a high dose of FUra/CF we don't get liver toxicity.

Dr. Houghton: I think that is probably predictable but just in terms of tumors that have metabolic characteristics that may be favorable for this interaction, primary hepatomas may fall into that category.

Dr. Bertino: In tissue culture with a hepatoma cell line we have seen good modulation but we have no in vivo data.

Dr. Houghton: Is there any clinical trial planned?

Dr. Bertino: Not that I know of, not yet, but maybe.

Dr. Rustum: I believe the people from Genoa did the first trial 2-3 years ago with 5-methyl, and I believe it was negative.

Dr. Mini: We observed in the CCRF-CEM cell in vitro system that fluorouracil and FdUrd cytotoxicity could be enhanced with concentrations of (6R,S)5-methyltetrahydrofolate which were basically the same as for CF. Of course the synergism was maximum at very high concentrations, in the range of 10-100 μM of the (6R,S) form. In regard to the clinical studies, it might be that lack of the synergy observed was due to the dose of 5-methyltetrahydrofolate used in the clinic.

Dr. Hakala: We also found that 5-methyltetrahydrofolate was identical to 5-formyltetrahydrofolic acid, provided that you had 100 μM ascorbic acid in the cell culture medium to maintain its stability. We got identical potentiation of FUra with both these compounds.

Dr. Fritz Peters: I have both a comment and a question. The comment is on the question of Dr. Paul Spears about the salvage by nucleosides. For the salvage of nucleosides the concentration of nucleosides in plasma is important, but more important is the concentration of the nucleosides in the tumor itself. Both Dr. James Darnowski (Yale) and our group demonstrated that the concentration of uridine is much higher in tumor than in normal tissue. We don't know the concentration of TdR in the tumor but it might also be higher than in plasma. This might be different for different tumors and thus affect the potentiation by CF of FUra. I think this is something which has to be investigated in the future. The question is about the schedule you used for the antitumor activity of FUra. Did you use a single i.v. push of FUra or did you repeat it several times?

Dr. Rustum: The studies I have shown here used a single dose. If you give multiple doses then the MTD dose of FUra is about 25 mg instead of 100 mg with a single dose. We have done these studies by multiple doses daily x5, infusion for 5 days, and single dose; we have done all kinds of schedules and doses.

Dr. Fritz Peters: Maybe that explains the difference between our results with colon 38 and 26 because we used weekly administration of FUra/CF. Considering your data on the retention of inhibition of TS, I think this schedule would be more appropriate because as long as you have inhibition of TS by FdUMP then you don't need to give FUra again. When the enzyme is coming back to its normal levels, you should give the FUra again.

Dr. Rustum: I agree. The purpose of the present studies is not to optimize chemotherapy. The plan is to keep things simple (with a single dose) to see what differences there are between the various schedules and modalities. I agree fully with you that this may not necessarily be the optimal therapeutic schedule for a curative regimen, but that was not the intent of these studies.

Dr. Galivan: There's an additional point with regard to hepatoma cells. We've looked at the folate levels in various hepatoma cells and if we compare them to literature data concerning MCF7 cells or other types of tumors, the hepatoma cells appear to be able to accumulate larger amounts of total folates. This is reflected in a higher level of all pools and that also may be relevant to their capacity to quickly metabolize the CF. They have a fairly high level of folylpolygluta-mate synthetase, that's the reason.

Audience: Was your comment about the failure of CF to effect the incorporation of FUra into RNA based on bolus treatment with FUra or infusion?

Dr. Rustum: In mice, we looked at a single i.v. push. We have not looked at the incorporation of FUra into RNA under conditions of con-tinuous infusion for 5 days.

Audience: Do you think it is possible that continuous infusion might provide increased RNA incorporation under those circumstances?

Dr. Rustum: It may. However in separate studies, we tried to compare inhibition of TS by FUra and the amount of incorporation into RNA under conditions of 5 day continuous infusion vs i.v. push. In the study by Danhauser in my laboratory, we saw more incorporation into RNA but also a stable pool of FdUMP and inhibition TS was more pro-longed; at least in these tumors there was no correlation between the antitumor activity and the amount of FUra incorprated into RNA. The correlation seemed to be more toward inhibition of TS as the important determinant of response to FUra.

Dr. Santi: I'm wondering if a sufficiently well developed system is available that can cleanly and clearly distinguish by modulation of FUra, say with CF or MTX, the RNA effect from the TS effect. By dis-tingush, I mean can you clearly convert by modulation between pure TS effects by FUra to pure RNA effects.

Dr. Hakala: We tried to do that by showing the total metabolism of FUra in the presence and in the absence of CF. And the fact is that the vast majority of FUra goes into FUTP no matter what, in the cells which we studied; and it is just a tiny little fraction which goes into FdUMP. Certainly if you look at FdUrd the situation is reversed. I don't remember whether I looked in that case whether CF would affect the metabolism. As far as FUra metabolism, we found no effect.

Dr. Rustum: Other data from Dr. Hakala's laboratory concerning rescue with thymidine may also be relevant. Following FUra treatment, the Hep2 cell wasn't rescued by thymidine while the S180 cell was; but when CF was added to this, both cell lines were rescued now by TdR indicating the site of action was shifted from RNA in the Hep2 cells to TS in presence of CF.

Dr. Hakala: Yes, the site of action was shifted because the presence of CF allowed FdUMP to inhibit TS and make it significant. This occurred even though the FdUMP content was the same with or without CF.

Dr. Mittelman: I think the clinical trial that was performed by several groups including our own, with the concomittant administration of thymidine with large doses of FUra, indicated quite clearly that all we saw was toxicity and no clinical benefit.

Dr. Rustum: Parallel with this toxicity there was an increase of FUra incorporation into RNA and a decrease of the pool of FdUMP in tumor tissue.

Dr. Bertino: That was complicated because thymidine blocked metabolism.

Dr. Rustum: Yes, but the point is that we shifted the site of action to potentiate the incorporation into RNA in the colon tumor. Under these conditions we potentiated the toxicity but not the therapeutic efficacy of FUra.

Dr. Peters: This shifting of toxicity with thymidine indicates of course that FUra is incorporated into RNA. This suggested a concept which we are exploiting in our lab and in the clinic in Amsterdam, a combination of FUra with uridine. We can demonstrate in patients that delayed uridine administration lowers the toxicity of FUra. In cell culture we subsequently demonstrated that the incorporation of FUra into RNA was inhibited by uridine. When uridine was able to reverse cytotoxicity then the incorporation of FUra into RNA was also decreased. This may be a future combination (FUra/CF with uridine) that might decrease toxicity since in all studies so far, one only looked at the FUra effect on TS in tumors, but not in normal tissues such as bone marrow and the gut.

Dr. Rustum: Certainly the use of uridine is an interesting concept.

Dr. Mittelman: Some years ago, people at Memorial gave FUR, the ribo-side, and in that trial they saw greatly enhanced toxicity but no clinical benefit.

Dr. Rustum: In the model system, if you compare FU, FUdR and FUR, you find significantly more FUra incorporation into RNA with FUR and yet the antitumor activity of the 3 agents is identical although toxicity is greater with FUR.

PHARMACOKINETIC ANALYSIS OF (6S)-5-FORMYLTETRAHYDROFOLATE
(1-CF), (6R)-5-FORMYLTETRAHYDROFOLATE (d-CF) AND 5-METHYL-
TETRAHYDROFOLATE (5-CH$_3$-THF) IN PATIENTS RECEIVING CONSTANT
i.v. INFUSION OF HIGH-DOSE (6R,S)-5-FORMYLTETRAHYDROFOLATE
(LEUCOVORIN) [1]

J.A. Straw[2] and E.M. Newman[3]

[2]Department of Pharmacology, George Washington
        University, Washington, D.C. 20037
[3]Division of Pediatrics, City of Hope National
        Medical Center, Duarte, Ca. 91010

INTRODUCTION

    The biochemical rationale for the combination of leu-
covorin and fluorouracil presumes that administration of
large doses of leucovorin will increase the endogenous
pools of active folates and enhance the formation and/or
stability of the thymidylate synthase-FdUMP-methylenetetra-
hydrofolate complex (1). A knowledge of the pharmacokinetic
behavior of leucovorin and its active metabolite is essential
if one is to select doses of leucovorin which will produce
adequate plasma levels of active folates.

    Leucovorin calcium is the soluble calcium salt of (6RS)-
5-formyltetrahydrofolate (d,1-CF). The commercially available
products are prepared by chemical rather than enzymatic
reduction and therefore consist of equal amounts of the
diastereoisomers. It is generally accepted that only the
natural (1) isomer is active as a cofactor (2). Furthermore,
previous studies have demonstrated that the diastereoisomers
have independent pharmacokinetic behavior, and any attempt
to describe their pharmacokinetics must treat the diastereoisomers as separate chemical entities (3). In this paper we
describe observations on the pharmacokinetics of the diastereoisomers studied during and after constant infusion
of high doses of leucovorin given over a 5.5 day period.

MATERIALS AND METHODS

    Eleven patients enrolled in phase II clinical trials
received leucovorin 500 mg/m^2/day for 5.5 days. These patients
also received 5-fluorouracil 370 mg/m^2 by i.v bolus daily
for 5 days beginning 24 hours after leucovorin infusion was
started.

_____

[1]Supported by NIH grant BRSG SO7RR-05471 and a grant from
Lederle Laboratories to the City of Hope National Medical
Center.

[2]To whom requests for reprints should be addressed.

Protocol

The dose of leucovorin for each 12 hr (250 mg/m^2) was dissolved 1 l of 5% dextrose and infused into a peripheral vein at 85 ml/hr using an IMED pump. The solution was protected from light during the infusion. Blood samples were taken from the opposite arm prior to the infusion, at 10,20 and 30 min; 2,4,6 and each 24 hr during the infusion; and at the same time points for the first 6 hr after the end of the infusion. In 6 of the patients, urine was collected for two 24 hr periods during steady-state.

Chemicals

Culture media were obtained from Difco Laboratories,Detroit,Mi. d,l-CF and d,l-5-CH3-THF used for HPLC standards were purchased from Sigma Laboratories, St.Louis, Mo. l-CF used as the standard for the microbiological assays was generously provided by R.Moran, Childrens Hospital of Los Angeles. Other chemicals and solvents were of standard laboratory grade except for the solvents used for HPLC which were HPLC grade.

Analytical Procedures

Plasma and urine samples were analyzed for biologically active folates using a semi-automated method (4). l-CF was measured directly, using Pediococcus cerevisiae, and 5-CH$_3$-THF was measured by Lactobacillus casei bioassay of appropriate HPLC fractions as previously described (5). In addition the urine samples were subjected to HPLC analysis using a step-gradient system in which 10 ml of 1.6 mM tetrabutylammonium hydroxide(TBA) in 10% methanol, pH 2.0 was used to elute ascorbic acid and other interfering substances followed by 1.6 mM TBA in 30% methanol, pH 4.1, to elute and separate the folates. The system used a 10 micron C-18 column and detection at 294 nm and gave superior separation of folic acid from the reduced folates than the method previously described (3). The concentrations of d-CF in plasma and urine samples were calculated as the difference between total CF and l-CF as determined by the biological assay.

Data Analysis

1.The concentration versus time data from start of the infusion to 6 hours post infusion for d-CF and 2 hours post-infusion for l-CF was fit to the following equation for constant infusion and first order decay for a one compartment model using PCNONLIN (Statistical Consultants, Lexington,Ky.).

Eq. 1. $C(T) = (D/TI)/Vd/K(EXP(-KTSTAR) - EXP(-KT))$

Where: D = total dose
       TI = time of infusion
       TSTAR = T - TI for T >TI   and TSTAR = 0 for T < TI
       Vd = volume of distribution
       K = elimination rate constant

The dose was taken as 1/2 the infusion rate of d,l-CF and the parameters Vd and K were varied to achieve the best fit. Clp was calculated as the product of Vd and K.

2. The concentration versus time data for 5-CH3-THF from start of the infusion to 6 hours post-infusion was fit to a two compartment model described by the following system of equations.

Eq. 2. $d(5\text{-}CH3\text{-}THF)_1/dt = KFC - (K10+K12)(5\text{-}CH3\text{-}THF)_1 + K21(5\text{-}CH3\text{-}THF)_2$

Eq. 3. $d(5\text{-}CH3\text{-}THF)_2/dt = K12(5\text{-}CH3\text{-}THF)_1 - K21(5\text{-}CH3\text{-}THF)_2$

Where: $(5\text{-}CH3\text{-}THF)_1$ = the concentration in compartment one; $(5\text{-}CH3\text{-}THF)_2$ = the concentration in compartment two; and the input function (KFC) is the elimination rate constant for l-CF times the fraction of l-CF metabolized to $5\text{-}CH_3\text{-}THF$ times the plasma concentration of l-CF at time "t" as described by Eq.1 above.

The parameters varied to obtain the best fit were the micro rate constants K10, K12, and K21 and F, the fraction of l-CF metabolized to $5\text{-}CH_3\text{-}THF$. The parameter F, was constrained to be ≤ the fraction of l-CF excreted unchanged in urine and ≥ the fraction excreted as $5\text{-}CH_3\text{-}THF$. The volume of compartment 1 (Vc) was assumed to be the same as the Vd of l-CF. This assumption implies that 5-CH3-THF is produced in and removed from a pharmacokinetic compartment identical to that defined by the pharmacokinetic behavior of l-CF. Clp was calculated as the product of K10 and Vc. The steady-state volume of distribution (Vdss) was calculated from the formula: Vdss = Vc(1 + k12/k21).

3. Urinary clearance was calculated for 24 hour excretion during steady-state using the equation: Clr = amount excreted/unit time/m^2/plasma concentration. Non-renal clearance (Clnr) was calculated as the difference between Clp and Clr.

RESULTS

Table 1 shows the pharmacokinetic parameters calculated for the three compounds in 11 patients. d-CF achieved a steady state plasma concentration of 41.7 μM which was associated with a half life of greater than 6 hours, a relatively low plasma clearance and a small volume of distribution. In contrast the natural isomer had a half-life of only 45 minutes, achieved a plasma concentration of 3 μM and had a large plasma clearance. Its volume of distribution was approximately one and one half times that of d-CF. The metabolite of l-CF, $5\text{-}CH_3\text{-}THF$, had a steady-state plasma concentration of 5.4 μM and a half-life of 10 hours. The plasma half life of $5\text{-}CH_3\text{-}THF$ was much more variable than that of the other two compounds due to two patients with extremely long half lives. The median half life was 7.75 hours. Plasma clearance was intermediate between that of d-CF and l-CF whereas the volume of distribution was much greater than that of either of the other two folates. The parameter "F", obtained by computer fit as described in methods, was 0.63 ± .14 which implies that 63% of the infused dose of L-CF was converted to $5\text{-}CH_3\text{-}THF$.

Table 1. Pharmacokinetic parameters obtained in 11 patients receiving leucovorin by constant i.v. infusion at a dose of 500 mg/m^2/24 hours for 5.5 days.

	C_{ss} (μM)	$t_{\frac{1}{2}}$ (min)	Clp (ml/min/m^2)	Vdss (1/m^2)
d-CF	41.7[a] ± 16	385 ± 164	9.2 ± 3.3	4.5 ± 1.0
1-CF	3.0 ± 0.75	45 ± 15.6	123 ± 36	7.6 ± 2.2
5-CH$_3$-THF	5.4 ± 2.3	600 ± 402	46 ± 18	23 ± 13

[a]Mean ± S.D.

Table 2 shows the urinary excretion data obtained in 6 of the patients. For d-CF, 94% of the infused dose was recovered unchanged in the urine and nonrenal clearance (Clnr) was not significantly different from zero. However, we cannot exclude the possibility that small amounts of d-CF entered the normal folate pathways or were eliminated by other routes.

Thirty two % of the infused dose of 1-CF was recovered unchanged in the urine, and an additional 47% was accounted for in the urine as 5-CH$_3$-THF. Attempts to identify the remaining 21 % of the infused 1-CF using HPLC and microbiological assay were unsuccessful. However, traces of a compound which eluted with the same Rf as folic acid were present in some urine samples.

Table 2. Urinary excretion data in 6 patients receiving leucovorin by constant i.v. infusion at a dose of 500 mg/m^2/24 hours for 5.5 days.

	% in urine	Clr (ml/min/m^2)	Clnr (ml/min/m^2)
d-CF	94[a] ± 6.3	8.3 ± 1.4	0.5[b] ± 0.3
1-CF	32 ± 7.9	47 ± 17	97 ± 27
5-CH$_3$-THF	47 ± 10	32 ± 11	15.5 ± 17

[a]Mean ± S.D.
[b]Not significantly different from zero.

DISCUSSION

The findings presented here support previous reports that the pharmacokinetics of d-CF and l-CF differ considerably(3) and that during constant infusion of leucovorin, d-CF is the predominant folate present in plasma (5). Jolivet and Bertrand reported at this symposium that the affinity for transport of l-CF in human lymphoblastic CCRF-CEM cells was 30 to 45 times greater than that for d-Cf. in the constant infusion studies reported here the steady-state concentration of d-CF was about 14 times that of l-CF. Therefore it is possible that d-CF was taken up into cells. Our pharmacokinetic studies do not exclude this possibility. However, the observation that d-CF was almost completely recovered unchanged in the urine and the fact that d-CF appeared to be distributed in a single small compartment argue against extensive tissue uptake of the inactive isomer.

The plasma concentration vs time data for l-CF was adequately fit by a one compartment model with first order elimination. This implies that it achieved rapid equilibrium with a central compartment which probably consists of plasma and highly perfused tissues. Because there was no evidence of a second slowly equilibrating compartment it would appear that plasma l-CF is not in equilibrium with a form of tissue folates which reappear in plasma as l-CF.

The plasma concentration vs time data for $5-CH_3-THF$ required a two compartment model to achieve an adequate fit to the data. This implies that $5-CH_3-THF$ is produced in a compartment that is in rapid equilibrium with plasma and that it is also in equilibrium with a more slowly equilibrating compartment. The pharmacokinetic significance of the second compartment is that the relatively large volume of distribution results in a long half life, even though plasma clearance is quite high. The possible physiological (therapeutic) interpretation of the second compartment is that it represents a pool of reduced folates that are in equilibrium with plasma $5-CH_3-THF$. This pool could be $5-CH_3-THF$ or its polyglutamates or could equally well be other reduced folates that are converted to $5-CH_3-THF$ before they are detected in plasma. This suggests that plasma concentrations of $5-CH_3-THF$ are indicative of tissue stores of reduced folates but that the plasma concentrations of l-CF are only indirectly related to tissue pools of reduced folates in that l-CF is the precursor of $5-CH_3-THF$.

REFERENCES

1. Moran, R.G. and Keyomarsi, K. Biochemical Rationale for the Synergism of 5-Fluorouracil and Folinic Acid. NCI Monographs No.5:159-162, 1987.

2. Blakley, R.L. The Biochemistry of Folic Acid and Related Pteridines, p. 82. New York: American Elsevier Publising Co., 1969.

3. Straw, J.A., Szapary, D., and Wynn W.T. Pharmacokinetics of the Diastereoisomers of Leucovorin after Intravenous and Oral Administration to Normal Subjects. Cancer Res. 44:3114-3119,1984

4. Newman, E.M. and Tsai, J.F. Microbiological Analysis of 5-Formyltetrahydrofolic Acid and Other Folates Using an Automatic 96-Well Plate Reader.Analytical Biochem. 154: 509-515, 1986.

5. Straw, J.A., Newman E.M., and J.H. Doroshow Pharmaco-kinetics of Leucovorin (d,l,-5-Formyltetrahydrofolate) After Intravenous Injection and Constant Intravenous Infusion. NCI Monographs No. 5:41-45, 1987.

THE ROLE OF THYMIDYLATE SYNTHASE IN THE RESPONSE TO FLUOROPYRIMIDINE-FOLINIC

ACID COMBINATIONS

Sondra H. Berger*, Stephen T. Davis*, Karen W. Barbour, and
Franklin G. Berger

Departments of Basic Pharmaceutical Sciences* and Biology
University of South Carolina, Columbia, SC 29208

ABSTRACT

A panel of human colorectal tumor cell lines has been examined to
determine the role of TS in the response to fluoropyrimidine antimetabolites.
Among these cell lines, the response to FdUrd does not correlate with the
levels of TS. In cell lines HCT 116 and RCA, which are poorly responsive to
FdUrd, structural alterations in TS have been identified. In HCT 116, two TS
polypeptides are present: a common form, occurring in all the cell lines and
a variant form. The variant TS polypeptide has a reduced affinity for the TS
ligands, FdUMP and $CH_2H_4PteGlu$, relative to the common TS polypeptide.
Clonal populations of HCT 116 that overproduce each form have been isolated.
Clones that overproduce the variant polypeptide are 4-fold less responsive to
TS-directed cytotoxic agents than those that overproduce the common; thus,
the presence of the variant TS is associated with a reduced response to TS-
directed cytotoxic agents. The response of cell line RCA to FdUrd is dependent upon the extracellular CF concentration: response increases as CF is increased. RCA contains a TS enzyme with reduced affinity for $CH_2H_4PteGlu$,
relative to cell line C, which is sensitive to FdUrd at all CF concentrations. Both cells form high chain-length polyglutamates of $CH_2H_4PteGlu$ at
CF concentrations in which the response to FdUrd differs by 4-fold. In RCA,
the TS structural gene is variant, relative to the other cell lines. This
variation may underlie the altered enzyme affinity for $CH_2H_4PteGlu$ and
the sensitivity to modulation of FdUrd response by CF.

INTRODUCTION

The enzyme TS (EC 2.1.1.45) catalyzes the reductive methylation of dUMP
by $CH_2H_4PteGlu$ in the synthesis of dTMP. TS is inhibited by the fluoropyrimidine metabolite, FdUMP, which, in the presence of $CH_2H_4PteGlu$,
forms a covalent ternary complex with the enzyme that is extremely stable.
Thus, cytotoxicity resulting from the TS-directed actions of fluoropyrimidines is expected to be governed by the intracellular levels of TS enzyme,
FdUMP, and $CH_2H_4PteGlu$ and by the kinetic properties of the enzyme. In
fact, alterations in each of these four parameters have been associated with
reduced response to fluoropyrimidines (1-4).

The relationship between TS and response to fluoropyrimidines has frequently been assessed with FdUrd, since TS is a primary target of this agent.
While contributing significantly to elucidation of determinants of response

in cells in culture, the relevance of such studies to the clinical setting has been questioned, since FUra, not FdUrd, is utilized in the therapy of solid tumors. The cytotoxicity of FUra is derived from inhibition of TS and from the formation of fraudulent RNA; the relative contribution of these mechanisms to the clinical utility of FUra is unclear. Recent studies in patients with carcinomas of the GI tract have revealed that the administration of CF with FUra increases the clinical response significantly, relative to FUra alone (5). This combination is designed to enhance TS-directed action, since CF is thought to serve as a source of intracellular $CH_2H_4PteGlu$. This would indicate that TS plays a role in the response of human colorectal carcinoma to FUra and provides a rationale for investigations aimed at assessing the role of TS in the response to FdUrd and fluoropyrimidine-CF combinations.

A panel of seven human colorectal tumor cell lines has been utilized to examine the relationship between TS and the response to fluoropyrimidines. These cell lines vary in differentiation status, growth rate, drug sensitivity, and tumorigenicity (6); thus, they may be representative of the spectrum of colon tumor phenotypes encountered clinically. Three of the cell lines, HCTs 116, 116a, and 116b, are derived from the same primary tumor and, thus, reflect intratumoral heterogeneity. The other four cell lines, MOSER, RCA, C, and CBS, were derived from separate tumors. These cell lines have been characterized with respect to TS enzyme, mRNA, and gene structure, and the response to FdUrd and/or FdUrd-CF combinations. In two of the cell lines, structural variations in TS have been identified that are associated with reduced response to TS-directed cytotoxic agents.

MATERIALS AND METHODS

Cell Culture and Growth Studies. The human colorectal cell lines were maintained as monolayers in Dulbecco's modified Eagle medium supplemented with 10% FBS[1]. All growth studies were carried out in T-25 flasks inoculated with 100,000 cells. Drug-supplemented medium was added 24 hr after inoculation. Growth was continued for 5-6 cell generations, after which relative growth was measured by protein determination. For studies of the relationship between TS levels and FdUrd response, growth sensitivity to continuous FdUrd was determined in maintenance medium. For growth analysis of HCT 116/200 clones, cell lines were exposed continuously to RPMI 1640 medium supplemented with 5% FBS, FdUrd, 10μM CF, and 100 μM dIno[2]. For CF modulation studies, cells were depleted for 12 d in folate-free RPMI 1640 medium supplemented with 5% charcoal-stripped FBS and 100 μM hypoxanthine, 30 μM thymidine, and 30 μM glycine; folate-depleted cells were inoculated into CF-containing medium for 24 hr prior to 3 hr exposure to FdUrd-CF. The FdUrd was removed and the cells grown in CF-supplemented medium.

FdUrd-resistant HCT 116 cells were selected by adaptation to stepwise increases in drug concentration between 10 and 200 nM. The HCT 116/200 population was subcloned in conditioned medium supplemented with 15% FBS; the cloning efficiency was 70%.

Ternary Complex Formation. TS enzyme levels were determined in subconfluent cells by incubating 100,000 x g cell extracts with [6-^{3}H] FdUMP and $CH_2H_4PteGlu$ (7). A modified assay in which FdUMP was increased by 10-fold was carried out to ensure complete titration of TS in cell extracts.

TS enzyme structure was determined by incubating cell extracts with [^{32}P] FdUMP and $CH_2H_4PteGlu$ under conditions described previously (7),

---

[1] FBS, fetal bovine serum
[2] dIno, deoxyinosine

except that the FdUMP was increased 10-fold. [^{32}P] FdUMP was prepared by in-cubating [γ-^{32}P] ATP with FdUrd in the presence of partially purified E. coli thymidine kinase (8). The labelled ternary complexes were denatured in 6M urea and separated by isoelectric focusing in 9M urea-4% acrylamide gels containing 0.67% (vol/vol) each of Ampholines pH 4-6, 6-8, and 3.5-10 (9). After electrophoresis, the gels were fixed, dried, and subjected to autoradiography at -70°C.

A folate binding assay, which is a modification of the TS ligand binding assay (7), was developed to determine the levels of intracellular folates that stimulate ternary complex formation with TS in vitro. The assay con-tains 10 pmol L. casei TS (R.B. Dunlap, University of South Carolina), 30 pmol [6-^{3}H] FdUMP, 37 mM sodium ascorbate, and 0.1-3.2 pmol $CH_2H_4PteGlu$ or ascorbate extract in 0.1 ml total volume. Complexes were allowed to form for 1 hr at 30°C: total complexes were determined by the charcoal binding procedure (7); covalent complexes were determined after heating at 90°C in 1% sodium dodecyl sulfate by centrifugal elutriation on Sephadex G-50. Fol-ates were extracted from cells by heating at 90°C in 50mM Tris-HC1-1% ascorbate, pH 7.4. The extraction efficiency was 93%.

The glutamyl chain-length distribution of intracellular $CH_2H_4PteGlu_2$ was determined by forming ternary complexes among ascorbate extracts, [^{32}P]

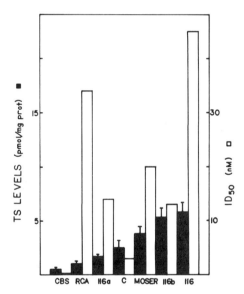

Fig. 1. TS levels and FdUrd sensitivity. TS levels in cell extracts were deter-mined by ternary complex formation utili-zing [^{3}H] FdUMP and $CH_2H_4PteGlu$ as des-cribed in Materials and Methods. The height of the solid bars represents the mean TS level, with the error bars in-dicating the S.D. The growth sensitivity to continuous FdUrd was determined as described in Materials and Methods. The height of the open bars represents the average ID_{50} value (concentration of FdUrd required for 50% inhibition of growth relative to control growth).

FdUMP, and partially purified human HEp-2/500 TS (10) using the folate binding assay conditions. The complexes were denatured, separated by isoelectric focusing, and detected by autoradiography as described for TS enzyme structure determination. The migration of the complexes formed with intracellular $CH_2H_4PteGlu$ was compared to that of complexes formed with pteroylpolyglutamate standards reduced enzymatically with L. casei dihydrofolate reductase to (6S) $H_4PteGlu$ forms (11), then converted to $CH_2H_4PteGlu$ polyglutamates with formaldehyde.

TS Sequences in Nucleic Acids. Total RNA and DNA were isolated from the colorectal cells as described previously (10). TS-specific sequences in RNA and DNA were analyzed by Northern and Southern analyses, as described previously (10). The TS probe was a gel-purified 750 base pair fragment of plasmid pMTS-3, which has been described previously (10).

RESULTS AND DISCUSSION

The TS levels and response to FdUrd in colonic tumor cell lines is depicted in Figure 1. It is immediately apparent that no consistent relationship exists between TS concentration and FdUrd response, even among the three cell lines isolated from the same tumor (HCTs 116, 116a, and 116b). That the enzyme levels determined in vitro reflect the in situ situation is indicated by analysis of TS mRNA levels, which parallel enzyme levels (data not shown). Two cell lines, namely HCT 116 and RCA, demonstrate a significant deviation between TS levels and FdUrd response, relative to the other cell lines. The data indicate that parameters other than TS levels are determinants of response to FdUrd.

One parameter that may influence FdUrd response is the structure of the TS enzyme. Structural variation in the TS polypeptide may alter enzyme affinity for FdUMP and $CH_2H_4PteGlu$ (4). TS structure was analyzed by isoelectric focusing gel electrophoresis of ternary complexes formed in cell extracts in vitro. As is shown in Figure 2, all the cell lines produce a polypeptide in common; in addition, HCT 116 contains an additional polypeptide that is more basic than the common form. That the two forms are not the result of

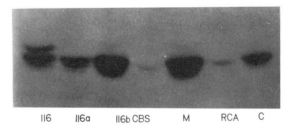

116   116a   116b CBS   M   RCA   C

Fig. 2. Isoelectric focusing gel electrophoresis of TS ternary complexes. Cell extracts were incubated with $[^{32}P]$ FdUMP and $CH_2H_4PteGlu$ under conditions in which TS is limiting. The resulting ternary complexes were subjected to isoelectric focusing gel electrophoresis and detected by autoradiography as described in Materials and Methods. The intensity of complexes does not reflect the relative abundance of TS in cell extracts.

population heterogeneity was demonstrated by subcloning parental HCT 116 cells; all clonal derivatives contain both TS forms (D. Eagerton and S. Berger, unpublished results).

The presence of two TS polypeptides in HCT 116 could be due to two TS structural genes or to a single gene which generates two polypeptide charge forms as a consequence of differential transcription and/or processing of TS mRNA. In order to distinquish between these possibilities, the parental cells were subjected to FdUrd under conditions that allow for selection of resistance due to TS gene amplification. The rationale for such an approach derived from previous studies in cells that are heterozygous for a selectable gene: amplification of only one allele of the gene was observed within any cell of the selected population (12). Thus, if two TS gene alleles are present in HCT 116 cells, cloned cells resistant to FdUrd by gene amplification should overexpress one or the other, but not both, TS forms. If a single gene is present and the two forms are derived from differential processing, all amplified cells should contain both forms. The electrophoretic analysis of representative clonal populations resistant to 200 nM FdUrd is shown in Figure 3. The clonal population designated 10 overproduces the common form of TS, while the clone designated 11 overproduces the variant form. The enzyme overexpression in all clones was a consequence of gene amplification, as determined by Southern blot analysis (data not shown). These data indicate that the two TS forms are derived from separate TS genes. The uncloned HCT 116/200 population, shown for comparison, is indicative of the relative abundance of the amplified phenotypes as well as other FdUrd resistant phenotypes.

The existence of populations that differentially overexpress TS allows for elucidation of the relationship between response to TS-directed cytotoxic agents and TS structure. Growth studies were carried out in FdUrd-containing medium supplemented with CF and dIno; the inclusion of CF and dIno maximizes TS-directed cytotoxicity by increasing the availability of $CH_2H_4PteGlu$ for ternary complex formation (S. Berger, unpublished results). Two clones of each amplification phenotype were utilized for cytotoxicity studies; all four clones express similar levels of TS. As is observed in Table 1, clones 11 and 15, which overproduce the variant TS, are 4-fold more resistant than clones 9

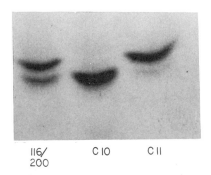

116/
200   C 10   C 11

Fig. 3. Expression of TS forms in HCT 116/200 cells. [^{32}P]-labelled ternary complexes formed in extracts of HCT 116/200 clone 10, clone 11, and uncloned population were analyzed as described in the legend to Fig. 2. The intensity of complexes reflects the relative abundance of TS in the extracts.

Table 1. Characteristics of HCT 116/200 Clonal Cell Lines

Cell[a] Line	FdUrd[b] ID_{50} (nM)	FdUMP[c] EC_{50} (nM)	$CH_2H_4PteGlu$[c] EC_{50} (μM)
Clone 9	25	ND[d]	ND
Clone 10	26	10	10
Clone 11	102	140	30
Clone 15	94	ND	ND

[a] Clones 9 and 10 overproduce the common form of TS by 15-fold; clones 11 and 15 overproduce the variant TS by 15-fold.

[b] Cells maintained in drug-free medium for 2 wk were exposed continuously to FdUrd-CF-dIno as described in Materials and Methods. The ID_{50} is the concentration of FdUrd required for 50% inhibition of cell growth, relative to control growth. The numbers are the average of 1 determination carried out in triplicate.

[c] Ternary complexes were formed in mixed extracts of clones 10 and 11 under conditions in which either [^{32}P] FdUMP or $CH_2H_4PteGlu$ is varied. The complexes were denatured and separated by isoelectric focusing as described in Materials and Methods. The EC_{50} is the concentration of ligand required for 50% maximal ternary complex formation. The EC_{50} was estimated from autoradiograms after densitometric analysis.

[d] ND, not determined.

and 10, which overproduce the common form. Thus, the presence of the variant TS is associated with reduced response to TS-directed cytotoxic agents.

The biochemical basis for the response difference was examined by estimating the concentration of FdUMP and $CH_2H_4PteGlu$ required for 50% maximal ternary complex formation (EC_{50}) in mixed extracts of clones 10 and 11. The data in Table 1 reveal that the apparent affinity of the variant TS for both FdUMP and $CH_2H_4PteGlu$ is reduced. Although it is clear that the two forms differ significantly in affinity for the ligands involved in ternary complex formation and that this difference is associated with the response difference, these data are preliminary. Because the analyses were carried out in cell extracts, it is unlikely that they reflect the absolute affinity of the purified enzymes for FdUMP and $CH_2H_4PteGlu$. Studies are in progress to purify the two enzymes for kinetic analyses and for elucidation of sequence variation by peptide mapping. In addition, we have isolated cDNA sequences corresponding to both TS mRNAs for sequence analyses and for functional tests in in vitro and in vivo systems.

A second mechanism which could underlie reduced response to FdUrd is reduction in either the intracellular level or the extent of polyglutamation of $CH_2H_4PteGlu$. This possibility was examined in two cell lines, RCA and C, which differ significantly in response to FdUrd (Figure 1). The cells were depleted of folates for 12 d, after which the response to FdUrd was determined at varying CF concentrations. As is shown in Table 2, the response of RCA to FdUrd is potentiated 10-fold by increasing the CF concentration 1000-fold, while the response of C is enhanced 4-fold over this concentration range. Both cells approach a similar ID_{50} at 10 μM CF. Thus, RCA is more sensitive than C to modulation of FdUrd response by CF.

The biochemical basis for the difference in response to CF modulation of FdUrd cytotoxicity was examined by analyzing the intracellular levels of folates that stimulate ternary complex formation with TS. The levels of total TS folate co-substrates (folates that stimulate covalent and non-covalent

Table 2. TS Folate Co-substrates and FdUrd Sensitivity

Cell Line	CF Conc. (M)	FdUrd[a] ID_{50} (μM)	Total TS Folate[b] Co-substrates (pmol/mg prot)	$CH_2H_4PteGlu$[c] Levels (pmol/mg prot)
C	10^{-8}	0.11 (2)	1.1 ± 0.5 (4)	0.11 ± 0.08 (4)
RCA	10^{-8}	0.38 (2)	ND[d]	ND
C	3×10^{-8}	0.09 (2)	2.9 ± 0.1 (4)	0.32 ± 0.10 (4)
RCA	3×10^{-8}	0.33 (2)	1.2 ± 0.5 (4)	0.20 ± 0.04 (4)
C	10^{-7}	0.04 (2)	7.4 ± 1.7 (4)	1.54 ± 0.16 (3)
RCA	10^{-7}	0.11 (2)	5.2 ± 0.4 (4)	0.69 ± 0.06 (4)
C	10^{-5}	0.03 (2)	12.0 ± 0.6 (4)	3.18 ± 0.11 (4)
RCA	10^{-5}	0.04 (2)	8.3 ± 0.4 (4)	2.03 ± 0.40 (3)

[a] Folate-depleted cells were exposed to FdUrd for 3 hr as described in Materials and Methods. The ID_{50} is the concentration of FdUrd required to inhibit cell growth by 50% with respect to controls. The data are the mean ± S.D. The number of separate determinations, each carried in triplicate, is shown in parentheses.

[b] Total TS folate co-substrates comprise the folates that stimulate formation of covalent and non-covalent ternary complexes with [3H] FdUMP and L. casei TS as described in Materials and Methods. The data are mean values ± S.D. The numbers in parentheses represent the number of separate determinations carried in triplicate.

[c] The $CH_2H_4PteGlu$ levels comprise the folates that stimulate formation of covalent complexes with [3H] FdUMP and L. casei TS. The data are mean values ± S.D. The numbers in parentheses represent the number of separate determinations.

[d] ND, not detected.

complexes) and of $CH_2H_4PteGlu$ (folates that stimulate covalent complexes) were determined in extracts of each cell line exposed to various CF concentrations. At all CF concentrations, C accumulated higher levels of intracellular TS folates than RCA (Table 2). Furthermore, the cells differ in the levels of intracellular TS folates required to promote equivalent TS-directed cytotoxicity (Table 2).

The differential response to intracellular TS folates may be due to a differential capacity to form higher glutamyl chain-length derivatives of $CH_2H_4PteGlu$. Since the affinity of most TS enzymes for $CH_2H_4PteGlu$ increases with increasing glutamyl chain-length (13), a reduction in folylpolyglutamate levels could have significant effects on TS inhibition by FdUMP. The levels and distribution of $CH_2H_4PteGlu$ polyglutamates were determined in RCA and C after exposure to various CF concentrations. Shown in Figure 4 is the electrophoretic pattern of ternary complexes formed in vitro with endogenous $CH_2H_4PteGlu$. As also shown in Table 2, the levels of total ternary complexes stimulated by intracellular $CH_2H_4PteGlu$ are higher in C than in RCA at all concentrations of CF; however, there is no detectable reduction in the proportion of ternary complexes stimulated by higher chain-length polyglutamates in RCA extracts. In fact, the proportion of higher chain-length polyglutamates is greater in RCA than in C at CF concentrations below 10^{-7} M. Thus, it would appear that the proportion of $CH_2H_4PteGlu$ polyglutamates is not limiting the interaction of FdUMP with the RCA TS.

An alternative possibility for the differential TS-directed response to equivalent intracellular $CH_2H_4PteGlu$ is that the TS enzyme in RCA has a reduced affinity for $CH_2H_4PteGlu$. The enzymes from RCA and C were partially purified and the EC_{50} values for FdUMP and $CH_2H_4PteGlu$ for maximal ternary complex formation were determined. No difference in the apparent EC_{50} values for FdUMP was detected between the enzymes (data not shown); the RCA enzyme required 3-fold higher $CH_2H_4PteGlu$ for maximal ternary complex formation, as determined by the in vitro folate binding assay (data not shown) and by gel electrophoretic analysis (Figure 5). Thus, reduced affinity of RCA TS for $CH_2H_4PteGlu$ may underlie the reduced TS-directed response of these cells to intracellular $CH_2H_4PteGlu$. It is of interest that RCA contains variation in the TS structural gene, which has not been detected in the other colorectal cell lines (data not shown). Whether the TS structural variation is associated with the functional alteration is a possibility currently under investigation.

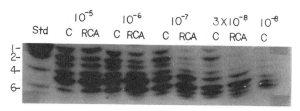

Fig. 4. Glutamyl chain-length distribution of ternary complexes formed with endogenous folates. Cellular folates were extracted as described in Materials and Methods after exposure of RCA and C to various CF concentrations. Ternary complexes were formed among human TS, [^{32}P] FdUMP, and extracted folates under conditions in which folate is limiting; the complexes were separated by isoelectric focusing gel electrophoresis and detected as described in Material and Methods. Complexes formed with $CH_2H_4PteGlu$ derivatives containing 1, 2, 4, and 6 glutamyl residues were utilized as standards.

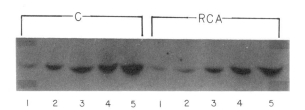

Fig. 5. Kinetics of $CH_2H_4PteGlu$ binding to TS enzymes from RCA and C. TS partially purified from RCA or C was incubated with excess [^{32}P] FdUMP and varying concentrations of $CH_2H_4PteGlu$; the resulting ternary complexes were analyzed by isoelectric focusing gel electrophoresis as described in the legend to Fig. 2. The concentrations of $CH_2H_4PteGlu$ utilized were: lane 1, 19 nM; lane 2, 38 nM; lane 3, 76 nM; lane 4, 190 nM; and lane 5, 380 nM.

These studies indicate that this panel of human colorectal tumor cells is an excellent model system for elucidation of the extent of variation that exists in response to TS-directed cytotoxic agents; moreover, it is useful for mechanistic studies of the interaction between CF and fluoropyrimidines. The identification of structural alterations in TS associated with reduced response to fluoropyrimidines is of particular utility to the prediction of clinical response to TS-directed chemotherapy. In this regard, future directions are aimed at determining whether such variations exist in the human population and at assessing whether they are genetic determinants of clinical response to FUra-CF combinations.

REFERENCES

1. J.L. Grem and P.H. Fischer, Alteration of fluorouracil metabolism in human colon cancer cells by dipyridamole with a selective increase in fluorodeoxyuridine monophosphate levels, Cancer Res. 46:6191 (1986).
2. B. Ullman, M. Lee, D.W. Martin, Jr., and D.V. Santi, Cytotoxicity of 5-fluoro-2'-deoxyuridine: requirement for reduced folate cofactors and antagonism by methotrexate, Proc. Natl. Acad. Sci. USA 75:980 (1978).
3. W.L. Washtien, Thymidylate synthase levels as a factor in 5-fluorodeoxyuridine and methotrexate cytotoxicity in gastrointestinal tumor cells, Mol. Pharmacol. 21:723 (1982).
4. A.R. Bapat, C. Zarow, and P.V. Danenberg, Human leukemic cells resistant to 5-fluoro-2'-deoxyuridine contain a thymidylate synthetase with lower affinity for nucleotides, J. Biol. Chem. 258:4130 (1983).
5. N.J. Petrelli and A. Mittelman, An analysis of chemotherapy for colorectal carcinoma, J. Surg. Oncol. 25:201 (1984).
6. M.G. Brattain, A.E. Levine, S. Chakrabarty, L.C. Yeoman, J.K.V. Willson, and B. Long, Heterogeneity of human colon carcinoma, Cancer Metas. Rev. 3:177 (1984).
7. R.G. Moran, C.P. Spears, and C. Heidelberger, Biochemical determinants of tumor sensitivity to 5-fluorouracil: ultrasensitive methods for the determination of 5-fluoro-2'-deoxyuridylate, 2'-deoxyuridylate, and thymidylate synthetase, Proc. Natl. Acad. Sci. USA 76:1456 (1979).
8. D. Ayusawa, K. Iwata, T. Seno, and H. Koyama, Conditional thymidine auxotrophic mutants of mouse FM3A cells due to thermosensitive thymidylate synthase and their prototrophic revertants, J. Biol. Chem. 256:12005 (1981).
9. P.H. O'Farrell, High resolution two-dimensional electrophoresis of proteins, J. Biol. Chem. 250:4007 (1975).
10. S.H. Berger, C.-H. Jenh, L.F. Johnson, and F.G. Berger, Thymidylate synthase overproduction and gene amplification in fluorodeoxyuridine-resistant human cells, Mol. Pharmacol. 28:461 (1985).
11. D.G. Priest, K.K. Happel, and M.T. Doig, Electrophoretic identification of poly-γ-glutamate chain-lengths of 5,10-methylenetetrahydrofolate using thymidylate synthetase complexes, J. Biochem. Biophys. Meth. 3:201 (1980).
12. J.A. Lewis, J.P. Davide, and P.W. Melera, Selective amplification of polymorphic dihydrofolate reductase gene loci in Chinese hamster lung cells, Proc. Natl. Acad. Sci. USA 79:6961 (1982).
13. C.A. Allegra, B.A. Chabner, J.C. Drake, R. Lutz, D. Rodbard, and J. Jolivet, Enhanced inhibition of thymidylate synthase by methotrexate polyglutamates, J. Biol. Chem. 260:9720 (1985).

DISCUSSION OF DR. S. BERGER'S PRESENTATION

Dr. Rustum: As you know there is a lot of clinical interest in both FdUrd and FUra and, at least under certain conditions, they seem to behave differently in terms of toxicity. I wonder whether your cell lines with different phenotypes respond similarly to modulation of FUra and FUdR by CF.

Dr. Berger: We've looked at both the 116 and RCA. With FUra, RCA cytotoxicity is highly modulated by CF; in the case of 116, FUra cytotoxicity does not seem to be affected by CF, certainly at high CF. The 116 seems to be resistant. The question is, "Is TS the target of FUra at low CF". We don't know that yet.

Dr. Moran: You presented data that says that the proteins are different and you've concluded from some of your selection of resistant cell lines that the genes are actually different and that is responsible for the resistance. Do you have any RFLP analysis or any data that there are actually two forms of genomic structures that end up coding for TS; do you have any direct evidence for that? It would be terribly important in terms of, if nothing else, developing a screen to find out which variant is present in a particular tumor.

Dr. Berger: We've looked at at least a half dozen enzymes but we have yet to find an RFLP. That's not surprising since that's sometimes like looking for a needle in a haystack. We're going to continue to look for an RFLP. We also can make a specific oligonucleotide probe to the region of difference which can actually differentiate between the 2 genes. That's what we're going to do with the cDNA probe. However, right now since we do have $[P^{32}]$FdUMP, we can pick up the structural difference in small biopsies, milligram samples, because of the extreme sensitivity of the $[P^{32}]$FdUMP.

Dr. Kalman: I wonder about that biphasic curve. What seems interesting about it is that there is something else happening with these cells which is that at very low concentrations of CF you, in fact, have higher polyglutamates in higher proportion. I wonder if you would like to comment whether there may be an underlying connection there. That is, the cell lines which display FdUrd sensitivity at very, very low concentrations seem to also accumulate very high chain length polyglutamates at very low concentrations.

Dr. Berger; All we know is that the affinity for the monoglutamate seems to be different between the 2 enzymes. What happens with the polyglutamates is certainly one of the experiments we're going to do once we purify the enzymes. All we can say now is that there's a differential response to methylenetetrahydrofolate monoglutamate and what appears to be the most likely difference between the 2 cell lines is an affinity alteration for that monoglutamate. Will that be magnified for the polyglutamate, we don't know.

Dr. Arbuck: Have you been able to identify this variant yet in fresh human tumor samples?

Dr. Berger: No, one of the first things we want to do is a population study. That's why it will be good to have an RFLP where you can get DNAs on blots and determine whether it's present in the human population. Unfortunately, we don't have that right now but that is certainly where we're going.

Dr. Bertino: We recently showed the same kind of situation in a colon cell line for dihydrofolate reductase where there seem to be 2 genes present and one of them is amplified, which is a variant gene which is more resistent to MTX than the sensitive gene. We found the mutations responsible for the resistance. Do you think your mutation comes from the development of the tumor, because this is a tumor which is induced by carcinogen, or do you think maybe it's a polymorphism which is endogenous in the population, i.e., this is something that normal people have.

Dr. Berger: I can't even rule out the possibility that it was selected during cell culture from the primary tumor. We just don't know what the origin of the variation was. In this regard, it's very interesting that colonic tumors often have monosomy for chromosome 18, and TS is on chromosome 18. If you have heterozygosity for TS and you have 2 different types of TS present in the population segregating out, then you have the chance, if you're going to get loss of one of the chromosome 18, either to select out a patient who could be very sensitive or patient which can be very non-responsive. We don't know and that is certainly why we want to go to the human population to find it.

Dr. Daneberg: Did you say the cells are cross-resistant to FUra?

Dr. Berger: Yes, I think the ID_{50} for 116 cells for FUra is around 200–300 μM. They have a real resistance to FUra.

TUMOR CELL RESPONSES TO INHIBITION OF THYMIDYLATE SYNTHASE [1]

Richard G. Moran[2], Khandan Keyomarsi, and Ramesh Patel

Departments of Pediatrics (RGM) and Biochemistry (RGM,KK)
University of Southern California

Division of Hematology/Oncology
Children's Hospital of Los Angeles (RGM,RP)
Los Angeles, CA 90027

ABSTRACT

Whether inhibition of thymidylate synthase is lethal to a population of tumor cells depends upon three factors: 1) the dependence of the cells upon *de novo* synthesis of thymidine nucleotides; 2) the length of time enzyme is inhibited and the requirement for thymidine nucleotides during this period; and 3) the biochemical responses of the cells to the initial inhibition of enzyme, many of which interfere with maintenence of thymidylate synthase in an inhibited state. Following inhibition of thymidylate synthase, deoxyuridylate accumulates, as does the cellular content of thymidylate synthase. In addition, the initially formed enzyme-inhibitor complexes dissociate. These biochemical sequelae alter the effectiveness of the blockade of thymidylate synthase in a time-dependent, continuously-changing manner. Whether cell kill occurs depends on whether the dynamic balance of these factors allows a sufficiently low enzymatic activity to be maintained for a long enough period of time.

An analysis of this interaction of factors leads us to the conclusions that efficient tumor cell kill with fluoropyrimidines is best attained by combination with reduced folate cofactors and inhibitors of deoxypyrimidine biosynthesis. Each of these agents modifies the response of tumor cells with the result that the fluorodeoxyuridylate-induced inhibition of thymidylate synthase is maintained. This analysis also suggests that folate analogs inhibitory to thymidylate synthase are more compatible than pyrimidine

---

[1] This work was supported in part by USPHS grant CA-36054 from the National Cancer Institute. RGM is a Scholar of the Leukemia Society of America.

[2] To whom correspondence should be addressed at: Division of Hematology/Oncology, Children's Hospital of Los Angeles, 4650 Sunset Blvd, Los Angeles, CA 90027

analogs with inhibition of thymidylate synthase as an approach to cancer chemotherapy.

INTRODUCTION

The fluorinated pyrimidine 5-fluorouracil (5-FU)[1] and its 2'-deoxyribonucleoside (FdUrd) have been the focus of considerable attention as chemotherapeutic agents for the treatment of carcinomas of the gastrointestinal tract. 5-FU has been the agent of choice for colorectal carcinoma for > 25 years- a remarkable fact. It is even more remarkable that 5-FU is, to this day, most often used as a single agent for the treatment of this (these) disease(s). Yet, the frequency of objective responses of colorectal carcinomas to this agent is only modest (7-19 % in different studies- see other contributions to this volume) and complete responses of metastatic colorectal carcinomas induced by this drug are very rare.

The 5-FU metabolite, 5-fluoro-2'-deoxyuridine-5'-monophosphate (FdUMP), is a tight-binding inhibitor of thymidylate synthase (TS) and is a prototypical example of a mechanism-based enzyme inhibitor (1). FdUMP follows the initial steps in the sequence of interactions with TS that occurs with 2'-deoxyuridine-5'-monophosphate (dUMP) during the enzymic reaction leading to the synthesis of thymidylate. During these steps, dUMP (or FdUMP) becomes covalently attached to both TS and the folate cofactor used for this reaction, $5,10\text{-}CH_2\text{-}H_4PteGlu_n$. Thereafter, in the normal reaction, TS catalyzes the transfer of a hydride ion to the 5-position of dUMP, a reaction which appears to obligatorily involve cleavage of the nucleotide-enzyme bond and the concommittant loss of the 5-hydrogen of dUMP. This hydride transfer is not possible for FdUMP due to the stability of the -C-F bond. Thus, TS is trapped as a covalently-bound ternary complex (TC) with nucleotide and cofactor.

It is commonly assumed that, because this TC involves covalent attachment of enzyme to inhibitor, FdUMP inhibition of TS is an irreversible phenomenon. This assumption is directly contradicted by a substantial body of evidence demonstrating the dissociation of this complex with the regeneration of catalytically active TS. Given that TS catalyzes the formation of TC, the principle of microscopic reversibility dictates that, in theory, this protein would also be capable of catalyzing the reverse reaction, namely, the regeneration of free enzyme. We have recently reported (2) that this reversal occurs in intact leukemic cells at a rate that would limit cell kill by FdUMP.

In this manuscript, we analyze the consequences of the reversibility of the formation of TC to therapeutics of tumors based on inhibition of TS. A case is made that the dynamics of dUMP synthesis, TS synthesis, folate cofactor levels, and the rate of cell death resultant from TMP deprivation should all be considered in order to understand how cells are killed by inhibition of TS with pyrimidine analogs. Some of the biochemical responses of tumor cells that make pyrimidine analog-based TS inhibition difficult should enhance inhibition of TS by folate analogs.

---

1 The abbreviations used were: 5-fluorouracil, 5-FU; 5-flouro-2'-deoxyuridine, FdUrd; 2'-deoxyuridine-5'-monophosphate, dUMP; 5-fluoro-2'-deoxyuridine-5'-monophosphate, FdUMP; thymidylate synthase, TS; ternary complex, TC; $5,10\text{-}$methylenetetrahydrofolate with an unspecified polyglutamyl side chain, $5,10\text{-}CH_2\text{-}H_4PteGlu_n$; thymidine-5'-monophosphate, TMP; 10-propargyl-5,8-dideazafolic acid, CB3717; methotrexate, MTX.

RESULTS

Accumulation of dUMP

After the inhibition of thymidylate synthesis either by a direct inactivation of TS by fluoropyrimidines or by an indirect effect consequent to inhibition of dihydrofolate reductase by methotrexate, dUMP accumulates in dividing tumor cells (3-5). In some cell types, e.g. the CCRF-CEM human lymphoblastic leukemia cell (Fig. 1), this effect can be quite pronounced. Exposure of CCRF-CEM cells to a cytotoxic (Fig 1B, inset) concentration of 5-FU results first in progressively higher degrees of inhibition of TS activity (Fig 1A) followed by the accumulation of dUMP (Fig. 1B). Prior to inhibition of TS, the dUMP concentration in these cells was found to be 5-10 μM; after 11 hours of exposure to 30 μM 5-FU, the dUMP content of these cells was equivalent to a concentration of 1.2 mM. It is notable that, following the accumulation of dUMP in these cells, free FdUMP was detected and inhibition of TS did not intensify, so that free TS and free FdUMP coexisted in these cells.

Why does dUMP accumulate in mammalian cells after inhibition of TS ? A review of the literature reveals that the two enzymes responsible for the biosynthesis of dUMP, ribonucleoside diphosphate reductase and deoxy-cytidylate deaminase, are subject to feedback regulation by deoxyribo-nucleoside triphosphates but not by dUMP (6,7). As a result, following a block of utilization of dUMP due to inhibition of thymidylate synthesis, dUMP could accumulate to substantial concentrations. The levels of dUMP will accumulate until a second (usually minor ?) pathway of loss becomes important or until the accumulating metabolite becomes inhibitory to some other cellular

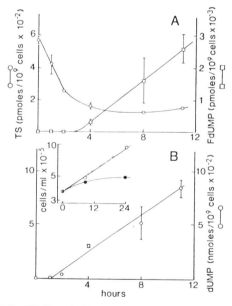

Figure 1 Levels of TS, dUMP and FdUMP in CCRF-CEM cells after exposure to 5-FU. (A) TS (O) and FdUMP(□) levels are shown as a function of time during continuous exposure of CCRF-CEM cells to 30μM drug. (B) dUMP (O) levels were determined on acetic acid extracts. Inset, mean cell numbers of duplicate control (O) or drug-treated (O) cultures as a function of time. Reproduced from reference 4 with the permission of Proc. Natl. Acad. Sci. USA.

process. Jackson (5) has shown that nucleotidase activity is an important function that limits dUMP accumulation in some cell types, and that deoxyuridine is found at substantial levels in the extracellular growth medium of such cells after inhibition of TS. A more complete analysis of the process of dUMP accumulation and the apparent differences among cell types would be important. For instance, analysis of dUMP levels in a number of human colorectal carcinomas (8) following 5-FU indicated that dUMP did not accumulate in spite of substantial inhibition of TS. This observation remains unexplained but potentially of paramount importance.

Level of TS activity compatible with tumor cell growth and cell kill

Taking the size of the human genome as 3×10^9 nucleotide base pairs for a diploid cell, the rate of synthesis of TMP that would allow DNA synthesis at a rate compatible with a generation time of 25 hrs would be 3.3 pmoles min^{-1} per million cells or about 0.042 nmol of TMP supplied per min per mg of cytosolic protein. This calculation assumes, of course, that all of the cells in a tumor mass are actively traversing the cell cycle. Nevertheless, it allows one to ask whether TS is present in tumor cells in excess. A brief survey of some recent publications that report TS levels per mg of soluble protein (or, per g of tissue, assuming about 40 mg cytosolic protein per g of tissue) indicates that the levels of TS range from 0.06 nmol per min per mg of protein for mouse L1210 cells (9) and 0.4 nmoles TMP per min per mg of protein for CEM cells (10) to between 0.13 and 2.5 nmol per min per mg protein for a series of murine cononic tumors (11). That is, the levels of TS present in these tumor cells range from just barely enough to suffice DNA synthesis to about 40 times that necessary for DNA synthesis. If this extrapolation is correct, in some tumors, TS would have to be inhibited > 95 % (relative to the level originally present) before any effect on tumor cell growth would be evident. Presumably, much higher levels of inhibition would be required for the initiation of tumor cell death. In addition, in other cell types for which the TS level is barely sufficient for cell growth, inhibition of cell growth should be parallel to inhibition of TS. Nevertheless, it seems clear that it cannot be assumed that there should be a direct relationship between inhibition of TS and inhibition of cell growth.

In the course of some recent studies (2,12) that sought to relate inhibition of TS to inhibition of mouse L1210 cells in culture, we found evidence that cell growth required only a fraction of the TS levels present in these cells. When these cells were exposed to low concentrations of FdUrd, growth was initially inhibited, but it subsequently recovered and resumed the same rate as in parallel control cultures. Measurement of TS in these cells during inhibition of growth and recovery demonstrated that the growth resumed at a time when the total free TS levels per cell were only 10-15 % of pretreatment levels (2). This indicated to us that 85-90 % inhibition of TS would be required in order to inhibit the growth of these cells at all. This is analogous to the situation with inhibition of dihydrofolate reductase by methotrexate: Goldman and his colleagues (13,14) have demonstrated that near complete inhibition of dihydrofolate reductase is insufficient to affect cell growth and DNA synthesis. In order to have effect on DNA synthesis by MTX, dihydrofolate reductase must be completely inhibited and must be kept completely inhibited.

For any cell line for which a high level of inhibition of TS is required in order to affect DNA synthesis, there are several practical problems that arise. Perhaps the most important is the experimental determination of residual TS levels after exposure to fluoropyrimidines. If 90 % inhibition of TS allows 100 % cell growth but 95 % inhibition of TS results in a 50 % inhibition of growth, then it often becomes very important to distinguish between 10 % and 5 % enzyme levels. The most widely used assay for TS levels relies on the titration of free TS binding sites with ^{3}H-FdUMP as a measure of enzyme(4,15).

74

Yet, using this assay, it is often found that it is difficult or seemingly impossible to completely inhibit all TS. For instance, the data of Fig 1A indicates that TS can be inhibited to a point at which growth stops and dUMP accumulates, but free TS is still found in these cells. Subsequent to these previously published results, it was suggested by Spears et al. (8) that the ^{3}H-FdUMP binding assay we used for these experiments can allow the exchange of label with FdUMP present in inhibited TS complexes to the extent of 13 % of TC. They concluded that low levels of free enzyme found following 5-FU using this technique are erroneous and that the free enzyme found in this experiment was an artifact. A reinvestigation of this effect in our laboratory indicates to us that exchange of ^{3}H-FdUMP with TC during such assays is only a problem when these assays are performed under alkaline conditions (as in ref. 11), and that the results shown in Fig. 1 (which assayed TS at pH 7.4) do not overestimate free TS by more than 2 or 3 percent. It is a question of some importance whether these residual TS binding sites represent free enzyme or are the result of some unrecognized artifact. Nevertheless, it would not seem prudent and seems to be unwarranted to report TS data after exposure to 5-FU by correcting free enzyme levels by subtracting 13 % of the bound values (11). This 13 % is the critical region of TS levels to distinguish cells that will respond to 5-FU and those that will not. Of course, this technical problem becomes even more significant to the interpretation of results when data is drawn from human tumor biopsy data, when only a small percentage of the samples contain enough TS so that these measurements exceed 2-5 times background levels (see Allegra et al, this volume).

Levels of 5,10-CH$_2$-H$_4$PteGlu$_n$ in tumor cells

Several studies have demonstrated that the growth-inhibitory potency and the cytotoxicity of fluoropyrimidines can be substantially increased by exposure of tumor cells to high concentrations of reduced folates (12,16-18). For instance, when mouse L1210 cells were exposed to either 5-FU or FdUrd for

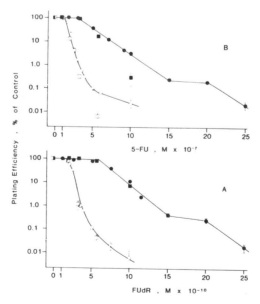

Figure 2. Cytotoxicity of FUdR (A) and of 5-FU (B) in the presence (open symbols) or absence (closed symbols) of 10^{-5} M folinic acid. L1210 cells were exposed to fluoropyrimidines and folinic acid for 72 hrs. and then plated in soft agarose in the absence of drugs. Colonies were counted 10 days later. Reproduced from reference 12 with the permission of Cancer Research.

three days in the presence of folinic acid (5-CHO-H$_4$PteGlu, leucovorin) a concentration of either drug that was without effect in the absence of reduced folates was 99-99.8 % cytotoxic in the presence of 10^{-5} M folinic acid (Fig 2). While this effect is quite striking, it is only relevant over a limited concentration range. Thus, at a concentration of 5-FU greater than 25 µM or a concentration of FdUrd greater than 25 nM, tumor cell kill would be equivalent in the presence or absence of reduced folates. The fact remains, however that these concentrations (or, more correctly, the equivalent exposure under a more clinically relevant dosage schedule) may be unattainable *in vivo* without undue host toxicity, and that the effect of folinic acid may be to decrease the drug exposure at which significant tumor cell kill occurs.

The biochemical basis of this synergism has recently been investigated in this laboratory. The originally proposed hypothesis that folinic acid augmented the cytotoxicity of the fluoropyrimidines by enhancing the stability of the ternary complex was compatible with the results of this study. Thus, exposure of leukemic cells to increasing concentrations of folinic acid resulted in an expansion of the cellular pools of 5,10-CH$_2$-H$_4$PteGlu$_n$ and did so over exactly the range of folinic acid concentrations that extended the inhibition of cell viability by 5-FU. The rate of recovery of cellular TS was found to directly reflect the ability of the cells to proliferate in the presence of FdUrd either in the presence or absence of folinic acid. Thus, the key difference between cells exposed to FdUrd alone and cells exposed to drug in the presence of folinic acid was the rate and extent of recovery of active enzyme. In cells exposed to FdUrd alone, this recovery was found to be due to both synthesis of new enzyme and to the dissociation of enzyme that was initially involved in ternary complex. In cells exposed to FdUrd and folinic acid, the rate of dissociation of ternary complexes was too slow to be a factor in the recovery of free TS.

Time , hours

0   1.5   3   6   9   12   18   24   30   36

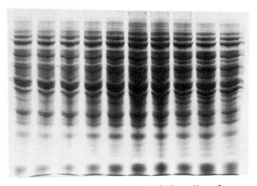

Figure 3. Accumulation of protein in L1210 cells after exposure to FdUrd and folonic acid. L1210 cells were exposed to 7 x 10^{-10} M FdUrd and 10^{-5} M folinic acid for 36 hrs. At the indicated times, the amount of cytosolic protein in 5 x 10^6 cells was analyzed on a 10 % stacking SDS polyacrylamide gel and stained with Coomassie Blue. For details, see reference 2.

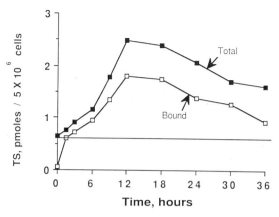

Figure 4. Accumulation of TS in L1210 cells as TC following exposure to FdUrd and folinic acid. L1210 cells were exposed to 7 x 10^{-10} M ^{3}H-FdUrd in thge presence of 10^{-5} M folinic acid as in Fig. 3. Aliquots of cultures were removed at the indicated times and the cellular content of TS bound to drug ( ) and total cellular TS ( ) was determined as described in ref 2. The horizontal line indicates the basal level of TS found in cells at time zero. Each point represents the mean of duplicate determinations.

Accumulation of TS in cells undergoing thymine-less death

When the proliferation of mammalian tumor cells is interrupted by FdUrd, 5-FU, or by several other inhibitors of the synthesis of precursors of DNA, DNA synthesis stops but the content of protein per cell increases. As shown by the data of Fig 3, this accumulation of protein per cell continues for 12 hours in mouse L1210 cells, a period equivalent to one generation time. This phenomenon is well known from other studies of the characteristics of "thymine-less death"(19-21) and has been called "unbalanced growth". This term is only partially accurate because the number of cells present does not increase with time, but rather the size of the cells increases in parallel to the total content of protein. An interesting question was raised by the data of Fig 3: what were these proteins, and what was their normal function in the cell? One of these proteins turned out to be TS. The amount of TS per cell continuously increased over the interval up to 12 hours after exposure to FdUrd (Fig4), although the excess enzyme was immediately inactivated by intracellular FdUMP with the formation of TC. The total content of TS increased, and this increase was entirely accounted for by an increased amount of bound TS. However, because all of this enzyme was capable of dissociation back to free TS (in the absence of folinic acid), the increased TC in essence formed a reservoir of enzyme which was capable of generating free TS and terminating inhibition of DNA synthesis. In addition, once this enzyme accumulates, it must be maintained inactive in order to have a continued effect on cell growth. Thus, if the level of total TS increases 5-fold following exposure to 5-FU, in a cell type that has a 20-fold excess level of TS over that required for DNA synthesis, then a 95 % inhibition of enzyme will be without effect, and the minimally effective level of enzyme inhibition would be 99 %. This effect would exacerbate the difficulty of maintaining the tumor cells in a state that will lead to cell death using fluoropyrimidines. Of course, it would also potentially lead to a misinterpretation of the situation if it is observed that a 99 % inhibition of TS is not cytotoxic to a tumor cell population.

DISCUSSION

When tumor cells are exposed to 5-FU, a sequence of events is initiated. The synthesis of 5-fluorouridine-5'-triphosphate leads to the incorporation of the 5-FU base into all RNA species. The metabolism of FdUrd or 5-FU to FdUMP leads to inhibition of TS. At a sufficiently high level of drug exposure, these effects lead to cell death, as can be easily demonstrated in cultured cells. However, during the treatment of tumors *in vivo*, the constraints of normal tissue damage restricts the dose and duration of drug exposure that can be used. Hence, the response of the cell to the initial effects of these ultimate toxic metabolites and the relationship between drug effects and cell kill become of major importance to the efficacy of treatment.

The cytotoxic consequences of the accumulation of FdUMP depends in large part on the response of cellular metabolism to the initial inhibition of TS. Available information tells us that dUMP accumulation is a necessary result of decreased utilization and a continuing (or, even, increased) synthesis of this metabolite. The lack of accumulation of dUMP in some studies (8) is a fascinating observation that may explain the large differences in sensitivity of different tumors to 5-FU. It is important that TS interacts with dUMP (or FdUMP) first, then with $5,10-CH_2-H_4PteGlu_n$ and that the affinity of dUMP and FdUMP for TS (in the absence of folates) is not significantly different (22,23). Thus, the accumulation of dUMP would be a factor that tends to protect any TS made after exposure to drug from inhibition by FdUMP or any TS that reappears due to dissociation of TC. However, other factors are in the equation, and whether sufficient TS activity is reinstituted in time to prevent cell death is the result of the balance of these factors.

These factors would be:
1. the rate of dissociation of the ternary complex to a TS-cofactor binary complex;
2. the rate of dissociation of a TS-cofactor binary complex back to free TS compared with the rate of reassociation of cofactor with the binary complex;
3. the rate of association of dUMP with free TS compared with the rate of association of FdUMP with free TS;
4. the rate of synthesis of new enzyme;
5. other factors that determine how long a tumor cell must be held without TTP in order to initiate cell death.
Whereas 1. and 4. appear to be invariant, or at least beyond therapeutic manipulation, factors 2. and 3. can be modified to decrease the fluoropyrimidine exposure necessary to achieve cell kill. Thus, exposure of tumor cells to excess exogenous folinic acid has been shown to expand the cellular pools of $5,10-CH_2-H_4PteGlu_n$(2). As a result, the rate of overall dissociation of ternary complex in intact cells has been shown to decrease by a large factor (2), presumably due to an increased rate of reassociation of binary complex with reduced folate. We have also found that the therapeutic efficacy (24) and the cytotoxicity (25) of the fluoropyrimidines is greatly enhanced by inhibitors of deoxyuridylate nucleotide synthesis, such as hydroxyurea. We presume, but have not yet proven, that this effect is the result of interference with the accumulation of dUMP subsequent to TS inhibition with a resultant shift in the balance of factors in 3.

The requirement for the continued inhibition of TS over a period of multiple hours in order to induce cell kill is a severe limitation to fluoropyrimidine therapy. This is particularly the case in view of what appears to be excess levels of TS in some cell types and the ability of the response of tumor cells to reinstate enzyme activity. This leads us to the conclusion that fluoropyrimidine therapy of neoplastic diseases should routinely involve the coadministration of folinic acid and/or hydroxyurea. The fact that the toxicity of 5-FU to normal tissues is not changed by folinic acid treatment in proportion to the increased antitumor activity has not been addressed and remains difficult to explain. However, others (26,27) have also shown that the administration of uridine to mice allows higher doses of 5-FU to be administered without toxicity, while the antitumor effects of 5-FU are unchanged by uridine. It is tempting to suggest that inhibition of TS using fluoro-pyrimidines will be most effective only with the coadministration of several other agents (folinic acid, hydroxyurea, and uridine) to maintain the effects against tumor and minimize the effects against the host.

A second approach to inhibition of TS as a therapeutic modality would be to use folate antimetabolites instead of pyrimidine analogs. A model TS inhibitor that is an analog of the folate cofactor, 10-propargyl-5,8-dideazafolate (CB3717)(28), has been shown to have characteristics that would circumvent some of the limitations of 5-FU (29). Like FdUMP, CB3717 forms a tightly-bound complex with TS, but, unlike FdUMP, this complex includes a mole of dUMP(30). Hence, as dUMP accumulates after TS blockade, the inhibition of TS by CB3717 would be enhanced. Likewise, the cytotoxicity of CB3717 is greatest when cellular folate cofactor levels are low (29). Hence, the low levels of $5,10\text{-}CH_2\text{-}H_4PteGlu_n$ in human tumors which limit the activity of 5-FU, would promote the activity of CB3717. An additional advantage of folate analogs for TS inhibition is that they would not be incorporated into RNA and DNA. Hence, not only would their activity against tumor cells be easier to monitor, but analogy with other folate analogs would suggest that they would have very low or nonexistent mutagenic or carcinogenic activities.

REFERENCES

1. Heidelberger, C., Danenberg, P.V., and Moran, R.G. (1983) Adv. Enzymol. 54, 57-119.

2. Keyomarsi, K. and Moran, R.G. (1988) J. Biol. Chem., submitted.

3. Myers, C.E., Young, R.C., and Chabner, B.A. (1975) J. Clin. Invest. 56, 1231-1238

4. Moran, R.G., Spears, C.P., and Heidelberger, C. (1979) Proc. Natl. Acad. Sci., USA. 76, 1456-1460.

5. Jackson, R.C. (1978) J. Biol. Chem. 253:7440-7446.

6. Lorenson, M.Y., Maley, G.F., and Maley,F. (1967) J.Biol.Chem. 242: 3332-3344.

7. Moore, E.C. and Hurlbert, R.B. (1966) J.Biol. Chem. 241: 4802-4809.

8. Spears, C.P., Gustavsson, B.G., Mitchell, M.S., Spicer, D., Berne, M., Bernstein, L., and Danenberg, P.V. (1984) Cancer Res. 44: 4144-4150.

9. Jackman, A.L., Alison, D.A., Calvert, A.H., and Harrup, K.R. (1986) Cancer Res. 46:2810-2815.

10. Lockshin, A., Moran, R.G., and Danenberg, P.V. (1979) Proc. Natl Acad. Sci., USA. 76, 750-754.

11. Spears, C.P., Shahinian, A.H., Moran, R.G.,, and Heidelberger, C. (1982) Cancer Res. 42, 450-456.

12. Keyomarsi, K. and Moran, R.G. (1986) Cancer Res. 46, 5229-5235.

13. Goldman, I.D., (1974) Mol. Pharmacol. 10, 257-274

14. White, J.C., and Goldman, I.D. (1976) Mol. Pharmacol. 12, 711-719

15. Santi, D.V., McHenry, C.S., and Perriard, E.R. (1974) Biochemistry 13: 467-470

16. Ullman, B., Melinda, L., Martin, D.W., and Santi, D.V (1978) Proc. Natl. Acad. Sci. U.S.A. 75, 980-983

17. Evans, R.M., Laskin, J.D., and Hakala, M.T. (1981) Cancer Res. 41, 3288-3295

18. Evans, R,M., Laskin, J.D., and Hakala, M.T. (1980) Cancer Res. 40, 4113-4122

19. Cohen, L.S., and Studzinski, G.P. (1967) J. Cell Physiol. 69, 331-340

20. Rueckert, R.R., and Mueller, G.C. (1960) Cancer Res. 20, 1584-1591

21. Maaløe, O., and Hanawalt, P.C. (1961) J. Mol. Biol. 3, 144-155

22. Lockshin, A., and Danenberg, P. V. (1981) Biochem. Pharmacol. 30, 247-257

23. Galivan., J. H., Maley, G.F., and Maley, F. (1976) Biochemistry 15: 356-362.

24. Moran, R.G., Danenberg, P.V., and Heidelberger, C. (1982) Biochem.Pharmacol.31, 2929-2935.

25. Unpublished observations.

26. Klubes, P., Cerna, I., and Meldon, M.A. (1982) Cancer Chemother. Pharmacol. 8: 17-21.

27. Martin, D.S., Stolfi, R.L., Sawyer, R.C., Speigelman, S., and Young, C.W. (1983) Cancer Res. 43, 4653-4661

28. Jones, T.R., Calvert, A.H., Jackman,A.L., Brown, S.J., Jones, M., and Harrap, K.R. (1981) Eur. J. Cancer 17: 11-19.

29. Jackson, R.C., Jackman, A.L., and Calvert, A.H. (1983) Biochem. Pharmacol. 32: 3783-3790.

30. Pogolotti, A. L., Danenberg, P.V., Santi, D.V. (1986) J. Med. Chem. 29: 478-482.

DISCUSSION OF DR. MORAN'S PRESENTATION

Dr. P. Houghton: You've hit on about every mechanism that one encounters that makes FUra not work. I wonder if in fact one's generalizing rather too much from the L1210 cell.

Dr. Moran: That's a legitimate comment and it's difficult to answer. I think it's a very dangerous possibility and I'd like to see it repeated, perhaps in some xenografts.

Dr. P. Houghton: From our experience dUMP accumulation seems to be very specific to the tumor line that we're looking at amongst human colorectal tumors.

Dr. Moran: So you have some lines where it accumulates and some lines where it does not.

Dr. P. Houghton: Right, and the sensitive lines are the lines that show low TS activity to start with so we can inhibit about 75% of the activity, that already starts from a very low level, which again supports what you're saying that there's some critical level that one has to achieve in terms of restricting TMP biosynthesis before one sees an effect. The same line doesn't accumulate dUMP either.

Dr. Moran: Clearly the cell line that you choose is going to modify the conclusions you can draw but what we're trying to do here is determine if the mechanism works and if it works how much of an effect does it have on therapeutics.

Dr. Rustum: The results you presented here with L1210 resemble the results of Maire Hakala with Hep-2 cells with and without CF. In comparing S-180 cells and Hep-2 cells, the extent of inhibition and duration of inhibition of TS was clearly the determining factor in modulation of FUra cytotoxicity. Maire and Sondra Berger have looked at dUMP and FdUMP concentrations, polyglutamate formation, and level of TS in S-180 and Hep-2 cells and found that FdUMP in the resistant cells (Hep-2) was much higher than in the sensitive cells, but that dUMP was not very different. Polyglutamates were higher in the sensitive cells than the resistant ones. However, to the point of the dUMP concentration, if you change the pool of dUMP by 2 to 10-fold when you have a high concentration of FdUMP, you really have to alter the ratio by approximately 1,000-fold to make a dent in the effect of FdUMP on TS. In all the experiments that I am aware of, the alteration of dUMP concentration through treatment with FUra or FdUrd does not approach this degree of modulation. So the ratio of FdUMP to dUMP is an extremely high one and changing the dUMP concentration I don't think is going to be critical factor in determining sensitivity to FUra.

Dr. Moran: You do or you do not?

Dr. Rustum: I do not.

Dr. Moran: You do not.

Dr. Rustum: I do not.

Dr. Moran: Oh, I do.

Dr. Houghton: I do, too.

Dr. Rustum: Well, let's see where the data are. Dr. Hakala has demonstrated very nicely that you can alter the pool of FdUMP without necessarily altering the therapeutic activity of FUra. I don't think it's going to make a difference and I have not seen the data today to demonstrate that dUMP concentrations are very critical, the most important determinant for sensitivity of FUra. Maybe I missed it.

Dr. Moran: No I don't think anyone has shown it.

Dr. Rustum: Then tell us about it.

Dr. Moran: There are two things that amaze me when I look at this data. One thing is, in those lines that accumulate dUMP, it goes to an enormous concentration. Number 2, there is a big variation between cell lines in how high the dUMP goes before it starts diffusing out of the cell or getting broken down to nucleosides and things. Another thing that amazes me when I look at the data is that to have enough methylenetetrahydrofolate present to form complex and to have more than enough FdUMP and still to have free enzyme, is amazing.

Dr. Rustum: I agree with that. However, when you change the dUMP concentration you still have a very high concentration of FdUMP. If you measure the ratio of FdUMP to dUMP under various condition and correlate that with the change of toxicity I think you're going to see a very poor correlation.

Dr. Moran: Well, I don't want to argue in the absence of data in particular, but I don't think the final story is in.

Dr. Houghton: I think accumulation of dUMP is actually very important when one is dealing with bolus administration of a drug where FdUMP may be present for a relatively short period of time.

Dr. Priest: This is with regard to the accumulation of tetrahydro-folates and may be relevant in the L1210 system. We've been using the ternary complex assay to look at not only methylenetetrahydro-folate but also 4 other reduced folates, by cycling; those are di-hydrofolate, tetrahydrofolate, 5-methyl and 10-formyltetrahydro-folate. If we change the folate level in the medium, we see essentially the same thing that you do with regard to accumulation of methylenetetrahydrofolate; by simply adding up those individual folates we can see a change of about 25-fold in the total with only about a 4-6-fold change in the methylenetetrahydrofolate. I was going to point out that the preponderance of that total appears to occur in the 5-methyl and the 10-formyl pools. They change dramatically; the other 3 pools change only minimally.

Dr. Moran: Why can't you make more 5,10-methylenetetrahydrofolate poly-glutamates? Is it a case of saturating FPGS; what is limiting the amount to which you can push that pool up?

Dr. Priest: I'm sorry I don't know the mechanism. I suspect it has something to do with the regulation of the pools in general. If we go low we see a disappearance of the 10-formyl and 5-methyl. If we go high, we see a striking appearance and I don't know what the mechanism is.

82

Dr. Schilsky: We've been conducting a clinical trial in patients with advanced head and neck cancer in which we administer hydroxyurea, FUra, and CF simultaneously with radiation therapy. The combination is well-tolerated in terms of its systemic toxicity and the entire treatment program is a very highly active program in producing tumor regressions. Obviously, it's difficult in tumor regression to dissect what is the effect of the chemo, the radiation and the combination but it is certainly possible to give those 3 drugs in combination. We give approximately 2-3 gm/day of hydroxyurea in divided dose along with 300 mg/m^2 of CF orally and in divided dose and a continuous infusion of FUra at 600 mg/m^2/day. That is tolerated with only moderate bone marrow suppression and some mucositis in the irradiated field.

Dr. Greco: In the initial part of your talk, you showed a growth assay of the cytotoxicity of FUra/CF. You thought it curious, it being so small, that this combination is so effective clinically. Then you showed pictorial results of a clonogenic assay. You then went on to a different topic and I was waiting for the punch line. As you know the merits of clonogenic versus growth assays are quite controversial and interpretation isn't so clear. Could you supply your conclusion to the comparison of those 2 experiments?

Dr. Moran: I thought it was self-evident, that's why I didn't comment on it. I think the conclusions are that when you run growth inhibition assays you see particles, but a lot more of those particles are dead if you treat it with FdUrd or FU plus CF than in any case of drug alone. That's all.

Dr. Greco: If you would have done a clonogenic assay where you seed a low density of cells and then pretend you're doing a clonogenic assay with one set of plates and a growth assay with another set, what results would you anticipate then?

Dr. Moran: I don't quite understand the experiment you're suggesting, but with clonogenic assays the interpretation gets very muddy if there's any drug in the agarose. You've got to run them after drug treatment rather than during; otherwise you have a combination of cell kill and growth inhibition. Run that by me again if you would.

Dr. Greco: A type of assay where you seed a low density of cells. You can then look at clusters of cells and call those colonies or you could do some sort of a growth assay on what you had. Just so you have a very low density. What do you anticipate you would get?

Dr. Moran: You see the synergism with both endpoints. I think you get struck in the face with it more if you're looking at cell kill rather than growth inhibition. There the effects are very clear.

SELECTIVITY OF CF AND 5-FLUOROURACIL: CRITICAL ROLE OF POLYGLUTAMYLATION

Janet A. Houghton, Larry G. Williams, Siebold S.N. deGraaf, Saeed Radparvar, Irving W. Wainer, John R. Rodman and Peter J. Houghton

Departments of Biochemical and Clinical Pharmacology, and Pharmacokinetics, St. Jude Children's Research Hospital Memphis, TN 38101

INTRODUCTION

Earlier studies from these laboratories have indicated that in human colon adenocarcinoma xenografts, the mechanism of intrinsic resistance to 5-fluoropyrimidines may be a consequence of low levels of CH_2-H_4PteGlu in tumor cells. Thus, after administration of FUra or FdUrd, the inhibitory complex between FdUMP, CH_2-H_4PteGlu and TS may form relatively slowly, or may dissociate quite rapidly (1,2). Due to the influence of CH_2-H_4PteGlu on the stability of the ternary complex, leucovorin, a stable form of reduced folate, has been used in cultured cells (3) and clinically (4,5) to attempt to increase the pool of CH_2-H_4PteGlu, the stability of the ternary complex, and the inhibition of TS. However, preclinical studies that document the fate of leucovorin in neoplastic tissues are currently lacking.

Intracellularly, reduced folates exist as polyglutamate forms with glutamate residues linked through the γ-carboxyl groups (6). Polyglutamates of CH_2-H_4PteGlu containing up to seven glutamate residues have increased affinity for thymidylate synthase. However, the influence of polyglutamylation of the cofactor on the formation and stability of the ternary complex remains poorly characterized. Polyglutamylation of CH_2-H_4PteGlu may be important for increasing the velocity of binding of [6-^{3}H]FdUMP to thymidylate synthase (7,8), for reducing the rate at which the nucleotide dissociates from the enzyme (7,9), or for binding the folate at lower concentration (7).

We therefore examined the concentration of CH_2-H_4PteGlu$_n$ and H_4PteGlu$_n$ in tumors, the distribution of polyglutamate forms, and have characterized the interaction of CH_2-H_4PteGlu$_n$ in formation and stability of the FdUMP-TS-CH_2-H_4PteGlu complex using enzyme purified from a human colon adenocarcinoma xenograft. In addition, the xenograft models have been used to examine the modulation of CH_2-H_4PteGlu$_n$ and H_4PteGlu$_n$ pools within tumors relative to levels of the active [6S]isomer of 5-CHO-H_4PteGlu when host mice were infused with [6R,S]5-CHO-H_4PteGlu at different rates of administration.

MATERIALS AND METHODS

Tumor Lines

The characteristics of HxELC$_2$, HxGC$_3$ and HxVRC$_5$ human colon adenocarcinoma xenografts have been described previously; line HxELC$_2$ has shown some sensitivity to treatment with 5-fluoropyrimidines, whereas HxGC$_3$ and HxVRC$_5$ tumors were intrinsically resistant (10).

Inhibition of Thymidylate Synthase

The degree and duration of TS inhibition was determined in three human tumor xenograft lines after the i.p. administration of FUra at a dose level of 100 mg/kg, using an assay based upon the release of ^{3}H from [5-^{3}H]dUMP, as described previously (11).

Determination of the Pools of CH$_2$-H$_4$PteGlu$_n$ and H$_4$PteGlu$_n$

A catalytic assay was employed to determine the endogenous concentrations of the combined pool of CH$_2$-H$_4$PteGlu$_n$ and H$_4$PteGlu$_n$ in the presence of excess formaldehyde using L. casei thymidylate synthase, [5-^{3}H]dUMP and tumor extracts as the source of reduced folates, as described previously (12).

Distribution of Polyglutamates of CH$_2$-H$_4$PteGlu and H$_4$PteGlu

Determination of the distribution of polyglutamate forms of the combined pool of CH$_2$-H$_4$PteGlu$_n$ and H$_4$PteGlu$_n$ and the pool of CH$_2$-H$_4$PteGlu$_n$ was based upon the technique described by Priest and Doig (13). Ternary complexes formed between [6-^{3}H]FdUMP (125 nM), excess L. casei TS and CH$_2$-H$_4$PteGlu$_n$ from tumor extracts were electrophoresed on 9% polyacrylamide non-denaturing gels and fluorograms prepared as described previously (12).

Analysis of Ternary Complexes by SDS Gel Electrophoresis

Tumor extracts, heat-treated in the presence of excess formaldehyde, were incubated with [6-^{3}H]FdUMP (125 nM) and excess L. casei TS prior to denaturation in 0.1% SDS and analysis by SDS gel electrophoresis according to the method of Laemmli (14). Fluorograms were prepared after gel drying as previously described (12).

Stability of the FdUMP-Thymidylate Synthase-CH$_2$-H$_4$PteGlu$_n$ Ternary Complex

Complex was formed with [6-^{3}H]FdUMP (100 nM), [6R]CH$_2$-H$_4$PteGlu$_n$ (1.5 to 10 μM) and TS (27.2 to 40 nM [6-^{3}H]FdUMP binding sites) purified from a human colon adenocarcinoma xenograft at 37° over 45 min, as described previously (12). Complexes were subsequently diluted, and their stability determined at 37° in the presence of unlabeled FdUMP (100 μM), and various concentrations of the species of [6R]CH$_2$-H$_4$PteGlu$_n$ used to form the complex. Charcoal adsorption was used to terminate reactions. [6R]CH$_2$-H$_4$PteGlu$_{1-6}$ were synthesized from PteGlu$_{1-6}$ as previously described (12).

Plasma Pharmacokinetics of [6S]CF in Mice

Fifty-six non-tumor-bearing immune-deprived mice received [6R,S]5-CHO-H$_4$PteGlu at a dose level of 500 mg/m^2 either by i.v. bolus injection or 24 hr infusion. A blood sample of 0.5 to 0.8 ml was obtained from each mouse. Following bolus injection, the sampling schedule was from 5 min to 24 hr. Plasma concentrations of [6S]CF were determined by enantioselective HPLC analysis, as previously described (15) with a lower limit of detection of 0.5 μg/ml. Pharmacokinetic parameters were estimated using an open two-compartment model with elimination from the central compartment. Parameters were identified by means of the least squares method (with weighting according to inverse variance of the estimates), and were subsequently used for the simulation of plasma concentration-time profiles for the various dose regimens (16).

[6R,S]CF Infusions in Tumor-Bearing Mice

Host mice were infused with CF at different intensities of administration; CF was administered at 500 mg/m^2 by i.v. bolus injection, or by i.v. infusion over 4 or 24 hr. At various times during, and post infusion, mice were killed, tumors were excised and processed as described to examine the modulation of pools of CH$_2$-H$_4$PteGlu$_n$ and H$_4$PteGlu$_n$.

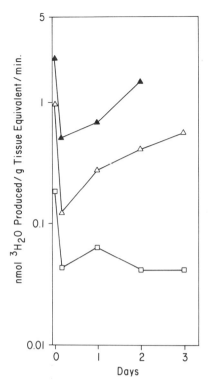

Fig. 1.   Inhibition of thymidylate synthase in ▲ HxVRC$_5$, △ HxGC$_3$ and □ HxELC$_2$ tumors after i.p. administration of FUra (100 mg/kg) to tumor-bearing mice.

RESULTS

The inhibition of TS was determined in three human colon adenocarcinoma xenograft lines (HxELC$_2$, HxGC$_3$, HxVRC$_5$) following a single i.p. administration of FUra (100 mg/kg) to tumor-bearing mice. Within 4 hr of drug treatment, TS was inhibited >75% in all lines, although the residual activity was lower in HxELC$_2$ (the line most sensitive to FUra); by 24 hr, TS activity began to recover in HxGC$_3$ and HxVRC$_5$ tumors (FUra insensitive), and continued for a further 2 days (Fig. 1). In HxELC$_2$ tumors, however, TS activity remained inhibited for at least 72 hr after FUra administration.

Table 1.   Concentrations of the Combined Pool of CH$_2$-H$_4$PteGlu$_n$ and H$_4$PteGlu$_n$ and Estimated Levels of the Pool of CH$_2$-H$_4$PteGlu$_n$

Tumor line	Concentration (nM; mean ± SD)[a]	
	CH$_2$-H$_4$PteGlu$_n$[b] + H$_4$PteGlu$_n$	CH$_2$-H$_4$PteGlu$_n$[c]
HxELC$_2$	499 ± 208	185
HxGC$_3$	968 ± 295	484
HxVRC$_5$	2709 ± 43	1693

[a]Results are the mean ± SD from 6 (HxELC$_2$), 4 (HxGC$_3$) and 2 (HxVRC$_5$) separate experiments.
[b]Determined from the catalytic release of ^{3}H from [5-^{3}H]dUMP.
[c]Estimated from data derived from fluorograms.

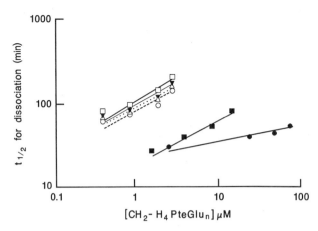

Fig. 2. Relationship between $t\frac{1}{2}$ for dissociation of the $[6\text{-}^3\text{H}]\text{FdUMP-TS-}$ $\text{CH}_2\text{-H}_4\text{PteGlu}_n$ complex and concentration of $[6R]\text{CH}_2\text{-H}_4\text{PteGlu}_n$, where n = ●—● 1, ■—■ 2, Δ....Δ 3, □—□ 4, o--o 5, ▼—▼ 6, using TS purified from HxVRC$_5$ tumors.

The concentrations of the combined pool of $\text{CH}_2\text{-H}_4\text{PteGlu}_n$ and $\text{H}_4\text{PteGlu}_n$ were determined in these tumors using a catalytic assay (Table 1). These were determined to range from 0.5 μM in HxELC$_2$ tumors to 2.7 μM in line HxVRC$_5$. From data obtained after gel electrophoresis of $[6\text{-}^3\text{H}]\text{FdUMP-TS-}\text{CH}_2\text{-H}_4\text{PteGlu}_n$ ternary complexes, the pool of $\text{CH}_2\text{-H}_4\text{PteGlu}_n$ was estimated to range from approximately 0.2 to 1.7 μM, respectively.

Subsequently, HxELC$_2$ and HxGC$_3$ tumors were examined for the % distribution of polyglutamate species of $\text{CH}_2\text{-H}_4\text{PteGlu}$ and H_4PteGlu (Table 2). The pentaglutamate was the predominant species in each tumor line for both the combined pool, and the pool of $\text{CH}_2\text{-H}_4\text{PteGlu}$ (52% to 65%), with the hexaglutamate as the second most prominent species (26% to 33%); tri- and tetra-glutamate forms (0.6% to 6%) were also detected in both tumors, while the diglutamate was detected in some experiments, and absent in others. The distribution of polyglutamate species was similar between the two tumor lines.

Table 2. Percent Distribution of Polyglutamate Forms of $\text{CH}_2\text{-H}_4\text{PteGlu}$ and H_4PteGlu in HxELC$_2$ and HxGC$_3$ Tumors

Tumor line	Folate n =	% Distribution (mean ± SD)[a]				
		2	3	4	5	6
HxELC$_2$	$\text{CH}_2\text{-H}_4\text{PteGlu}_n$ + $\text{H}_4\text{PteGlu}_n$	0.3±1.0	0.6±1.0	2.8±1.4	63.2±4.5	33.1±5.5
	$\text{CH}_2\text{-H}_4\text{PteGlu}_n$	0.5±1.8	2.7±2.8	5.0±2.5	65.4±8.8	26.4±6.1
HxGC$_3$	$\text{CH}_2\text{-H}_4\text{PteGlu}_n$ + $\text{H}_4\text{PteGlu}_n$	0.7±1.7	3.2±2.3	4.8±2.3	57.9±5.1	33.4±8.0
	$\text{CH}_2\text{-H}_4\text{PteGlu}_n$	2.5±5.7	5.2±6.3	6.6±1.7	52.4±5.3	33.3±9.1

[a]Data represent the mean ± SD from 9 to 11 separate determinations.

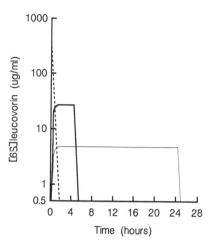

Fig. 3.   Simulated plasma concentration-time profiles for [6S]CF during and following 3 different i.v. administration schedules of [6R,S]CF (500 mg/m^2) in non-tumor-bearing mice. --- bolus injection, ▬ 4 hr infusion, ── 24 hr infusion.

Due to the presence of different polyglutamate forms of CH_2-H_4PteGlu in tumors, their influence on the stability of the [6-^{3}H]FdUMP-TS-CH_2-H_4PteGlu$_n$ complex was determined using TS purified from HxVRC$_5$ tumors. The relationship was derived for n = 1 to 6 (Fig. 2).   For [6R]CH_2-H_4PteGlu$_{3-6}$, a >200-fold lower concentration (0.9 to 1.6 μM) was required to stabilize the ternary complex with a t$\frac{1}{2}$ for dissociation of 100 min in comparison to the concentration required for [6R]CH_2-H_4PteGlu$_1$ (335 μM); an 18-fold lower concentration of [6R]CH_2-H_4PteGlu$_2$ (18.2 μM) compared to [6R]CH_2-H_4PteGlu$_1$ was required to yield a comparable level of stability.

To determine the influence of [6R,S]CF on the pools of CH_2-H_4PteGlu$_n$ and H_4PteGlu$_n$ and the distribution of polyglutamate species in tumors, [6R,S]CF (500 mg/m^2) was administered to mice bearing HxELC$_2$ tumors using 3 different intensities, namely i.v. bolus injection or 4 hr or 24 hr i.v. infusion.   The relationship between plasma levels of [6S]CF and intratumor

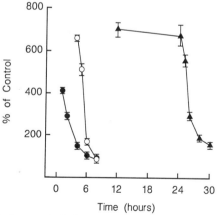

Fig. 4.   Effect of i.v. administration of [6R,S]CF (500 mg/m^2) in tumor-bearing mice on pools of reduced folates in HxELC$_2$ tumors as determined by the rate of catalytic release of ^{3}H from [5-^{3}H]dUMP; ● bolus injection, o 4 hr infusion, ▲ 24 hr infusion.

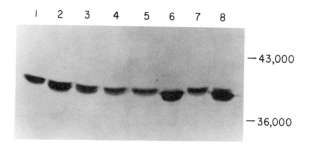

Fig. 5.   Analysis of [6-^{3}H]FdUMP-TS-CH$_2$-H$_4$PteGlu$_n$ complexes by SDS gel electrophoresis.   Heat-treated extracts were prepared in the presence of excess formaldehyde from HxELC$_2$ tumors during and following a 4 hr i.v. infusion of [6R,S]CF (500 mg/m^2) in tumor-bearing mice.   Extracts or standards of CH$_2$-H$_4$PteGlu$_n$ were incubated with [6-^{3}H]FdUMP (125 nM) and L. casei TS prior to denaturation in 0.1% SDS and gel electrophoresis.   Extracts, lanes: 1 (time 0); 2 (4 hr); 3 (5 hr); 4 (6 hr); 5 (8 hr).   Standards, lanes: 6 (CH$_2$-H$_4$PteGlu$_1$); 7 (CH$_2$-H$_4$PteGlu$_6$); 8 (mixture).

pools of reduced folates catalytically active in the TS reaction were also examined.   Simulated plasma concentration-time profiles for [6S]CF following i.v. bolus injection or 4 hr and 24 hr infusion of [6R,S]CF in non-tumor-bearing mice are shown in Fig. 3.   After i.v. bolus injection of [6R,S]CF, the plasma concentration of [6S]CF declined rapidly with a $t\frac{1}{2}\alpha$ of 3.5 min and a $t\frac{1}{2}\beta$ of 11.4 min.   At 5 min, the plasma concentration was $\approx$1 mM.   During a 24 hr infusion, steady state concentrations ($\approx$10 μM) were reached within 60 min.   Upon cessation of CF administration, levels declined rapidly.   Plasma concentration-time profiles were also simulated for [6S]CF after 4 hr i.v. infusion of [6R,S]CF (Fig. 3); the steady state concentration was $\approx$60 μM.   Levels of [6S]CF determined in plasma samples from tumor-bearing mice administered each [6R,S]CF regimen, were found to be close to the simulations shown in Fig. 3.

The effect of dose intensity of [6R,S]CF (500 mg/m^2) on pools of reduced folates determined by catalytic assay were subsequently determined in HxELC$_2$ tumors (Fig. 4).   Levels of reduced folates were 409% of control 1 hr after i.v. bolus injection of [6R,S]CF, and declined rapidly thereafter, reaching control levels after a further 5 hr.   At the end of a 4 hr infusion, reduced folate concentrations were 660% of control, at which point levels again decreased rapidly, reaching control values after a

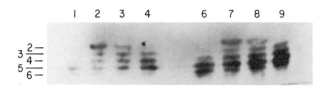

Fig. 6.   Analysis of polyglutamates of CH$_2$-H$_4$PteGlu (lanes 1-4) and the combined pool of CH$_2$-H$_4$PteGlu + H$_4$PteGlu (lanes 6-8) in extracts derived from HxELC$_2$ tumors by electrophoresis of [6-^{3}H]FdUMP-TS-CH$_2$-H$_4$PteGlu$_n$ complexes on 9% polyacrylamide non-denaturing gels.   Tumors were excised during and following a 4 hr i.v. infusion of [6R,S]CF (500 mg/m^2) in tumor-bearing mice.   Time 0 (lanes 1, 6); 4 hr (lanes 2, 7); 5 hr (lanes 3, 8); 8 hr (lanes 4, 9).

further 4 hr. By 12 hr into a 24 hr infusion of [6R,S]CF, reduced folates in $HxELC_2$ tumors had reached 700% of control, and were maintained at this level until the end of the infusion, at which time levels declined rapidly, as observed for the other two CF regimens, approaching control values by 6 hr post infusion.

When ternary complexes formed between [6-^{3}H]FdUMP, L. casei TS and CH_2-H_4PteGlu$_n$ (derived from the combined pool of CH_2-H_4PteGlu$_n$ and H_4PteGlu$_n$ in extracts of $HxELC_2$ tumors) were analyzed by SDS gel electrophoresis, complexes electrophoresed with a mw between 36 and 43 Kd. After the administration of [6R,S]CF in all regimens, a lower mw species was detected that disappeared as reduced folate pools decreased in tumors. Figure 5 illustrates results obtained during and after a 4 hr infusion of [6R,S]CF in $HxELC_2$ tumors. In this study, the lower mw species was observed on fluorograms at the end of the infusion and 1 hr post infusion, but was considerably less prominent after a further 1 to 3 hr. Ternary complexes formed with either [6R]CH_2-H_4PteGlu$_1$ or [6R]CH_2-H_4PteGlu$_6$ were also electrophoresed under the same conditions, the former eluting with a lower mw than the latter (Fig. 5).

Polyglutamate forms of CH_2-H_4PteGlu$_n$ and H_4PteGlu$_n$ were determined on the same samples (Fig. 6). CH_2-H_4PteGlu$_2$ was maximally elevated by the end of the infusion, and had decreased after a further 1 hr. At these times, the triglutamate was also elevated; CH_2-H_4PteGlu$_4$ predominated to the greatest extent by 4 hr post-infusion. The extent of elevation was CH_2-H_4PteGlu$_2$ > CH_2-H_4PteGlu$_3$ > CH_2-H_4PteGlu$_4$. Also after cessation of infusion, CH_2-H_4PteGlu$_5$ appeared to increase as levels of the shorter polyglutamate forms dissappeared. For the combined pool, the maximal elevation in di- to tetra-glutamates was detected at the end of the infusion; however, by 4 hr post-infusion, the diglutamate had disappeared, and the pentaglutamate was increased. Data from i.v. bolus injection of [6R,S]CF yielded predominant changes in the di- and tri-glutamates at 1 to 2 hr post injection, with no detectable effect on the pentaglutamate. Following a 24 hr i.v. infusion of [6R,S]CF, increases in the di-, tri- and tetra-glutamates were maximal by the end of infusion or shortly following the infusion. Upon cessation of infusion, the trend was similar to that observed for the 4 hr infusion, in that the shorter polyglutamate chain length forms decreased as levels of the pentaglutamate increased.

DISCUSSION

In three human colon adenocarcinoma xenografts, the in vivo sensitivity of tumors to FUra has correlated with the degree and duration of inhibition of thymidylate synthase (Fig. 1; 11). However, in these tumors (10), and in colorectal adenocarcinomas in patients (17), responses to FUra are transient. Consequently, the combined pool of CH_2-H_4PteGlu$_n$ and H_4PteGlu$_n$ was determined by catalytic assay, and the pool of CH_2-H_4PteGlu$_n$ estimated in xenografts. The combined pools were determined to range from 0.5 to 2.7 μM, and for CH_2-H_4PteGlu$_n$ alone, in the order of 0.19 to 1.7 μM (Table 1; 12). The presence of a high proportion of intracellular folates as polyglutamates (90%) had been shown to be important in enhancing the antithymidylate effect of FUra in cultured cells (18). However, in human colon xenografts, the distribution of polyglutamate species within the pools of CH_2-H_4PteGlu and H_4PteGlu appeared similar, irrespective of the sensitivity of tumors to FUra, the predominant species consisting of the penta- and hexa-glutamates (Table 2; 12).

Due to the detection of CH_2-H_4PteGlu$_{2-6}$ within tumors, their influence on the stability of the [6-^{3}H]FdUMP-TS-CH_2-H_4PteGlu$_n$ complex was determined (Fig. 2; 12). Clearly, concentrations of CH_2-H_4PteGlu$_1$ (>300 μM) or CH_2-H_4PteGlu$_2$ (>18 μM) required to stabilize the complex would be considerably higher than those achievable physiologically. However, CH_2-

$H_4PteGlu_{3-6}$ stabilized complexes at a >200-fold lower concentration than required for CH_2-$H_4PteGlu_1$. Nonetheless, at physiological concentrations of CH_2-$H_4PteGlu_n$ present in tumors, these would be suboptimal for stabilizing the ternary complex to a level that would cause significant and prolonged inhibition of TS in human colon adenocarcinomas (several hours). Consequently, to achieve greater and more prolonged inhibition of TS, it would be desirable to not only increase the pool of CH_2-$H_4PteGlu$, but to increase the concentrations of the longer polyglutamate chain length forms for optimization of the interaction between FdUMP, TS and CH_2-$H_4PteGlu$.

Based upon these initial studies, [6R,S]CF was administered to tumor-bearing mice as a potential precursor of CH_2-$H_4PteGlu_n$ and $H_4PteGlu_n$. One tumor line ($HxELC_2$) was studied in detail. The objectives of the study were to 1) relate plasma pharmacokinetics of reduced folates to intratumor changes in folate pools, and 2) determine the optimal schedule or intensity for administration of CF based upon the elevation of reduced folate pools in tumors, and the formation of polyglutamate species of CH_2-$H_4PteGlu$ and $H_4PteGlu$ containing 3 to 6 glutamate residues.

The time course of the active [6S]isomer of CF in plasma was studied initially. This reduced folate reached high concentrations (≈ 1 mM at 5 min), and was rapidly eliminated with a terminal half-life of ≈ 11.4 min. Plasma concentrations of [6S]CF >15 μM were maintained for 1 hr, as were levels achieved clinically (>10 μM) following an i.v. bolus injection of [6R,S]CF (200 mg/m^2), although the α (t$\frac{1}{2}$ = 20 min; 5) and β (t$\frac{1}{2}$ = 32-122 min; 4,5,19) half-lives for elimination of [6S]CF were longer than observed in the mouse. For the 4 hr and 24 hr infusions in mice, steady-state concentrations of [6S]CF reached 60 μM and 10 μM, respectively, followed by rapid elimination from plasma. For the 24 hr infusion, [6S]CF levels were slightly higher in the mouse than achieved for continuous infusion at the same dose level in patients (≈ 4.5 μM; 4).

Of interest, however, were the effects of the different schedules of administration of [6R,S]CF (500 mg/m^2) on reduced folates catalytically active in the TS reaction. These appeared maximally elevated at 660% to 700% of control during the infusion schedules of 4 hr or 24 hr duration, and rapid decline in levels followed cessation of drug administration. From in vitro studies, 10 μM [6S]5-CHO-$H_4PteGlu$ has been optimal in potentiating FUra cytotoxicity in cultured cells (3), and in this study, plasma levels of [6S]CF were maintained at ≥ 10 μM during the course of both the 4 hr and 24 hr infusions. Clearly, however, i.v. bolus administration of [6R,S]CF had a more transient effect on reduced folates within tumors than either infusion schedule. Of importance was the observation that changes in the intratumor reduced folate pools correlated with the presence and maintenance of [6S]CF in plasma.

Administration of [6R,S]CF to tumor-bearing mice also affected the distribution of polyglutamates of CH_2-$H_4PteGlu$ and $H_4PteGlu$ in $HxELC_2$ tumors. Data from the 4 hr i.v. infusion schedule demonstrated increases in the di- to tetra-glutamates by the end of the infusion or shortly after cessation of infusion, the degree of elevation being inversely related to the number of polyglutamate residues. However, after stopping the infusion, a trend was observed that as the lower polyglutamate chain length forms declined, the pentaglutamate was observed to increase. This effect was not seen after i.v. bolus injection of [6R,S]CF, but was observed following the 24 hr i.v. infusion. It is not yet clear, however, whether the elevation in shorter polyglutamate forms during infusion was preventing the formation of the pentaglutamate, and hence whether it would be necessary to stop the infusion before this species was increased.

These studies have therefore suggested that 1) the duration of elevation of reduced folate pools is determined by the length of the [6R,S]CF infusion period, and 2) that the duration of administration of [6R,S] CF should be prolonged, at least beyond i.v. bolus injection, to allow the longer polyglutamate chain length forms of CH_2-H_4PteGlu and H_4PteGlu to be synthesized for optimization of the interaction between FdUMP, TS and CH_2-H_4PteGlu. Future studies will determine 1) the relationship between changes in reduced folate pools and inhibition of TS, and 2) the relationship between TS inhibition and increased cytotoxicity.

Supported by NCI grant CA 32613 and by American Lebanese Syrian Associated Charities.

REFERENCES

1. J. A. Houghton, S. J. Maroda, J. O. Phillips, and P. J. Houghton, Biochemical determinants of responsivenss to 5-fluorouracil and its derivatives in xenografts of human colorectal adenocarcinomas in mice, Cancer Res. 41:144 (1981).
2. J. A. Houghton, P. M. Torrance, S. Radparvar, L. G. Williams, and P. J. Houghton, Binding of 5-fluorodeoxyuridylate to thymidylate synthase in human colon adenocarcinoma xenografts, Eur. J. Cancer Clin Oncol. 22:505 (1986).
3. R. M. Evans, J. D. Laskin, and M. T. Hakala, Effect of excess folates and deoxyinosine on the activity and site of action of 5-fluorouracil, Cancer Res. 41:3288 (1981).
4. E. Newman, J. Doroshow, M. Bertrand, P. Burgeson, D. Villacorte, D. Blayney, D. Goldberg, B. Carr, L. Leong, K. Margolin, G. Cecchi, and R. Staples, Pharmacokinetics of high-dose folinic acid (dl-CF) administered by continuous intravenous (iv) infusion, Proc. Am. Assoc. Cancer Res. 26:158 (1985).
5. D. Machover, E. Goldschmidt, P. Chollet, G. Metzger, J. Zittoun, J. Marquet, J.-M. Vandenbulcke, J.-L. Misset, L. Schwarzenberg, J. B. Fourtillan, H. Gaget, and G. Mathé, Treatment of advanced colorectal and gastric adenocarcinomas with 5-fluorouracil and high-dose folinic acid, J. Clin. Oncol. 4:685 (1986).
6. R. L. Kisliuk, Pteroylpolyglutamates, Mol. Cell Biochem. 39:331 (1981).
7. C. J. Allegra, B. A. Chabner, J. C. Drake, R. Lutz, D. Rodbard, and J. Jolivet, Enhanced inhibition of thymidylate synthase by methotrexate polyglutamates, J. Biol. Chem. 260:9720 (1985).
8. D. G. Priest, and M. Mangum, Relative affinity of 5,10-methylenetetrahydrofolylpolyglutamates for the Lactobacillus casei thymidylate synthetase-5-fluorodeoxyuridylate binary complex, Arch. Biochem. Biophys. 210:118 (1981).
9. P. V. Danenberg, and A. Lockshin, Tight-binding complexes of thymidylate synthetase, folate analogs, and deoxyribonucleotides, Adv. Enz. Regul. 20:99 (1982).
10. J. A. Houghton, and P. J. Houghton, On the mechanism of cytotoxicity of fluorinated pyrimidines in four human colon adenocarcinoma xenografts maintained in immune-deprived mice, Cancer 45:1159 (1980).
11. J. A. Houghton, K. D. Weiss, L. G. Williams, P. M. Torrance, and P. J. Houghton, Relationship between 5-fluoro-2'-deoxyuridylate, 2'-deoxyuridylate, and thymidylate synthase activity subsequent to 5-fluorouracil administration, in xenografts of human colon adenocarcinomas, Biochem. Pharmacol. 35:1351 (1986).
12. J. A. Houghton, L. G. Williams, S. Radparvar, and P. J. Houghton, Characterization of the pools of 5,10-methylenetetrahydrofolates and tetrahydrofolates in xenografts of human colon adenocarcinoma, Cancer Res., in press (1988).
13. D. G. Priest, and M. T. Doig, Tissue folate polyglutamate chain length determination by electrophoresis as thymidylate synthase - fluorodeoxyuridylate ternary complexes. Meth. Enzymol. 122:313 (1986).

14. U. K. Laemmli, Cleavage of structural proteins during the assembly of the head of bacteriophage T4, <u>Nature (London)</u> 227:680 (1970).

15. I. W. Wainer, and R. M. Stiffin, Direct resolution of the stereoisomers of leucovorin and 5-methyltetrahydrofolate using a bovine serum albumin high-performance liquid chromatographic chiral stationary phase coupled to an achiral phenyl column, <u>J. Chromatogr</u>. 424:158 (1988).

16. D. Z. D'Argenio, and A. Schumitzky, A program package for simulation and parameter estimation in pharmacokinetic systems, <u>Comp. Progr. Biomed</u>. 9:115 (1979).

17. J. M. Gilbert, Adjuvant chemotherapy of large bowel cancer, <u>Cancer Treat. Rev</u>. 9:195 (1982).

18. M.-B. Yin, S. F. Zakrzewski, and M. T. Hakala, Relationship of cellular folate cofactor pools to the activity of 5-fluorouracil, <u>Mol. Pharmacol</u>. 32:190 (1983).

19. J. A. Straw, D. Szapary, and W. T. Wynn, Pharmacokinetics of the diastereoisomers of leucovorin after intravenous and oral administration to normal subjects, <u>Cancer Res</u>. 44:3114 (1984).

DISCUSSION OF DR. HOUGHTON'S PRESENTATION

Dr. DeLap: Extrapolating from what you presented, it appears that one might be able to swamp the capacity of the system to create long chain polyglutamates with a sufficiently excessive dose of 6S-CF. In essence this would achieve the counterproductive goal of generating a smaller proportion of long chain polyglutamates which might not be as effective in stabilizing the ternary complex for long periods of time. Is that a reasonable extrapolation

Dr. Houghton: It is an interesting idea and we plan to look at the relationship between the dose of CF administered and how that affects polyglutamate chainlength forms. Also how perturbation in these pools ultimately is going to correlate with TS inhibition. It could raise some quite interesting questions.

Dr. Kalman: Throughout the previous discussions, it became clear that a number of parameters are different in different cell lines such as dUMP pools, accumulation, etc. I want to comment on something which is quite similar and that is we have looked at the stability of the L.casei enzyme ternary complex, using a spectrophotometric assay of their stabilities after isolation. We observe precisely the same kind of pattern which you find. Up to 3 glutamate residues you have very marked changes in stability and beyond that you don't see much effect; there is no question that polyglutamate forms in a bacterial ternary complex are just as stable as you have shown for the mammalian TS.

Dr. Houghton: It seems that the crucial phase is converting 5,10-methylenetetrahydrofolate through to the triglutamate. That seems, I think, to be very important.

METHODS FOR THYMIDYLATE SYNTHASE PHARMACODYNAMICS:
SERIAL BIOPSY, FREE AND TOTAL TS, FdUMP AND dUMP,
AND H_4PTEGLU AND CH_2-H_4PTEGLU ASSAYS

Colin Paul Spears and Bengt G. Gustavsson

University of Southern California Comprehensive Cancer Center
Cancer Research Laboratory
1303 N. Mission Road, Los Angeles, CA 90033

University of Göteborg, Department of Surgery
Östra Hospital, Göteborg, Sweden

ABSTRACT

   This report details our methods for performance of the major parameters related to quantitation of TS inhibition resulting from fluoropyrimidine administration to patients, methods equally applicable to preclinical studies. Sampling of tumors before and after drug treatment is done by 4 mm disposable punch biopsy or forceps biopsy via subcutaneous tunneling. Homogenates are prepared using N_2 or polytron-mincing. Cytosolic free TS is measured by either the tritium-release method for small biopsies or by [^{3}H]FdUMP ligand-binding. FdUMP and dUMP are separated by DEAE-cellulose column and measured by competitive binding and [^{14}C]dTMP synthesis by the Moran methods. Total, post-FUra TS is measured by pre-incubation dissociation of FdUMP-bound TS after neutral charcoal removal of cytosolic ligands. H_4PteGlu and CH_2-H_4PteGlu are measured by the Priest method using L. Casei TS. The materials and methods are described in sufficient detail to permit wide application of this approach.

INTRODUCTION

   Thirty years of clinical experience with FUra have failed to result in little consensus of progress regarding optimal dose and schedule, judging from the frequent use of the relatively dangerous 5-day bolus loading method reported in this Symposium. Addition of CF to FUra introduces an additional order of magnitude of complexities. We feel that a more efficient approach to improvement of fluoropyrimidine therapy is by direct study of patients' cancers, rather than just meticulous evaluation of host factors predictive of outcome. The methods described below have been in ongoing use in our laboratories for several years (1-6), and require only ordinary diligence for successful performance. By application of these methods we were the first to show that near abrogation of intratumoral free TS after bolus FUra may be a concomitant of response preclinically (2) and clinically (4), and that total TS changes (2,5,6) also correlate. More recently, we have found statistically significant correlations between acute and chronic TS inhibition and response, and total TS levels and survival, in tumors of patients with gastrointestinal malignancies treated with FUra without CF (7) and in serial biopsies of breast cancer in patients treated with FUra plus high-dose CF (8). Some of the single biopsy data showing correlation with FUra response are presented elsewhere in this volume.

BIOPSY METHODS

A Keyes 4-mm punch instrument (e.g., "Baker's Biopsy Punch," disposable, Baker/Cummins Key Pharmaceuticals, Miami, FL 33069) is most useful for exophytic superficial tumor or even subcutaneous disease. This yields 15-50 mg of tissue. The defect plugs with eschar within a day and heals completely, without suture, in 1-2 weeks.

Approaches to subcutaneous tumor include introducing a punch through a 1-2 cm incision directly over the tumor; and forceps biopsy (e.g., micro-ear forceps, Cat. AWF-5321, S and T Microsurgical, Accurate Surgical and Scientific Instruments Corp., Westbury, N.Y. 11590) biopsy via subcutaneous tunneling (with a trocar) through a 1-2 cm skin incision 2-3 cm distal from the tumor margin.

Biopsies are placed within 30 sec, in 1-ml polyvials, in a dry ice container, then stored at -80°C (Revco). We have always done the folate assays within 24 h of biopsy. The order of stability, in intact tissues, generally appears to be TS $>$ nucleotides $>$ folates. Tissue triage, TS and folate assays must be done on the day of homogenization.

EQUIPMENT

Spectrophotometer (UV/Vis) with water jacket; lyophilizer; conductivity/pH meter; polytron-type homogenizer; shaker bath; Pipetman variable pipettors; cold storage (-80°C or colder) cabinet.

MATERIALS

1. L. Casei TS. An ammonium sulfate preparation may be obtained from Biopure (Boston, MA 02111), at about 1200 mIU/ml. An alternative source may be from Dr. Daniel Santi, University of California, San Francisco. 1.0 I.U. is the amount of enzyme that will catalyze the formation of 1.0 μmole dTMP/min, and represents about 4.14 nmoles of TS based on [^{3}H]FdUMP-ligand binding of 1.7 binding sites/molecule TS. The Friedkin spectrophotometric assay (9) is used to follow TS activity during phosphocellulose column (10) purification. DHFR elutes early and TS, late. The TS fractions are pooled and stored at 4°C. Reactivation of TS inhibited by an accumulation of disulfides is done by periodic dialysis against 5 mM potassium phosphate buffer, pH 7.1, containing 20 mM 2-mercaptoethanol. Long-term storage of TS is best done by addition of an equal volume of glycerol and placing at -20°C. Freeze-thawing of purely aqueous stocks should be avoided. Serial dilution of enzyme, for the TS and folate assays, is done in Homogenization Buffer (see below) supplemented with 0.2% BSA.

2. Radioisotopes. [6-^{3}H]FdUMP, 18-20 Ci/mmole, and [5-^{3}H]dUMP, 18-20 Ci/mmole, are available from Moravek Biochemicals (Brea, CA 92621). Working stocks of both isotopes, stored at -20°, should be cleaned up of breakdown products of radiolysis within several weeks of use for lowest blanks; DEAE-cellulose (see below) is useful for this. [^{14}C] Formaldehyde, 40-60 mCi/mmole (NEN Research Products, Boston, MA 02118) is stored at room temperature to avoid cold-temperature polymerization to paraformaldehyde.

3. Charcoal. HCl-washed activated charcoal (Sigma) is suspended in a 10-fold (w/v) excess of deionized water at room temperature, centrifuged at 1000 x g, and the supernatant fine particles removed by aspiration; this is repeated twice. To stock charcoal as a 10% (w/v) suspension are added 2.5% (w/v) bovine albumin (we have used generic Sigma Fraction V; Cat. Nos. A3294 or

A7888 may be desirable) and 0.25% (w/v) dextran (Ave. M.W. 70,000, Sigma). This stock is "10% neutral charcoal" and may be kept at 4°C for a year or more. Acid charcoal is made by adding 60 ml H_2O and 10 ml of 3N HCl to 30 ml of neutral charcoal. The 3% acid charcoal is rapidly stirred in an ice-bath during use.

4.   DEAE-Cellulose Minicolumns. DEAE (cellulose N,N-diethylaminoethyl ether, Kodak Laboratory Chemicals, Rochester, N.Y. 14650) is swollen in 0.1 N NaOH during gentle stirring for 30 min at room temperature. On settling, the supernatant fine particles are aspirated; an excess of deionized water is added, the suspension stirred for 10 min then allowed to settle, and the supernatant again aspirated, this process being repeated 3 more times. An excess of 1 M NH_4HCO_3 buffer, pH 8.0 (at 4°C), is added to the washed, packed DEAE-cellulose; the suspension is mixed at room temperature for 1 h, and the supernatant removed after settling. Deionized H_2O is added and the slurry is poured into 5-ml pipette tips (with glass wool at the tips); the contracted 1-cm wide bed of material should be 4.0 cm high and be topped by Whatman No. 1 filter paper. The columns can be kept sterile by addition of 1 ml of 0.1% NaN_3 (note: mutagenic) for storage at 4°C. Prior to use, the columns are washed with 10 ml of H_2O.

5.   Tetrahydrofolate ($H_4PteGlu_1$). Although we have previously used enzymically-prepared material (1), for TS assays we now routinely use the Sigma product, using a separate 25-mg ampule for each day's work. A 2 mM primary stock of l-$H_4PteGlu_1$ is made by addition to 25 mg d,l-$H_4PteGlu_1$, (typically, "68% active in a formiminoglutamic acid transferase assay"), in order, 52 µl of 14.3 M 2-mercaptoethanol, 90 µl of 1 M Na ascorbate, pH 6.5, 17 µl of 37% (w/w) formaldehyde, and 7.96 ml of 0.2 M Tris-HCl buffer, pH 7.0. A 10-min incubation at room temperature (in the dark) allows completion of $\underline{l}$-CH_2-$H_4PteGlu_1$ formation. Dilutions are made in the same buffer mixture ("Folate Buffer"), with or without formaldehyde. Concentrations of $\underline{l}$-CH_2-$H_4PteGlu_1$ can be checked spectrophotometrically (11).

6.   Buffers. In addition to the Folate Buffer, above, are the Homogenization and Dissociation Buffers. The Homogenization Buffer, for 10 ml, consists of 61 mg 5'-CMP, 1 ml of 1N NaF, 28 µl 2-mercaptoethanol, 0.568 ml of 1 M Na ascorbate (pH 7.0) diluted to 10 ml with 0.2 M Tris-HCl buffer, pH 7.4. The 5'-CMP and NaF are present to eliminate the otherwise often severe effects of phosphatases. One should avoid the temptation to use phosphate anions (which can inhibit TS [12, 13]). The Dissociation Buffer is identical to the Homogenization Buffer except that 0.3 M NH_4HCO_3, pH 8.0 (at 4°C), is substituted for Tris-HCl, and 2% (w/v) gelatin (Sigma, approx. 60 Bloom) is present to reduce effects of proteases. Down adjustment of pH of stock NH_4HCO_3 is conveniently done with dry ice chips.

TISSUE HOMOGENIZATION

To portions of tumor biopsies, 10-100 mg, are added a 10- to 30-fold excess of Homogenization Buffer at 4°C. After scissors-mincing, homogenates at 4°C are prepared by the action of polytron-type rotating shearing blades (VirTishear, at the micro-generator 50-60 setting for 15-30 sec., using the 10-mm shaft). Pulverization of liquid N_2-frozen tissue with thrice freeze-thawing works equally well. Sonication (e.g., 100-watt bursts with the fine probe of a Braunsonic instrument) beyond 10 sec we find reduces $CH_2H_4PteGlu$ yields, even with aggressive cooling. Dounce and ground-glass homogenziation are gentle, but often inadequate for full yields of DNA and TS.

TISSUE TRIAGE

A 200 µl aliquot (or more) or the homogenate is immediately taken for heating for 15 min at 65°C to inactivate enzymes, then stored at -20°C prior to FdUMP/dUMP separation. Acetic acid extraction is unnecessary, and can lead to excessive conductivities after lyophilization. A 100 µl aliquot is taken for protein assay, or is added to perchloric acid for subsequent DNA and RNA assays by modified Burton and orcinol methods (2,14), respectively. Approximately 1 ml of homogenate is centrifuged at 4°C and 4000 x g for 20 min, and the cytosol assayed for TS and $CH_2-H_4PteGlu_1$ on the day of homogenization.

DEAE-COLUMN SEPARATION OF dUMP AND FdUMP

The heat-inactivated portion of homogenate is diluted with water to less than 1 mmHo conductivity and applied to a 1 x 4 cm column (above). Our present step gradient gives somewhat better separation using less salt than employed previously (1): in sequence at 4° are added 6 ml H_2O; 10 ml of 50 mM NH_4HCO_3, pH 7.5, which elutes nucleosides; 5 ml of 50 mM NH_4HCO_3, pH 8.0 dUMP then elutes with 5 ml of 50 mM NH_4HCO_3, pH 8.0 followed by 13 ml of 50 mM NH_4HCO_3, pH 8.5; FdUMP then is eluted with 10 ml of 100 mM buffer, pH 9.5. The FdUMP and dUMP fractions are lyophilized to complete dryness prior to reconstitution in 1 ml of 5 mM potassium phosphate buffer, pH 7.4.

TS ASSAYS

[^{3}H]FdUMP Ligand-Binding Assay. To 50 µl of 4000 x g cytosol on wet ice, in plastic test tubes in duplicate, are added 50 µl of Dissociation Buffer, 50 µl [^{3}H]FdUMP (5 pmoles or about 200,000 DPM of 18 Ci/mmole material) in H_2O, and 25 µl of 2 mM $CH_2H_4PteGlu_1$. The tubes are incubated at 30°C for 15 min, then 1.0 ml of 3% acid charcoal (rapidly stirring at 4°C) is added followed by pulse vortex mixing x 10. The tubes are centrifuged at 4°C for 25 min, and 0.8 ml of supernatant is taken for DPM determination (using 10 ml of RIA-Solve II, Research Products International, Mt. Prospect, ILL 60056). Backgrounds using Homogenization Buffer without tissue may be as low as 250 DPM, but twice this is highly useable. The sensitivity of this assay, 40-50 DPM/fmole TS, is limited not by this background but by the S.D.s of the replicates. Good technique with the Gilson Pipetman should result in an average S.D. of less that 30 DPM. The L. Casei enzyme is less stable at pH 8.0 than mammalian TS, so if this is used as a standard, Tris buffer at pH 7.4 is preferred. For total TS (cytosolic FdUMP-bound plus free TS), after Dissociation Buffer addition the tubes are incubated, tightly-capped, at 30°C for 3 hr prior to [^{3}H]FdUMP addition. This approach may be less successful for tissues from patients on leucovorin protocols; treatment of cytosols with an equal volume of 6% neutral charcoal to remove free (aromatic) ligands prior to the 3-h pre-incubation may be useful (15,16). Near-sterility during the 3-h dissociation incubation is done by prior 0.45 µm membrane filtration of cytosols. We have not found neutral charcoal to significantly decrease [^{3}H]FdUMP-titratable activity as reported (15). Correction for exchange-labeling of cytosolic ternary complex is done routinely (2). This factor becomes proportionately smaller for incubations shorter than 20 min, and is only about 5% if pH 7.4 conditions are used (where total TS is taken from the pre-FUra biopsy): true TS_f = (apparent TS_f - 0.05 TS_{tot})/0.95. Subsequent correction for dilution by cytosolic FdUMP is usually necessary for tissue FdUMP concentrations greater than 100 pmole/g.

[^3H_2O] Tritium-Release [^{3}H]dUMP Assay of TS Activity. This is the preferred assay for small (e.g., 10 mg) samples. Although L. Casei standards (usually 0.01 pmole/assay for tritium-release, and 0.1 pmole for [^{3}H]FdUMP-binding) are at least 40-fold higher by this method (about 1500 DPM/fmole), in practice this advantage may be substantially less due to isotope dilution by cytosolic dUMP. However, increased dUMP (when CH_2-H_4PteGlu$_1$ is in excess) also drives the reaction faster, so that, e.g., a 10-fold dilution of assay [^{3}H]dUMP by cytosolic dUMP results in only a 40 percent decrease in apparent TS activity. No correction for ternary complex dissociation is needed in our experience. A method similar to the Houghton modification (15) of Robert's assay that we have found useful is the following: to 50 µl of cytosol at 4°C are added 50 µl of [^{3}H]dUMP (5 pmoles or about 200,000 DPM of 18 Ci/mmole stock) in H_2O and 25 µl of 2 mM CH_2-H_4PteGlu$_1$; after incubation at 37°C for 10 min, 1.0 ml of ice-cold 3% acid charcoal is added. Backgrounds in the 4000 x g supernatants should be below 2000 DPM. Dissociation Buffer and 3-hr pre-incubation for total TS determination, for post-FUra treated tissues may be done as described above with results at least equal to those [^{3}H]FdUMP ligand binding.

FdUMP AND dUMP ASSAYS

These are done nearly precisely as described (1). [^{3}H]FdUMP should be in slight excess over L. Casei TS FdUMP binding sites (1.7 sites/molecule TS) to avoid negative intercepts on the FdUMP standard curve. Thus, it is not practical to use higher concentrations of ligands in order to allow shorter incubations. We typically use 0.15 pmoles TS and 0.5 pmoles [^{3}H]FdUMP per tube. The [^{14}C]TMP synthesis method for dUMP is essentially as described (except we use 1.95 ml of "Buffer A", p. 1456, Ref. 1). Also, separation of [^{14}C]TMP from remaining radioactivity may be done as for dUMP separation, above. However, smearing by [^{14}C]formaldehyde products can be a problem: following lyophilization of final [^{14}C]TMP, any residual "crystals" are an indication for redissolving product in H_2O and repeating the lyophilization.

CH_2-H_4PteGlu AND H_4PteGlu ASSAYS

The conditions of Priest's method (17-19), only slightly modified by us (20,21), use TS and FdUMP at concentrations not dissimilar from intratumoral levels of these ligands. To 50 µl of cytosol or Homogenization Buffer alone are added 50 µl of [^{3}H]FdUMP (20 pmoles, about 800,000 DPM), 4 pmoles of L. Casei TS in 25 µl of Homogenization Buffer (with 0.2% [w/v]BSA), and 25 µl of Folate Buffer (with or without formaldehyde). A useful quantity of CH_2-H_4PteGlu$_1$ for the standard is 1.0 pmole, which should give 10-20 DPM/fmole (about 50 percent of stoichiometric binding). The tubes are incubated at 37°C for 10 min, then 1.0 ml of ice-cold 3% acid charcoal added for separation of protein-bound radioactivity, as above. H_4PteGlu and CH_2-H_4PteGlu$_1$ concentrations are given by the results of tubes with and without formaldehyde, respectively (19). Results are expressed in monoglutamate equivalents. The no-folate binary-complex values, which are substantially higher (about 1500-2000 DPM) than the no-TS blanks, should be used for background subtraction from the specimen values. The binary-complex blanks, however, are occasionally greater than raw specimen values, presumably because of cytosolic dUMP that lowers the binary complex blank. This effect may be precisely quantitated (21) after results of FdUMP and dUMP assays are known: the raw DPMs are first corrected by substraction of the no-TS blank values; the decrease in the binary complex background caused by dUMP can be calculated (21) by dividing the apparent figure by (0.13 x ([dUMP]/[FdUMP])). This gives the true binary-complex background. Additional small correction for dilution of [^{3}H]FdUMP label by cytosolic FdUMP may be needed. A further complexity of this assay is the fact that excess dUMP can lead to consumption of low cytosolic CH_2-H_4PteGlu$_n$ during [^{3}H]FdUMP-TS binding. Addition of dUMP (20-100 pmoles) to paired assay tubes may be a useful test of the specificity of the assay for the presence of 5,10-methylene (20), and to assess effects of endogenous cytosolic dUMP on ternary complex formation. An increase in assay FdUMP to 50-100 pmoles may be useful to overcome the dUMP effects, and is currently under study.

An alternative assay has been described, using L. Casei TS and a $[5-^3]$dUMP tritium-release approach (22). Although in principle tritium may be released from $[5-^3H]$dUMP in the absence of 1-carbon transfer (23), we have found this to be a negligible effect. Standardization of this assay for the effects of cytosolic dUMP should be done, and presumably TS should be at least equal to cytosolic FdUMP concentrations.

INCORPORATION OF FUra INTO RNA

We have described a method for quantitation of the percent replacement of uracil in tissue RNA by non-radiolabeled FUra (14). This method requires at least 500 mg of tissue in most instances and is relatively labor intensive. FUMP is released from tissue RNA by alkali and converted to FUR by alkaline phosphatase. Periodate and $Na[^3H]BH_4$ treatment results in radiolabeled ring-opened FUR trialcohols which are then isolated.

FUra in RNA may be synergistic with TS inhibition by several mechanisms: (a) F-RNA provides a depot storage for slow release of FdUMP precursors (14); (b) There may be cell-cycle synergy; (c) F-RNA may block TS gene amplification or expression (accounting for the extreme laboratory rarity of TS-elevated FUra-resistant mutants, in contrast to FdUrd); and (d) F-RNA may also form "frozen" ternary complexes with RNA methylating enzymes (24).

REFERENCES

1. Moran, R.G., Spears, C., and Heidelberger, C. Biochemical determinants of tumor sensitivity to 5-fluorouracil: ultrasensitive methods for the determination of 5-fluoro-2'-deoxyuridylate, 2'-deoxyuridylate, and thymidylate synthetase. Proc. Natl. Acad. Sci. USA 76:1456-1460 (1979).

2. Spears, C.P., Shahinian, A.H., Moran, R.G., Heidelberger, C., and Corbett, T.H. In vivo kinetics of thymidylate synthetase inhibition in FUra-sensitive and -resistant murine colon adenocarcinomas. Cancer Res. 42:450-456 (1982).

3. Spears, C.P. Thymidylate synthetase inhibition in Peyton adenocarcinoma xenografts following bolus 5-fluorouracil. Exerpta Med. Int. Congr. Series 647:12-19 (1984).

4. Spears, C.P., Gustavsson, B.G., Mitchell, M.S., Spicer, D., Berne, M., Bernstein, L., and Danenberg, P.V. Thymidylate synthetase inhibition in malignant tumors and normal liver of patients given bolus intravenous 5-fluorouracil. Cancer Res. 44:4144-4150 (1984).

5. Berne, M.H.O., Gustavsson, B.G., Almersjö, O., Spears, C.P., and Frösing, R. Sequential methotrexate/5-FU: FdUMP formation and TS inhibition in a transplantable rodent colon adenocarcinoma. Cancer Chemother. Pharmacol. 16:237-242 (1986).

6. Berne, M., Gustavsson, B., Almersjö, O., Spears, C.P., and Waldenström, J. Concurrent allopurinol and 5-fluorouracil: 5-fluoro-2'-deoxyuridylate formation and thymidylate synthase inhibition in rat colon carcinoma and in regenerating rat liver. Cancer Chemother. Pharmacol. 20:193-197 (1987).

7. Spears, C.P., Gustavsson, B.G., Berne, M., Frösing, R., and Hayes, A.A. Mechanisms of innate resistance to thymidylate synthase inhibition after 5-fluorouracil. Cancer Res. 48: in press (1988).

8.   Spears, C.P., Leichman, G., and Muggia, F.M. Acute and chronic thymidylate synthase inhibition in serial breast cancer biopsies from patients treated with fluorouracil plus high-dose leucovorin (Submitted, 1988).

9.   Fridland, A., Langenbach, R.J., and Heidelberger, C. Purification of thymidylate synthetase from Ehrlich ascites carcinoma cells. J. Biol. Chem. 246:7110-7114 (1971).

10.   Sharma, R.K., and Kisliuk, R.L.   Quenching of thymidylate synthetase fluorescence by substrate analogs. Biochem. Biophys. Res. Commun. 64:648-655 (1975).

11.   Daron, H.H., and Aull, J.L.   A kinetic study of thymidylate synthase from Lactobacillus casei. J. Biol. Chem. 253:940-945 (1978).

12.   Galivan, J.H., Maley, G.F., and Maley, F. Factors affecting substrate binding in Lactobacillus casei thymidylate synthetase as studied by equilibrium dialysis. Biochem. 15:356-362 (1976).

13.   Lockshin, A., and Danenberg, P.V.   Biochemical factors affecting the tightness of 5-fluorodeoxyuridylate binding to human thymidylate synthase. Biochem. Pharmacol. 30: 247-257 (1981).

14.   Spears, C.P., Shani, J., Shahinian, A.H., Wolf, W., Heidelberger, C., and Danenberg, P.V. Assay and time course of 5-fluorouracil incorporation into RNA of L1210/0 cells in vivo. Mol. Pharmacol. 27:302-307 (1984).

15.   Houghton, J.A., Weiss, K.D., Williams, L.G., Torrance, P.M., and Houghton, P.J. Relationship between 5-fluoro-2'-deoxyuridylate, 2'-deoxyuridylate, and thymidylate synthase activity subsequent to 5-fluorouracil administration, in xenografts of human colon adenocarcinomas. Biochem. Pharmacol. 35:1351-1358 (1986).

16.   Fernandes, D.J., and Cranford, S.K. A method for the determination of total, free, and 5-fluorodeoxyuridylate-bound thymidylate synthase in cell extracts. Anal. Biochem. 142:378-385 (1984).

17.   Priest, D.G., Happel, K.K., and Doig, M.T. Electrophoretic identification of poly-γ-glutamate chain-lengths of 5,10-methylenetetrahydrofolate using thymidylate synthetase complexes. J. Biochem. Biophys. Methods 3:201-206 (1980).

18.   Priest,   D.G.,   and   Mangum,   M.   Relative   affinity   of   5,10-methylenetetrahydrofolylpolyglutamates   for   the   Lactobacillus   casei thymidylate   synthetase-5-fluorodeoxyuridylate   binary   complex.   Arch. Biochem. Biophys. 210:118-123 (1981).

19.   Doig, M.T., Peters, J.R., Sur, P., Dang, M., and Priest, D.G. Determination of mouse liver 5-methyltetrahydrofolate concentration and polyglutamate forms. J. Biochem. Biophys. Methods 10:287-294 (1985).

20.   Spears, C.P., Gustavsson, B.G., and Frösing, R. Folinic acid modulation of fluorouracil: kinetics of bolus administration. Invest. New Drugs 6: in press (1988).

21.   Spears, C.P., Hayes, A.A., Danenberg, P.V., Frösing, R., and Gustavsson, B.G. Deoxyuridylate effects on thymidylate synthase-5-fluorodeoxyuridylate-folate ternary complex formation (Submitted, 1988).

22. Houghton, J.A., Schmidt, C., and Houghton, P.J. The effect of derivatives of folic acid on the fluorodeoxyuridylate-thymidylate synthase covalent complex in human colon xenografts. Eur. J. Cancer Clin. Oncol. 18:347-354 (1982).

23. Pogolotti, A.L., Weill, C., and Santi, D.V. Thymidylate synthetase catalyzed exchange of tritium from [5-^{3}H]-2'-deoxyuridylate for protons of water. Biochem. 18:2794-2804 (1979).

24. Tseng, W.-C., Medina, D., and Randerath, K. Specific inhibition of transfer RNA methylation and modification in tissues of mice treated with 5-fluorouracil. Cancer Res. 38:1250-1257 (1978).

DISCUSSION OF DR. SPEARS' PRESENTATION

Dr. Rustum: The pharmacokinetic data of CF in man by 1 or 2 hour
infusion indicate a peak plasma concentration of folate is reached
about 1 - 2 hrs thereafter. You have removed biopsies somewhere
around 50 to 60 min after the treatment. Maybe at the time you are
biopsying these specimens it is too early. Have you looked for a
later specimen, say 24 hours after the dose?

Dr. Spears: That one patient who showed the bad reactions had a day 3
biopsy that showed only 40% enzyme inhibition, which perhaps is a
poor result. Perhaps she should still have 80% inhibition at day 3
similar to the Houghton data. It's a matter of practicality. You
take your baseline biopsies, post CF biopsies, post FUra biopsies;
the patient needs to go home.

Dr. Moran: I'd like to make two comments. The first one is that you
have demonstrated at least one patient where a very high level dUMP
seems to be giving you a problem with response. You've also seen low
tissue folates and difficulty pushing them up. Both of those are
going to give you problems with pyrimidine therapy aimed at TS. If I
can make a pitch for the CB-type compounds, if you have high dUMP, it
gets in the way of binding of FdUMP, but it's going to stimulate the
binding of CB3717. If you have low tissue folates it gets in the way
of FdUMP but it's going to stimulate the activity of CB3717. My
reading of it is all the factors that are getting in our way with
fluoropyrimidines are indications that we should be using folate
analogs.

Dr. Spears: The standard deviation between patient's dUMP values is
about 10 nmol/g so far with an average value of 25. One patient
showed 20-fold higher and clearly in that kind of case you would need
a totally individualized approach.

Dr. Moran: The second comment that I want to make is more of a techni
cal one. From the presentations that we had today, it is clear that
a lot of people are using binding of FdUMP to TS as an assay tissue
folates, tissue 5,10-methylene, presumably. I think we all agree
that in terms of sensitivity this is the way to go. It's a nice
system but it has some instrinic problems that I want to comment on
quickly. The major problem is the level of deoxyuridylate that
interferes with that assay. It's very, very low.

Dr. Spears: You can see that we have carefully quantitated that effect.

Dr. Moran: At the risk of being boorish, I want to repeat what you
just said, namely that you have to worry about competition between
tritium labeled FdUMP and tissue dUMP for binding to the enzyme.
That gets in the way for sure. dUMP in the presence of high levels
of enzyme and limiting levels of tetrahydrofolate is going to make
dTMP and it's catalytically destroying what you're trying to
measure. Janet Houghton, I think, was the only person to make comments about how to get around that problem. I think she was using a
5'nucleotidase to destroy the dUMP and something like this is
absolutely required.

Dr. Galivan: This is a brief comment in response more to Rick's comment and is related to the folate analog inhibitors of TS. We have, in fact, found in a tissue culture system that if one uses very low levels of dihydrofolate reductase inhibitors with a non-effective level of CB3717 that the dihydrofolate reductase inhibitors reduce the methylenetetrahydrofolate pools by about 80% and that this results in about a 10-fold enhancement of the activity of the CB3717. During this process, the dUMP pools do go up by about 30-fold; so by doing this you favor the formation of a ternary complex of the anti-folate TS inhibitor, dUMP and enzyme.

Dr. Spears: If the quinazolines were available I'd use them immediately. I gather that CB3717 is going to be supplanted by other quinazolines.

Dr. Galivan: That's correct. That is what I hear from the English group.

Dr. P. Houghton: Your data confirms the preclinical data that suggests that the pools of 5,10-methylenetetrahydrofolate and its polygluta-mates are extremely low in many human cancers. Since this is a substrate that is used by several enzymes and clearly it's way below the K_m TS reaction, physiologically the cell is almost setting itself up such that TMP production de novo is certainly not optimal under the unperturbed conditions.

Dr. Spears: You know we haven't made a distinction about the poly-glutamate state, so perhaps that may have some impact.

Dr. Houghton: With respect to K_m for the polyglutamates for the TS reaction, there is no difference.

Dr. Spears: Yet your V_{max} values are the same.

Dr. Houghton: The V_{max} values are the same and the K_m values are the same, but their levels in tissues are extremely low suggesting that conversion of dUMP to TMP would be suboptimal anyway.

THE TREATMENT OF METASTATIC BREAST CANCER

WITH 5-FLUOROURACIL AND LEUCOVORIN

C.J. Allegra, G.F. Egan, J.C. Drake,
S.M. Steinberg and S.M. Swain

Clinical Pharmacology Branch
Division of Cancer Treatment
National Cancer Institute
Bethesda, Maryland 20892

INTRODUCTION

The preclinical rationale for the use of 5-fluorouracil (5-FU) in combination with leucovorin has been well described in a number of articles [1]. Briefly, the formation and stability of the ternary complex formed between an active metabolite of 5-FU (FdUMP), thymidylate synthase (TS), and the reduced folate 5-10-methylene tetrahydrofolate is highly dependent on the concentration and polyglutamated state of the folate [2,3]. The addition of exogenous folate has been shown to enhance ternary complex formation, and thereby enzyme inhibition, in in vitro and in vivo investigations [4,5]. Inhibition of TS results in thymidylate deficiency and presumably cytotoxicity due to a diminished ability of cells to replicate and repair DNA. In light of the encouraging experience using 5-FU with leucovorin for the treatment of metastatic colon cancer [1], we sought to test this combination for the therapy of metastatic breast cancer wherein 5-FU is known to be an active agent. The objectives of our study were two-fold: 1) to assess the efficacy of 5-FU combined with leucovorin for the treatment of metastatic breast cancer, and 2) to determine the effect of leucovorin on the binding of FdUMP to TS in serial tumor samples obtained from patients undergoing therapy. This report represents a preliminary assessment of the efficacy and toxicity of the 5-FU and leucovorin combination and the biochemical studies relevant to the interaction of 5-FU with TS.

PATIENT CHARACTERISTICS

Of 54 patients entered on study, 50 are evaluable for response at the time of this preliminary report. Table 1 summarizes the salient patient characteristics. The majority of patients (67%) had visceral involvement with breast carcinoma, and one-half of the patients had two or more sites of disease involvement at the time of study entry. All patients had previously failed combination chemotherapy, and 90% had received prior 5-FU.

Table 1. Patient Characteristics

Age (median)	51
Performance status (median)	80
Prior therapy (%):	
5-FU	90
Combination chemotherapy	100
Radiation therapy	57

BIOCHEMICAL EVALUATION

Twenty patients with accessible tumor had serial tumor biopsies and biochemical measurements before and 24 hours after treatment with either 5-FU 375 mg/m^2 alone or 5-FU 375 mg/m^2 plus leucovorin 500 mg/m^2. Tumor samples were evaluated for the percent of total tumor TS that was bound by the administered drugs. All TS measurements were standardized to cytosolic protein. Total TS level and free TS levels were evaluated by standard TS binding assays using radiolabeled FdUMP in the presence of excess 5-10-methylene tetrahydrofolate [2,6]. The amount of radiolabeled FdUMP bound after a brief incubation with an aliquot of tumor cytosol served as a measure of free TS. A three-hour incubation of radiolabeled FdUMP with a separate aliquot of tumor cytosol (to allow for complete exchange of administered 5-FU [FdUMP] with the labeled compound) served as a measure of total TS. The fraction of TS bound was obtained by computing the difference between total and free enzyme levels and dividing by the total enzyme level. All measurements were performed on cytosol obtained from 4 mm punch biopsy samples that were frozen at $-70°C$ immediately upon harvesting.

TREATMENT REGIMEN

All patients were treated with the following regimen:

5-FU   375 mg/m^2/dx5
Leucovorin   500 mg/m^2/dx5 given 1 hr prior to the 5-FU

The regimen was administered at 21-day intervals.

RESULTS

Clinical Response

In 50 patients evaluable for response, we noted a complete (2 pts) plus partial (10 pts) response rate of 24%. An additional 28 patients had disease stabilization for greater than two cycles of therapy. The sites of disease response included liver (4), soft tissue (8), and bone (3). The overall survival of the entire group of patients was 8.3 months.

Toxicity

The prevalent toxicities observed occurred in the bone marrow and gastrointestinal tract. Table 2 summarizes the frequency of these toxicities. Myelosuppression alone was responsible for dose alterations in 38%

Table 2.   Toxicity

	Grades 3 & 4 (%)
MYELOSUPPRESSION	
Neutropenia	65
Thrombocytopenia	19
GASTROINTESTINAL	
Mucositis	33
Diarrhea	13*

*No grade 4 diarrhea.

of patients.   Overall, 76% of patients required dose reductions and 82% required a prolongation in the dose interval for recovery from toxicity.

Biochemical Evaluation

The mean TS activity for all samples was found to be 103 fmoles/mg. No correlation was noted between the tumor TS levels and the ultimate clinical outcome.   In three patients, paired tumor samples from treatment with and without leucovorin were evaluable.   The results are listed in Table 3 and demonstrate that the amount of TS in patient samples bound by the administered 5-FU 24 hours after the dose was markedly enhanced by the co-administration of leucovorin.   The ultimate clinical outcome was also correlated with degree of TS binding 24 hours after the 5-FU dose.   In four patients with partial responses, an average of 91% of the TS was bound by the administered drugs versus 30% in three patients with unresponsive disease.

DISCUSSION

The combination of 5-FU and leucovorin appears to be an active regimen for the treatment of metastatic breast carcinoma.   Twelve of 50 patients achieved an objective clinical response.   This result suggests that leucovorin can enhance the activity of 5-FU.   This is of particular importance in light of prior failure of combination chemotherapy in all patients and a 90% failure of prior therapy with 5-FU in combination regimens.   The primary toxicity noted in this patient population was myelosuppression,

Table 3.   Biochemical Evaluation

Patient	Leucovorin	% TS Bound 24 Hrs After 5-FU
1	−	49
	+	96
2	−	0
	+	84
3	−	52
	+	95

although a substantial degree of gastrointestinal toxicity was observed. Presumably, the predominance of myelosuppression reflects the heavy pre-therapy in the study population.

The biochemical evaluation of sequential tumor samples indicates that leucovorin enhances the stability of the formed ternary complex. Further, in a small number of samples it appears that the percent of tumor TS bound at 24 hours after 5-FU may be a useful predictive indicator of the ultimate clinical outcome.

Clearly, both the clinical results and biochemical correlates require additional exploration before definitive conclusions can be entertained. These results support further investigations of the 5-FU-leucovorin combination for breast cancer in both the salvage and primary therapeutic settings. Additional biochemical studies in tumor tissues are needed to establish predictive tests and as confirmation of the presumed biochemical modulations induced by the use of leucovorin.

REFERENCES

1. J.L. Grem, D.F. Hoth, J.M. Hamilton, S.A. King and B. Leyland-Jones, Overview of current status and future direction of clinical trials with 5-fluorouracil in combination with folinic acid, Cancer Treat. Rep. 71:1249-1264 (1987).
2. C.J. Allegra, B.A. Chabner, J.C. Drake, R. Lutz, D. Rodbard and J. Jolivet, Enhanced inhibition of thymidylate synthase by methotrexate polyglutamates, J. Biol. Chem. 260:9720-9726 (1985).
3. A. Lockshin and P.V. Dannenberg, Biochemical factors affecting the tightness of 5-fluorodeoxyuridylate binding to human thymidylate synthase, Biochem. Pharmacol. 30:247-257 (1981).
4. J.A. Houghton, S.J. Maroda, J.O. Phillips and P.J. Houghton, Biochemical determinants of responsiveness to 5-fluorouracil and its derivatives in xenografts of human colorectal adenocarcinomas in mice, Cancer Res. 41:144-149 (1981).
5. D. Santi, A biochemical rationale for the use of 5-fluorouracil in combination with leucovorin, in: "The Current Status of 5-Fluorouracil-Leucovorin Calcium Combinations," H.W. Bruckner and Y.M. Rustum, eds., Park Row Publishers, New York (1984).
6. R.G. Moran, C.P. Spears and C. Heidelberger, Biochemical determinants of tumor sensitivity to 5-FU: ultrasensitive methods for the determination of 5-fluoro-2'-deoxyuridylate, 2'-deoxyuridylate, and thymidylate synthase. Proc. Natl. Acad. Sci. USA 76:1456-1460 (1979).

DISCUSSION OF DR. ALLEGRA'S PRESENTATION

Dr. Moran: I was very interested in your comment that the total TS was going up after treatment. Did you normalize that per mg of protein?

Dr. Allegra: The data were normalized two ways, by milligram of cytosolic protein and also per wet weight of tissue. Either way the data are normalized you still see increases in TS.

Dr. Moran: You were saying about a 2 to 2.5-fold increase. Our experience has been with a homogenous population in cell culture; conditions where you can really manipulate things without the problems you have in the clinical samples. If we see a 2 to 2.5-fold increase in TS/mg tissue then the amount/cell was up above 5-fold, so you probably have really enormous increments. One of the important things you talked about today was the levels of TS in these tumor specimens being so low and just making it so difficult from a technical point of view to know whether what you have is real.

Dr. Allegra: I think you could get at that issue by numbers, actually, assuming that the same is true for FUra and FUra/CF/, and if you see differences.

Dr. Moran: I think this is very important particularly if the idea that I was trying to bring up in my talk is correct that you need to get 90 or 95% inhibition in order to have any effect. If that really is true then trying to determine <u>that</u> on someone's clinical samples is really a challenging job from just the technical point.

Dr. Allegra: Right.

Dr. Moran: Up until recently I didn't have any experience in trying to do these assays on clinical samples but Dr. Patel, a clinical fellow in my laboratory now, started to do some TS assays in childhood tumors. We were really bothered by the low levels of activity in even in some of these fast growing tumors. We found that we had to modify the technique that we used to use quite a bit in order to have results that made any sense. We used one of the modifications that Janet Houghton introduced with charcoal treatment and taking things down with TCA and that works nicely. I wanted to raise the point with you that if you're in a situation where you're not sure if the low numbers you're getting mean anything, the one control that's been very useful to us is the old trick that the hormone-binding people use of putting in a tremendous excess of cold FdUMP with your hot FdUMP. Of course if you do that you shouldn't have any binding unless it's non-specific. In doing that we found that using the assay with just charcoal absorption doesn't pass that test. You can still get radioactivity bound that is not a specific event. If you do charcoal and then TCA precipitation, that FdUMP high dilution control will be right down to your machine background.

Dr. Spears: Comment and a question. I very much appreciate your presentation. I've been waiting a long time to hear someone tell me about tumor biopsies. The backgrounds in tritiated FdUMP that has recently been recently been cleaned up on a DEAE column to get rid of radiolysis background products can be as low as 150 cpm. It is very common even with the cleanest FdUMP to have some very low enzymes. It seems perhaps unnecessary that you threw out a third of your data because they had low enzyme activity, they might have been some of your most interesting cases. The standard deviation over the background is I think more important. The background is not due to TS binding, it's due to something else. I don't know exactly what, but we have gone to the tritium release and it is substantially more sen-. sitive. The question I had was really a clinical one. Your FUra biopsies preceeded your FUra/CF biopsies. How do you know that the subsequent changes you saw weren't just part and parcel of the progression in response to FUra versus a CF effect? Do you have some stragegy for handling that clinical question?

Dr. Allegra: The biopsies were done on alternate cycles so that in some of the patients they had biopsies with FUra alone before they ever saw CF.

Dr. Spears: So it's a mixed group before and after?

Dr. Allegra: Exactly.

Dr. Clark: You've shown us a lot of data on TS enzyme levels, but we all know when you look at the histology of many of these tumors they're not all composed of tumor cells, there's a lot of fibroblast and the like. Have you made any attempts to look at the histology of the tumors that you're actually making your TS preps from to make sure that they are indeed reflective of tumor cells?

Dr. Allegra: I think that's an excellent point. There's some precedent for not doing that with estrogen receptors and progesterone receptors studies where it's simply standardized to the total cytosolic protein. You can devise other methods such as some sort of ratio of normal to malignant tissues. My feeling was that the non-malignant cells, the fat cells, the fibroblasts, etc., probably have very small amounts of TS; if you do biopsies on normal skin you can't measure any TS. So I think that the enzyme that we see is probably from malignant cells, but it's an assumption.

THYMIDYLATE SYNTHASE AND FLUOROURACIL

Kathryn M. Ivanetich and Daniel V. Santi

Departments of Biochemistry and Biophysics and
Pharmaceutical Chemistry, and the Biomolecular
Resource Center
University of California, San Francisco
San Francisco, California 94143

A knowledge of the catalytic mechanism of thymidylate synthase (TS), and its inhibition by 5-fluorodeoxyuridylate (FdUMP) was instrumental in developing the FUra-CF combination for cancer chemotherapy. The generation of the ideas which led to the current combination cleary demonstrates the importance of a fundamental knowledge of the interactions of inhibitors with their targets, and of how basic studies can be translated to clinical practice. The history of the development of the FUra-CF combination is a paradigm for the rational development of chemotherapeutic regimens. This report summarizes current knowledge of (a) the enzymology of the interaction of TS with FdUMP, (b) the 3-dimensional structure of TS, and (c) the effect of FUra on tRNA-uracil methyltranferase. Also, we suggest a possible molecular mechanism for the RNA effects of FUra.

INTERACTION OF TS WITH FdUMP

In the course of early studies on the catalytic mechanism of TS, it was found that FdUMP behaves as a mechanism-based inhibitor of this enzyme (1-3). In the presence of TS, CH_2-H_4folate and FdUMP, enzymic conversions occur up to the step normally associated with methyl transfer to the pyrimidine heterocycle, thereby trapping a covalent TS=FdUMP=CH_2--H_4folate complex. The covalent complex is an analog of a steady-state intermediate of the normal enzymic reaction, and has a Cys thiol of TS attached to the 6-position of FdUMP and the one carbon unit of the cofactor attached to the 5-position of the nucleotide (For a review see 4). This knowledge led to the suggestion that FUra and CF might be useful as a

Abbreviations: AdoMet, S-adenosyl methionine; CH_2-H_4folate, 5,10-methylenetetrahydrofolate; m5Urd, ribothymidine; PABA, para-aminobenzoic acid.

combination (5). Because of its importance in chemotherapy of neoplastic disease, the interaction of FdUMP with TS has been extensively studied. Furthermore, since the interaction mimics several steps in the normal enzymic reaction, it provides an approach towards studying individual steps of the reaction which are otherwise inaccessible. Now that the crystal structure of TS is known (6), this capability has taken on new importance. Following is a summary of the current status of our knowledge of the interaction of TS with FdUMP and CH_2-H_4folate.

Interaction of FdUMP with TS

The interaction of TS, FdUMP and CH_2-H_4folate (Scheme I) proceeds by an ordered mechanism (7). TS binds FdUMP first, and then CH_2-H_4folate to form a rapidly reversible, non-covalent ternary complex; this complex then undergoes unimolecular conversion to the covalent TS=FdUMP=CH_2-H_4folate complex.

An expanded reaction scheme is shown in Figure 1. (7,8). Subsequent to the ordered binding of substrate and cofactor leading to formation of the reversible, non-covalent ternary complex, enzyme catalyzed conversions occur that result in formation of a covalent bond between C-6 of the nucleotide and the thiol of the catalytic Cys of TS, and a covalent bond between C-5 of the nucleotide and the one carbon unit (i.e., CH_2-11) of the cofactor. The importance of this interaction to an understanding of catalysis is that it mimics several steps of the normal enzymic reaction, up to and including formation of the covalent adduct which is a stable analog of a steady state intermediate. We may reasonably assume that the individual chemical conversions in this interaction proceed in a sequence analogous to the normal enzymic reaction. As such, the FdUMP interaction provides an entree to studies of individual steps of catalysis that are otherwise inaccessible. Figure 1: Minimal mechanism for formation of the TS=FdUMP=CH_2-H_4folate covalent complex. Free TS (1) interacts with FdUMP to give the binary complex 2, and then with CH_2-H_4folate to give the non-covalent ternary complex 3. Protonation of N-10 of the cofactor results in the enzyme-bound FdUMP-iminium ion 4. Covalent bond formation between the catalytic thiol of TS and C-6 of FdUMP, and between the one carbon unit of the iminium ion and C-5 of FdUMP results in the stable covalent complex 5.

Chemical models and other studies have led to the generally accepted conclusion that the reactive form of CH_2-H_4folate is the 5-iminium ion (9,10) and that the reactive form of the nucleotide is a covalent dihydropyrimidine adduct that possesses enol/enolate character at the C-5 position (4,11). Further, secondary hydrogen kinetic isotope studies of the FdUMP interaction have permitted the placement of the putative intermediates relative to the rate determining step of the reaction (12). Some relevant points are as follows. (i) Covalent bond formation between the enzyme thiol and the C-6 of FdUMP occurs after the rate determining step. (ii) Formation of the bond between C-5 of FdUMP and the one-carbon unit of the cofactor occurs during or after formation of the FdUMP covalent adduct. (iii) Formation of the 5-iminium ion precedes thiol addition at C-6 of FdUMP and probably occurs at the rate determining step.

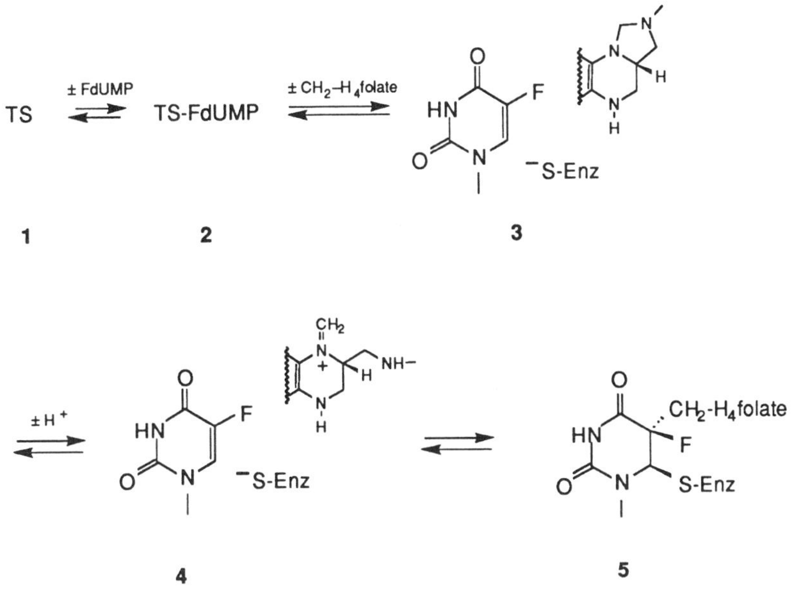

Figure 1. Minimal mechanism for formation of the TS=FdUMP=CH_2-H_4folate covalent complex. Free TS (**1**) interacts with FdUMP to give the binary complex **2**, and then with CH_2-H_4folate to give the non-covalent ternary complex **3**. Protonation of N-10 of the cofactor results in the enzyme-bound FdUMP-iminium ion **4**. Covalent bond formation between the catalytic thiol of TS and C-6 of FdUMP, and between the one carbon unit of the iminium ion and C-5 of FdUMP results in the stable covalent complex **5**.

Kinetics and Thermodynamics

The formation of the binary TS-FdUMP complex has been studied by several workers and dissociation constants under a variety of conditions have been reported (13,14). Likewise, the dissociation of FdUMP from the covalent TS=FdUMP=CH_2-H_4folate complex has been studied in detail (3,7,12) . The overall rates of formation of the covalent complex have been described but, because the conversion is so fast, the data are difficult to interpret (3,7); until recently (15),the kinetics of the overall formation of the covalent complex were indirectly determined and treated as a simple bimolecular reaction.

It is stressed that, with exception of formation of the binary complex and dissociation of the covalent complex, the kinetics and thermodynamics of the FdUMP interaction with TS are not trivial to measure experimentally. Many of the reactions are sufficiently fast that rapid kinetic measurements are required to obtain believable numbers, and these are only obtained after careful analysis of suitable equations (15). Likewise, the dissociation constant for the ternary covalent complex is so low, that it is not easily determined by direct equilibrium measurements. The simplest and most reproducible experimental parameter to measure is the rate of dissociation of the covalent complex, which has a half-life of hours, and reflects the "tightness" of the complex. For most comparative measurements, we recommend that this value be used as the most trustworthy one. Moreover, as described below, the first species to dissociate from the covalent complex is CH_2-H_4folate; as such, the extraordinarily low dissociation constant is a measure of dissociation of CH_2-H_4folate and *not* FdUMP.

The kinetics of formation of the covalent complex have recently been determined at several temperatures by semi-rapid quench methods (15). Combined data now permits calculation of every rate and equilibrium constant in the interaction. Conversion of the non-covalent ternary complex **3** (Figure 2)to the corresponding covalent complex **6** proceeds at a rate of 0.6 sec-1 at 25°, and the dissociation constant for loss of CH_2-H_4folate from the non-covalent ternary complex is ~1 uM. The equilibrium constant between the non-covalent **3** and covalent **6** ternary complexes is ~2 x 10^4, and the overall dissociation constant of CH_2-H_4folate from the covalent complex **6** is ~10^{-11} M. The conversion of the non-covalent ternary complex **3** to the covalent adduct **6** is about 12-fold slower than k_{cat} in the normal enzymic reaction. However, because the dissociation constant for CH_2-H_4folate from the non-covalent ternary complex is about 10-fold lower than from the TS-dUMP-CH_2-H_4folate Michaelis complex, the terms corresponding to k_{cat}/K_m are nearly equal. We proposed that some of the intrinsic binding energy of CH_2-H_4folate may be used to facilitate formation of the 5-iminium ion intermediate. We suggested that iminium ion formation is catalyzed by (*i*) general acid catalysis at N-10 of CH_2-H_4folate, and (*ii*) enzyme-induced perturbations of the 5-membered ring of the cofactor within the non-covalent TS-FdUMP-CH_2-H_4folate complex. The latter may involve hydrogen bonding of the enzyme general acid catalyst to N-10, perturbation of the PABA moiety of the cofactor, and strain on the 5-membered ring of the cofactor.

Figure 2 summarizes salient features of the current model (note: Structures in Figures 1 and 2 correspond to one another). Here, the enzyme is conformationally mobile and the reactants are relatively rigid. The most stable state of the free enzyme **1** does not optimally fit CH2-H4folate; binding of the nucleotide is required before the enzyme is accessible to the cofactor. We suggest that the binary enzyme-nucleotide complex **2** undergoes a conformational change towards **3**, a structure more complementary to the transition state for iminium ion formation.

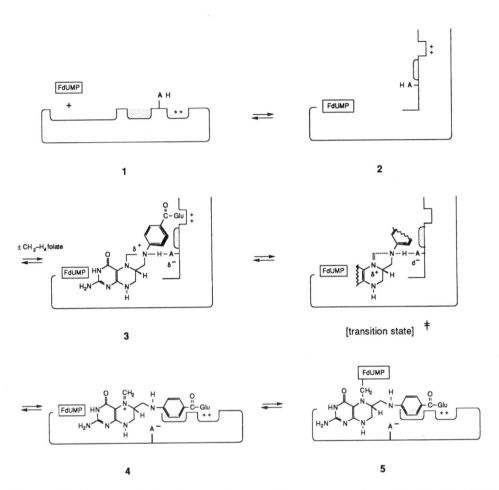

Figure 2. Proposed strain mechanism for conversion of CH2-H4folate to the 5-iminium ion in the TS-FdUMP(dUMP)-CH2-H4folate complex. A-H represents a proposed general acid catalyst of the enzyme which binds to N-10 and assists in cleavage of the N-10,CH2-11 bond of CH2-H4folate. The shaded area depicts a region of the enzyme with affinity for the PABA moiety of CH2-H4folate. **1** shows the stable form of the free enzyme which upon binding to FdUMP undergoes a conformational change to give the form of the enzyme **2** which can bind the cofactor. In the ternary complex **3** the N-10,CH2-11 bond is lengthened and weakened; the transition state is depicted for conversion of the imidazolidine ring of the cofactor to the 5-iminium ion, **4** represents the bound 5-iminium ion intermediate with the return of the more stable conformation of the enzyme, and **5** is the covalent TS=FdUMP=CH2-H4folate complex.

Hence, there is an apparent loss of intrinsic binding energy of CH_2-H_4folate upon formation of the non-covalent ternary complex. Within this complex **3**, the enzyme interacts with CH_2-H_4folate in a manner that alters the environment of the PABA group to increase the reactivity of the N-10,C-11 bond. This interaction could involve several factors. First, the basicity of N-10 of CH_2-H_4folate could be modified in a manner that could enhance protonation of N-10 and/or the reactivity of the N-10,C-11 bond. Second, the increased basicity of N-10 could enhance formation of a hydrogen bond to the putative general acid catalyst, A-H. Finally, reactivity could be increased by strain (lengthening) of the N-10,C-11 bond as the cofactor accommodates the transition state-like conformation of the enzyme. As the 5-iminium ion intermediate **4** is formed, several changes occur. (*i*) The enzyme adopts a conformation more like the lower energy state of the ground state. (*ii*) The hydrogen bond between TS and N-10 is broken because of the dramatically lower pKa (*ca*. 4 pH units) of N-10 when a positive charge develops on N-5 (9). (*iii*) The general catalyst of the enzyme is left as its conjugate base, A:. Finally, covalent bond changes occur to give the covalent complex **5** which has the PABA ring perturbed by the enzyme and has the hydrogen bond acceptor A: adjacent to N-10 as proposed from Raman resonance studies (16).

Perspectives

With a complete kinetic and thermodynamic description of all the steps in the reaction of FdUMP and CH_2-H_4folate with TS, and the recently reported 3-dimensional structure of the enzyme (6), we are now able to approach questions as to how each of these steps is catalyzed. In particular, we are looking forward to studies of how mutagenesis of specific amino acid residues of TS will affect individual steps of the reaction. Our proposal that enzyme-altered environment of the *p*-aminobenzoyl glutamate group effects reactivity of CH_2-H_4folate can also be tested with suitable chemically modified cofactor analogs and by in-depth studies of the *p*-aminobenzoyl glutamate chromophore perturbation. Finally, inquiries into the three dimensional structure of the TS=FdUMP=CH_2-H_4folate and/or related complexes may reveal whether our hypotheses on the binding of CH_2-H_4folate and on the mechanism of 5-iminium ion formation are correct. If so, there is good reason to hope that new folate analogs can be designed which resemble heretofore unidentified transition state or intermediate structures.

CRYSTAL STRUCTURE OF TS

In collaboration with R. Stroud, this laboratory has been engaged in attempts to obtain crystals of TS suitable for crystallography for over 10 years (17); only recently have we been successful. The X-ray structure of the native *L. casei* TS bound to inorganic phosphate has recently been reported (6). Details of the structure are presented in the cited paper and only a cursory description of features relevant to ligand binding and selectivity are described here.

TS crystallizes as a dimer of identical subunits having a two-fold axis of symmetry. All important secondary structural elements of TS are within highly conserved regions; thus, the core structure of *L. casei* TS will undoubtedly be similar to other TS's. The dimer interface is composed of an unusual 5-stranded b-sheet from both monomers. Each monomer has been separated into a small and large domain, separated by a cleft. The larger domain contains a) the b-strands of the dimer interface; b) a six-turn unusually hydrophobic a-helix, around which the large domain folds; and c) a shallow cavity which contains the active site. The small domain contains the *L. casei* insert (residues 90-139) which is found in no other species, a disordered region, and several a-helices.

An interesting, and possibly unique, feature of TS revealed by the crystal structure, is that several side chain residues of one monomer are shared by the other. This explains why catalytically active monomers of TS have not yet been isolated. Moreover, amino acid residues of one subunit contribute essential components of the active site of the other. For example, Arg 179 of one monomer provides the binding group for phosphate ion in the active site of the other monomer.

Of relevance to the present topic are amino acid residues within the active site. The cavity defined as the active site is lined by about 25 residues; 16 of these are conserved among TS of all species, and 8 of these have third functional groups on the side chain which could play roles in catalysis or binding. These include: C198; R218; S219; D221; Y233; H259; Y261; R178'; and R178. Importantly, they are also nucleophilic targets for potential covalent-bond forming inhibitors. That is, we anticipate that analogs of dUMP containing reactive functional groups (potential inhibitors) could be docked into the active site with the reactive moiety precisely juxtaposed to one of these groups for covalent bond formation.

Unfortunately, the structure of the native TS complex which has been solved does not appear appropriate for binding of substrates. We have ben unable to model either dUMP or CH_2-H4folate to the structure. We believe this is because of conformational changes which occur upon binding . Thus, to understand this enzyme, and to rationally design inhibitors by modeling technologies, structures of binary and ternary complexes will have to be determined. Clearly, it is important to direct efforts towards solution of the TS=FdUMP=CH_2-H4folate complex.

EXPRESSION OF TS IN HETEROLOGOUS SYSTEMS

Because of source limitations, most of the previous biochemical work on TS has been performed with the enzyme obtained from over-producing strains of methotrexate-resistant *L. casei*, in which the enzyme represents about 2 % of the total soluble protein (18-20). Studies of TS are now taking directions which require very large amounts (reagent quantities) of enzyme. In addition, it is an appropriate time to undertake studies of mutagenesis of TS to uncover more subtle aspects of structure/function. To these ends, several groups have been engaged in cloning the TS gene from various sources, and several high expression systems have been developed.

We have undertaken a program to express TS from various sources in heterologous systems as a source for large amounts of enzyme, and for mutagenesis studies. We have recently reported (21) the expression of the *L. casei* TS in *E. coli* in a system where 20% of the total protein is *L. casei* TS. This is some 10-fold higher expression than even the methotrexate resistant strain of *L. casei*, and provides an unlimited source of this protein. We also reported expression of the bifunctional TS-dihydrofolate reductase from the protozoan *Leishmania* in yeast and *E. coli* (22). To illustrate the power of such systems, we prepared over 4 grams of this protein which, only last year, was hardly available in milligram amounts. Currently, we are working on expression of the TS from human and *Plasmodium falciparum* with the objective of obtaining the amounts of protein necessary to perform structural studies.

FUra EFFECT ON tRNA-URACIL METHYL TRANSFERASE

tRNA (Ura-5)-methyltransferase catalyzes the S-adenosylmethionine (AdoMet)-dependent methylation of a specific Urd residue to form the m5Urd (ribothymidine) residue found in the TψC loop (loop IV) of all eubacterial and most eukaryotic tRNAs (Figure 3) thus far sequenced (23).

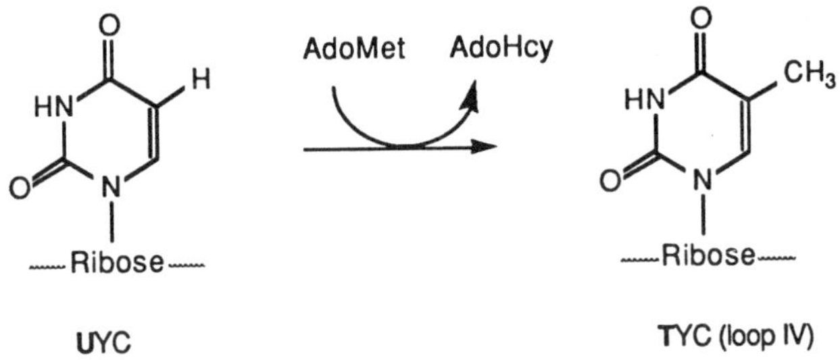

UψC   TψC (loop IV)

Figure 3. The overall reaction catalyzed by tRNA (Ura-5)-methyltransferase. The S-adenosylmethionine dependent methylation of the Urd of the UψC loop of tRNA to produe ribothymidine (TψC loop)

The similarity of the reaction catalyzed by this enzyme to thymidylate synthase (TS) suggests they may share mechanistic features. An early step in the reaction catalyzed by TS, the paradigm for this class of enzymes, is production of a 5,6-dihydropyrimidine intermediate. Michael addition of a cysteine thiol of the enzyme to carbon 6 of dUMP generates a covalent enzyme-substrate intermediate and serves to activate the 5 position for reaction with the electrophilic one carbon unit of the cofactor. An analogous mechanism has been demonstrated for tRNA (Ura-5)-methyltransferase (Figure 4).

It has been observed that tRNA in which Ura is extensively replaced by FUra is an inhibitor of tRNA (Ura-5)-methyltransferase activity, both *in vivo* (24,25) and *in vitro* (26). By analogy with TS, these results suggested to us that tRNA (Ura-5)-methyltransferase catalysis and inhibition by FUra-tRNA may proceed via nucleophilic catalysis.

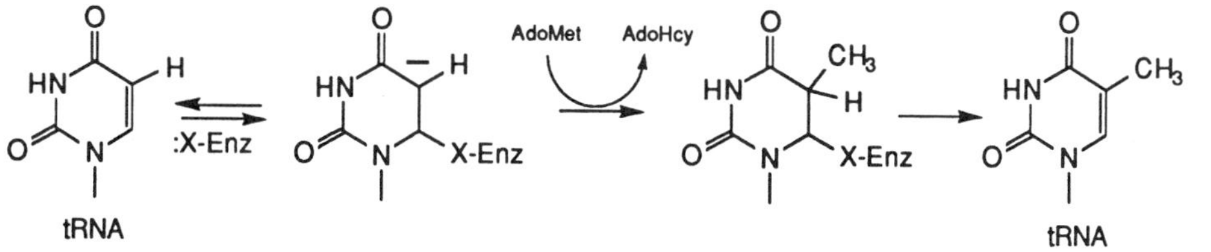

Figure 4. The mechanism of tRNA (Ura-5)-methyltransferase. After Michael addition of a nucleophile of the enzyme (presumably a Cys thiol) to form a covalent adduct, the methyl group of AdoMet is transferred to the covalent intermediate which, subsequent to elimination, provides methylated tRNA.

Inactivation of tRNA (Ura-5)-methyltransferase by FUra-tRNA

The inactivation of tRNA (Ura-5)-methyltransferase by FUra-tRNA in the presence of AdoMet provides further evidence for a covalent intermediate in catalysis (27). The proposed mechanism for this inactivation is shown in Figure 5. Here, an enzyme nucleophile adds to the 6-position of FUra within the substrate site of tRNA to provide an adduct which is subsequently trapped by AdoMet-dependent methylation at carbon 5. The ternary covalent complex is analogous to a steady state intermediate proposed in the normal enzymic reaction (Figure 4) and is similar in structure to that of the covalent complex formed between TS, CH_2-H$_4$folate, and 5-FdUMP. The methylated FUra-tRNA-enzyme covalent complex cannot break down to give product and regenerate the free enzyme, because the hydrogen at carbon 5 of the normal substrate has been replaced by fluorine; similarly, reversal of the reaction is highly unfavorable since

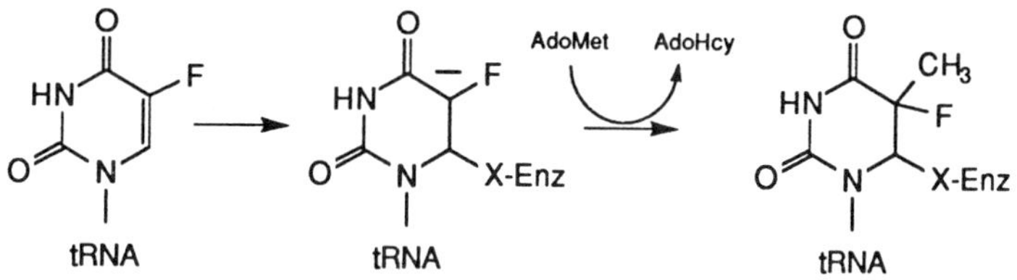

Figure 5. Mechanism of covalent complex formation between FUra-tRNA and tRNA (Ura-5)-methyltransferase. As in the normal catalytic reaction, the nucleophile of the enzyme attaches to the 6-position of the heterocycle. Methylation of this adduct results in a stable covalent complex since the C-F bond at position 5 cannot be broken.

it would require the energetically unfavorable cleavage of a carbon-carbon bond at the 5 position. Thus, we conclude that formation of the methylated FUra-tRNA-enzyme complex is irreversible.

SDS-PAGE analysis of tRNA (Ura-5)-methyltransferase before and after inactivation by FUra-tRNA and [^{3}H-Me]AdoMet supports the structure of the covalent complex proposed in **Figure 5**. The inactivated enzyme has a decreased electrophoretic mobility consistent with its proposed covalent link to tRNA, and is labelled by tritium derived from the methyl group of [^{3}H-Me]AdoMet. Treatment of the enzyme-tRNA complex with RNase results in an electrophoretic shift of the protein to a mobility almost identical to that of the enzyme before inactivation, but the inactivated enzyme is still labelled with tritium of the methyl group. In the absence of AdoMet isolable denatured complexes are not observed. It is evident from these results that FUra-tRNA is a potent and irreversible mechanism-based inhibitor of tRNA (Ura-5)-methyltransferase. Further, evidence has been obtained which implicates a Cys residue as the nucleophilic catalyst.

Possible RNA Effects of FUra

The inactivation of tRNA (Ura-5)-methyltransferase by covalent complex formation with FUra-tRNA may be directly relevant to the action of FUra. In addition to inhibition of TS by 5-FdUMP, the cytotoxic action of FUra is known to involve incorporation into RNA; the subsequent events which lead to significant biological effects remain controversial. From the present work, we can propose mechanisms which may contribute to the "RNA effect" of FUra. First, FUra-tRNA inhibition of tRNA (Ura-5)-methyltransferase will deplete the m5Urd in the TΨC loop of tRNA. However, hypomethylation at this site of tRNA in itself cannot be a major cell deficit since tRNA (Ura-5)-methyltransferase deficient mutants of *E. coli* (28) and yeast (29) are healthy; further, FUra-tRNA is functional in protein synthesis (30). In addition to m5U of the TΨC loop of tRNA, other modified pyrimidines of RNA are probably also formed by a mechanism involving transient covalent adducts between specific enzymes and the substrate pyrimidine residue (31). These include m5U of other RNA's, YUrd, m5C, and several other 5-alkylpyrimidines. Further, such modifications may involve tRNA, ribosomal RNA (32) and, in eukaryotic cells, the small nuclear RNAs (33). Hence, FUra could interfere with a variety of important enzymes and cellular processes, and hypomodification of one or more sites of one or more RNA's is an attractive contender for the RNA effect of FUra. Alternatively, or concomitantly, covalent FUra-RNA-enzyme complexes could play a direct role in the effects of FUra.

Proposal for FUra-AdoMet Modulation

As a final point, it is tempting to suggest experiments based on the mechanism of tRNA (Ura-5)-methyltransferase which might modulate the effect of FUra. We have shown that the inhibition of tRNA methylation by FUra requires AdoMet. It is possible that the intracellular concentration of AdoMet is not optimal for the FUra effect on RNA. Thus, it would be interesting to see whether agents which cause increased levels of AdoMet have an effect on FUra action. Conversely, since the RNA effect may be untoward toxicity, it would be interesting to ascertain what effects AdoMet depletion might have on FUra effects. This rationale is directly analogous to that used in the development of the FUra-CF regimen, and warrants consideration.

Acknowledgement. This work was supported by USPHS grant CA 14394 from the National Cancer Institute.

REFERENCES

1. D. V. Santi and C. S. McHenry, Proc. Natl. Acad. Sci. USA 69:1855-1857 (1972).
2. P. V. Danenberg, R. J. Langenbach, and C. Heidelberger, Biochemistry 13:926- (1974).
3. D. V. Santi, C. S. McHenry, and H. Sommer, Biochemistry 13:471-481 (1974).
4. D. V. Santi and P. V. Danenberg, Folates in Pyrimidine Nucleotide Biosynthesis in: "Folates and Pteridines," Vol. 1, R. L. Blakley and S. J. Benkovic, eds., John Wiley and Sons, New York (1984).
5. B. Ullman, M. Lee, D. W. Martin, and D. V. Santi, Proc. Natl. Acad. Sci. USA 75:980-983 (1978).
6. L. W. Hardy, J. S. Finer-Moore, W. R. Montfort, M. O. Jones, D. V. Santi, D. V. and R. M. Stroud, Science 235:448-455 (1987).
7. P. V. Danenberg, and K. D. Danenberg, Biochemistry 17:4018-4024 (1978).
8. Y-Z Lu, P. D. Aiello, and R. G. Matthews, Biochemistry 23:6870-6876 (1984).
9. R. G. Kallen and W. P. Jencks, J. Biol. Chem. 241:5845-5850 (1966).
10. S. J. Benkovic, Ann. Rev. Biochem. 49:227-251 (1980).
11. A. L. Pogolotti, Jr. and D. V. Santi, Bioorganic Chem. 1:277-377 (1977).
12. T. W. Bruice and D. V. Santi, Biochemistry 21:6703-6709 (1982).
13. C. A. Lewis, Jr. and R. B. Dunlap, Thymidylate Synthase and Its Interaction with 5-fluoro-2'-deoxyuridylate in "Topics in Molecular Pharmacology," A. S. V. Burgen and G. C. K. Roberts, eds., Elsevier/North Holland Biomedical Press (1981).
14. D. M. Mittelstaedt, and M. I. Schimerlik, Arch. Biochem. Biophys. 245:417-425 (1986).
15. D. V. Santi, C. H. McHenry, R. T. Raines, and K. I. Ivanetich, Biochemistry 26:8606-8613 (1987).
16. A. L. Fitzhugh, S. Fodor, S. Kaufman, and T. G. Spiro, J. Am. Chem. Soc. 108:7422-7424 (1986).
17. R. W. Koeppe, V. A. Pena, R. M. Stroud, and D. V. Santi, J. Mol. Biol. 98:155 (1975).
18. T. C. Crusberg, R. Leary, and R. L. Kisliuk, J. Biol Chem. 245:5292-5296 (1970).
19. R. P. Leary, and R. L. Kisliuk, Prep. Biochem. 1:47-54 (1971).

20. R. B. Dunlap, N. G. L. Harding, and F. M. Huennekens, _Biochemistry_ 10:88-97 (1971).

21. K. Pinter, V. J. Davisson, and D. V. Santi, _DNA_ 7:235-241 (1988).

22. R. Grumont, W. Sirawaraporn, and D. V. Santi, _Biochemistry_ 27:3776-378.(1988).

23. M. Sprinzl, J. Moll, F. Meissner, and T. Hartmann, _Nucleic Acids Research_ 13:r1-r49 (1985).

24. D. A. Frendewey and I. I. Kaiser, _Biochemistry_ 18:3179-3185 (1979).

25. K. Randerath, W. C. Tseng, J. S. Harris, L. -J.W. Lu, _Recent Results in Cancer Research_ 84:283-297 (1983).

26. D. A. Frendewey, D. M. Kladianos, V. G. Moore, and I. I. Kaiser, _Biochim. Biophys. Acta_ 697:31-40 (1982).

27. D. V. Santi and L. H. Hardy, _Biochemistry_ 26:8599-8606 (1987).

28. G. R. Bjork and F. C. Neidhardt, _J. Bacteriol._ 124:99-111 (1975).

29. A. K. Hopper, A. H. Furukawa, H. D. Pham, and N. C. Martin, _Cell_ 28:543-550 (1982).

30. E. S. Ramberg, M. Ishaq, S. Rulf, B. Moeller, and J. Horowitz, _Biochemistry_ 17:3978-3985 (1978).

31. D. V. Santi, Y. Wataya, and A. Matsuda, _in_: "Substrate Induced Irreversible Inactivation of Enzymes, N. Seiler, M.J. Jung, and J. Koch-Weser, J., eds., Elsevier, Amsterdam (1978).

32. G. R. Bjork, _in_: "Processing of RNA," D. Apirion, ed., CRC Press Inc., Boca Raton, Florida (1984).

33. H. Busch, R. Reddy, L. Rothblum, and Y.C. Choi, _Ann. Rev. Biochem._ 51:617-654 (1982).

DISCUSSION OF DR. SANTI'S PRESENTATION

Dr. P. Houghton: Dan, if I can ask you a question about your work with the tRNA. As you said, the work of Kurt Randerath has been largely forgotten. One of the problems I see with trying to potentiate that mechanism might be that in humans very major toxicity might result. In mice one can correlate toxicity more readily with RNA effects than one can with anti-thymidylate effects. What you're proposing may, in fact, increase toxicity to normal tissue. Is there any reason that that wouldn't happen do you think?

Dr. Santi: I'm suggesting it as a way of modulating the RNA effect. I really wouldn't have any response to that.

Dr. Danenberg: In the crystal structure of TS do you see any evidence for an asymmetric sub-unit arrangement?

Dr. Santi: The question was do we see any evidence for asymmetry in the dimer of the subunits in the crystal structure as previously indicated by biochemical studies. We don't see any. We're surprised at that and I don't know what the reason for that is. Maybe it's more subtle than the degree of resolution at this point.

MECHANISMS FOR CISPLATIN-FUra SYNERGISM AND CISPLATIN RESISTANCE IN HUMAN OVARIAN CARCINOMA CELLS BOTH IN VITRO AND IN VIVO

K.J. Scanlon, Y. Lu, M. Kashani-Sabet, J.x. Ma, and E. Newman*

Section of Biochemical Pharmacology, Medical Oncology and *Division of Pediatrics, City of Hope National Medical Center, Duarte, CA 91010

ABSTRACT

Cisplatin and FUra act synergisticly in human carcinomas. An increase in the availability of reduced folates necessary for tight binding of FdUMP to thymidylate synthase (TS) contributes to the enhanced cytotoxicity of this drug combination. The human ovarian A2780 cell line made three-fold resistant to cisplatin has been shown to have a three-fold elevation of m-RNA for dihydrofolate reductase (DHFR) and TS. However, this increase did not result from an amplification of the genes for these two enzymes. In contrast, ovarian carcinoma cells from patients who failed treatment with cisplatin and FUra have been shown to have both enhanced gene expression and increased gene copy number for DHFR and TS.

INTRODUCTION

Cisplatin is widely used alone or in combination for the treatment of carcinomas.[1] Unfortunately, despite initial responses, resistance to cisplatinum develops rapidly.[2] DNA has been considered an important site of action for cisplatin, and postulated mechanisms of resistance have focused on altered cisplatin-DNA interactions or increased thiol levels, which could inactivate the drug. However, neither mechanism is found universally. Both clinically and in tumor models, cisplatin does not behave like an alkylating agent. Patients who have failed treatment with alkylating agents are known to respond to cisplatin, and cisplatin resistant human tumor cells are not necessarily cross-resistant to alkylating agents.[1,2] Yet, cisplatin-resistant cells are cross-resistant to the antimetabolites, MTX and FUra in P388 mouse leukemia cells,[3] human squamous carcinoma cells,[4] and human ovarian carcinoma cells.[5,6] Also, L1210 mouse leukemia cells resistant to MTX are cross-resistant to cisplatin.[7] These studies suggest that tumor cells respond differently to cisplatin than to classic alkylating agents. There have been numerous papers demonstrating that cisplatin binds to DNA in cells.[1] It is not known which adducts are responsible for the antitumor activity of cisplatin. However, it is likely that the cells must repair these adducts to remain viable. After cisplatin-DNA complexes are excised, repair enzymes require a source of deoxynucleoside triphosphates. The TS cycle represents the sole de novo source for dTMP. An additional relationship between cisplatin and the TS cycle is indicated by studies demonstrating that cisplatin inhibits methionine transport into tumor cells.[8] A decreased accumulation of exogenous methionine may lead to increased intracellular metabolism, which in turn can enhance the tetrahydrofolate (H_4PteGlu) and 5,10-methylenetetrahydrofolate (CH_2-H_4PteGlu) pools at the expense of 5-methyltetrahydrofolate (5-CH_3-H_4PteGlu). The elevation of the CH_2-H_4PteGlu pool would also allow for an increase in dTMP synthesis. Thus the action of cisplatin at one site (methionine transport) may help to mitigate the damage induced by cisplatin at another site (DNA platination). The increase in the CH_2-H_4PteGlu pool may also account for the increased sensitivity to fluoropyrimidines in cells exposed briefly to cisplatin.[9] However, long term exposure to cisplatin stimulates m-RNA synthesis for DHFR, TS, thymidine kinase and also the fos oncogene.[6,10,11]

METHODS

Cell Culture Uptake Studies; Enzyme Assays

The human ovarian cell line, A2780,[12] was obtained from Dr. R. Ozols, National Cancer Institute and maintained in RPMI 1640 media with 10%(V/V) fetal calf serum as previously described.[5] The drug ED_{50} concentrations, the cellular accumulation of [195M]cisplatin and the activities of TS and DHFR were measured as previously described.[5,6]

Nucleic Acid Isolation and Blotting

Total RNA was extracted from tumor cells by using guanidinium isothiocyanate; m-RNA was purified by oligo(dT)-cellulose column chromatography; and DNA was purified using proteinase K and sodium dodecyl sulfate.[10] The cDNA clone for human TS was obtained from T. Seno (Saitama Cancer Center Research Institute, Saitama-ken, Japan).[10] The cDNA clone for human DHFR was obtained from G. Attardi (California Institute of Technology, Pasadena, CA).[10] The human c-fos oncogene (#41042) was obtained from American Type Culture Collection, Rockville, MD.

Patient material

Malignant ascites cells were obtained from three ovarian carcinoma patients (TS, DM, and MD) who had failed cisplatin and FUra treatment (submitted for publication).

RESULTS AND DISCUSSION

Synergy Studies

Exposure of A2780 cells for 60 min to the sequence of cisplatin (10 μM) for 30 min and then FUra (5 μM) for 30 min reduced cell growth to 24% ± 5.1% (Table 1). In contrast, at these same concentrations neither of the two drugs alone reduced cell growth below 86% of the control. The sequencing of FUra (5 μM) 30 min prior to the addition of cisplatin (10 μM) for 30 min resulted in only 41% ± 6.3% cell growth. The ED_{50}s for cisplatin for 1 hr and FUra for 2 hr were 16.5 μM and 32 μM, respectively. If inhibition of TS is critical for the cytotoxicity of this drug combination, then the addition of dThd to circumvent the need for de novo dTMP synthesis should protect the tumor cells from the synergistic action of the drugs. dThd alone for 1 hr at a concentration of 10 μM was not cytotoxic to the A2780 cells (Table 1). When 10 μM dThd was given in combination with cisplatin (10 μM) and FUra (5 μM), the cells were completely protected from the cytotoxic action of the cisplatin/FUra combination as cell growth reverted to control levels. dThd could not reverse the cytotoxic effects of either cisplatin or FUra alone. Thus, the biochemical basis for cisplatin and FUra synergy in human ovarian carcinoma cells involved the enhanced levels of the CH_2-H_4PteGlu pools that enabled binding of the FdUMP to TS.[9] Similar results have been obtained with a human colon carcinoma cell line, HCT8, except higher doses of cisplatin and FUra and longer exposure times were necessary for optimal synergy.[11]

Table 1.   Inhibition of A2780 cell growth by cisplatin and FUra

Concentration (μM)			
Cisplatin	FUra	dThd	% control growth
1	--	--	96
2	--	--	91
10	--	--	86
15	--	--	55
15	--	10	60
--	5	--	106
--	10	--	93
--	20	--	70
--	20	10	75
--	--	10	110
2	5	--	30
2	5	10	110
10	5	--	24
10	5	10	103

A2780 cells (5×10^3 cells) were exposed to cisplatin, dThd, and/or FUra under various conditions. The cells were pretreated for 30 min with cisplatin alone or with dThd, then FUra was added for 30 min. Thus, the A2780 cells were preincubated for a total of 60 min with the drugs, then incubated for 6 days in a drug-free medium. These experiments were performed in triplicate. The final cell number was 0.5-1.0 x 10^5 cells per culture in untreated cultures (100%). (Expanded from data in reference 9.)

Cross-Resistance in Cisplatin-Resistant Cells

The concentration of cisplatin needed to reduce cell proliferation by one half during 6 days subsequent to a 1 hr drug exposure was 16.5 and 52.5 μM, respectively, for A2780S and A2780DDP cells. A2780DDP cells were also collaterally resistant to MTX and FUra by 2.9- and 3.2-fold, respectively (Table 2).

Table 2. Inhibition of A2780 cell growth by cancer chemotherapeutic agents

EC_{50} (μM)

Compound	Exposure (hr)	A2780S	A2780DDP
Cisplatin	1	16.5	52.5
FUra	2	32	102.5
MTX	2	0.7	2.0

A2780 cells were plated and counted as previously described.[5]

Uptake Studies

One mechanism of how tumor cells become resistant to cancer chemo-therapeutic agents is a defect in the drug transport system. Uptake studies with [^{195M}Pt]cisplatin have been defined in A2780 cells. The 0-time point uptake of cisplatin in the A2780DDP cells exposed to 10 μM cisplatin was 22% less than in the A2780S cells, and the rates of uptake of cisplatin during the next 75 min were 2.0 ± 0.1 and 1.9 ± 0.1 pmol/min/mg protein for A2780S and A2780DDP cells, respectively.[4] This similarity of uptake was also evident in samples taken between 2 and 8 min and at concentrations of cisplatin as low as 2 μM (Figure 1). At 25 μM cisplatin, a concentration above the EC_{50} in the sensitive line, the initial rate of uptake was 18% lower in the A2780DDP cells than in the A2780S cells (data not shown). At higher concentrations (25-100μM) of cisplatin and longer exposure times (1 hr), large differences (<50%) of cisplatin accumulation have been noted between A2780S and A2780DDP cells. Similar observations have also been reported in the literature recently. However, it may be difficult to discriminate uptake from efflux and retention of cisplatin at these times and concentrations. Thus, it would appear that cisplatin uptake does not make a major contribution to the initial step of cisplatin resistance in A2780 cells.

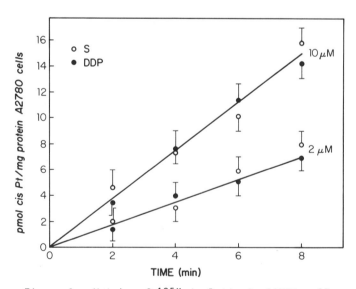

Figure 1. Uptake of ^{195M}cisplatin in A2780 cells

Table 3. Properties of extracts of A2780S and A2780DDP cells related to TS activity

Properties of A2780 cells*	A2780S	A2780DDP
TS (pmol/min/10^7cells)	170±6	420±20
FdUMP complex formed in vitro (pmol/10^7cells)	1.6±0.5	4.1±0.5
CH_2-H_4PteGlu (pmol/10^7cells)	2.9±0.4	7.2±0.5
H_4PteGlu (pmol/10^7cells)	2.2±0.3	4.8±0.5
FdUMP complex formed in intact cells (pmol/10^7cells)	1.8±0.5	3.1±0.2

*All analyses were performed as described in Materials and Methods using approximately 10^7cells for each sample. Reprinted, with permission, from Biochemical Pharmacology.[5]

Properties of the TS Cycle in A2780 Cells

The biochemical bases for cisplatin cross-resistance to antimetabolites are demonstrated in Table 3. TS activity as measured by the tritium release assay was increased 2.5-fold in cytosols from A2780DDP cells in comparison with cytosols from A2780S cells. Associated with this enhanced enzyme activity were increases in: (i) the capacity to complex [^{3}H]FdUMP in vitro in the presence of added folate cofactor and (ii) the levels of CH_2-H_4PteGlu and H_4PteGlu (Table 3). Incorporation of [^{3}H]FdUrd into the TS-FdUMP complex was 1.7 times higher in the resistant line than in the sensitive line (Table 3). HPLC of the acid-soluble material released by heating to 65° for 15 min confirmed that it was FdUMP; 97±7% of the radioactivity injected onto the HPLC column was recovered in the fractions of effluent collected, and 94±2% of the material recovered coeluted with the nonradioactive FdUMP standard. Thus, repeated challenges of cisplatin weekly for several months (1-3 months) can elevate the enzyme activity of the TS cycle.

Molecular Basis of Cisplatin Resistance

The molecular basis for cisplatin cross-resistance to antimetabolites is demonstrated in Figure 2. m-RNA analysis by Northern blot showed that the expression of TS and DHFR m-RNA was 3-5-fold increased in A2780DDP(R) cells compared with the m-RNA in A2780S cells (Fig. 2).[10] Expression of fos m-RNA in A2780S and A2780DDP(R) cells was also 3-5-fold increased in A2780DDP(R) cells. The increase in TS and DHFR m-RNA in A2780DDP cells was not associated with gene amplification as analyzed by Southern blot and DNA slot blot (Fig. 3). Similar data has been obtained from human colon carcinoma cells resistant to cisplatin.[11] The relationship between fos and the TS cycle has not yet been clearly defined. Both c-myc and c-fos expression have been shown to be enhanced in the presence of growth factors in mammalian cells.[13] These oncogenes (possibly nuclear proteins) may act as intermediates for a growth stimulator which increased DNA synthesis. A2780 cells resistant to cisplatin have elevated fos levels and the TS cycle is intimately involved in supplying an essential precursor for DNA synthesis and/or repair of DNA damage. DNA polymerase β may also act with the TS cycle for repair of cisplatin-induced DNA damage. This hypothesis is currently under investigation with tumor cells resistant to cisplatin in both in vivo and in vitro sources.

m·RNA expression in A2780 cells

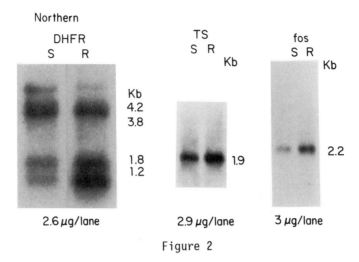

Figure 2

Based on this data from A2780 cells, three patients (TS, DM, and MD) with ovarian carcinoma were analyzed for gene amplification in response to cisplatin and FUra. Southern analysis of DHFR, TS and fos shows a 2-10 fold increase in the gene copies in resistant patient tumors (fig. 3, first 3 lanes) compared to the A2780 model system. Currently, we are collecting more appropriate controls of normal ovarian tissue and untreated ovarian carcinoma tissue for comparison of DNA and RNA from these ovarian carcinoma patients who have failed treatment.

DNA analysis of human ovarian carcinoma cells

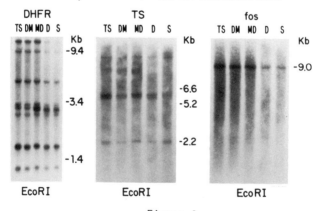

Figure 3

Cell samples from the patients (TS, DM and MD) also exhibited increased levels of m-RNA when compared to the A2780DDP cells(D) (Fig. 4). Unfortunately, the availability of the carcinoma tissue from these patients limited further analyses of RNA to only RNA slot blots. Recently, an in vitro enzymatic amplification assay has been developed to measure the increase in TS m-RNA expression from fresh cisplatin-resistant carcinoma cells.[14] The assay, which uses the Taq polymerase to amplify a 171 base sequence of TS m-RNA, has also shown 2-10 fold changes in TS m-RNA from cisplatin-resistant carcinoma cells from both in vivo and in vitro sources.

RNA analysis of
human ovarian carcinoma cells

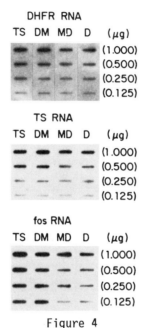

DHFR RNA

TS	DM	MD	D	(μg)
				(1.000)
				(0.500)
				(0.250)
				(0.125)

TS RNA

TS	DM	MD	D	(μg)
				(1.000)
				(0.500)
				(0.250)
				(0.125)

fos RNA

TS	DM	MD	D	(μg)
				(1.000)
				(0.500)
				(0.250)
				(0.125)

Figure 4

In contrast to the TS cycle genes and fos, the level of DNA and RNA did not change for the fms and erb-B genes in all the samples tested (data not shown). The oncogenes c-myc and H-ras were also elevated in these patient samples (submitted for publication). This is consistent with the published literature suggesting enhanced H-ras expression associated with cisplatin resistance in NIH 3T3 cells.[15] In addition, a normal rat liver epithelial cell line transfected with the activated H-ras oncogene causes a metabolic defect in the cells resulting in methionine dependence.[16] Thus, there appears to be a relationship between cisplatin resistance, oncogene expression (fos, H-ras and c-myc) and folate metabolism (TS cycle and methionine biosynthesis) and a possible role in the repair of cisplatin-DNA damage in cisplatin-resistant human carcinoma cells.

This notion of linking cisplatin to the TS cycle was previously initiated by the observation that cisplatin blocks methionine uptake into

133

tumor cells and perturbs folate metabolism.[5-11,17,18] Development of cisplatin resistance was concomitantly associated with a decreased requirement for exogenous methionine[17,18] and increased activity for the TS cycle.[5-7,9-11] The increase in CH_2-H_4PteGlu pool could result from enhanced endogenous methionine biosynthesis and could support the enhanced thymidylate synthesis needed for repairing cisplatin-DNA damage. This observation has been further strengthened by evidence for gene amplification of the TS cycle in ovarian carcinoma patients that have failed treatment with cisplatin/FUra. This phenomenon, observed both in cells in culture and in patient tumors, may be one relevant mechanism of cisplatin resistance. This does not preclude other mechansims of resistance, particularly at higher levels of resistance. The role of the fos oncogene in repair of cisplatin-induced DNA damage or another mechanism of resistance to cisplatin is as yet unclear; this area is currently being investigated in several types of human carcinoma from both in vitro and in vivo sources.

ACKNOWLEDGEMENTS

This work was supported by the American Cancer Society (Grant CH-265), Bristol-Myers Company and NIH Research Grants CA 33572 and CA22754. K.J.S. is a Scholar of the Leukemia Society of America. We wish to thank Dr. L. Leong and Dr. D. Blayney for providing the patient cells, Dr. J. Chen and Dr. H. Miyachi for their helpful suggestions and Ms. M. Schmidt for preparing the manuscript.

REFERENCES

1. B. Rosenberg, Fundamental studies with cisplatin, Cancer. 55:2303 (1985).
2. R. F. Ozols and R. C. Young, Chemotherapy of ovarian cancer, Sem. in Oncol. 11:257 (1984).
3. F. M. Schabel, H. E. Skipper, M. W. Trader, W. R. Laster, D. P. Griswold, and T. H. Corbett, Establishment of cross-resistance profiles for new agents, Cancer Treat. Rep. 67:905 (1983).
4. A. Rosowsky, J. E. Wright, C. A. Cucchi, J. L. Flatow, D. H. Trites, B. A. Teicher, and E. Frei, Collateral methotrexate resistance in cultured human head and neck carcinoma cells selected for resistance to cis-diamminedichloroplatinum(II), Cancer Res. 47:5913 (1987).
5. E. M. Newman, Y. Lu, M. Kashani-Sabet, V. Kesavan, and K. J. Scanlon, Biochemical basis for cisplatinum resistance in human ovarian carcinoma cells, Biochem. Pharm. 37:443 (1988).
6. Y. Lu, J. Han, and K. J. Scanlon, Biochemical and molecular properties of cisplatin resistance in A2780 cells grown in folinic acid, J. Biol. Chem. 263:4891 (1988).
7. K. J. Scanlon, M. Kashani-Sabet, A. R. Cashmore, M. Pallai, B. A. Moroson, and M. Saketos, The role of methionine in methotrexate sensitive and resistant mouse leukemia L1210 cells, Cancer Chemother. Pharm. 19:25 (1987).
8. K. J. Scanlon, R. Safirstein, H. Thies, R. B. Gross, S. Waxman, and J. B. Guttenplan, Inhibition of amino acid transport by cisplatin and its derivatives in L1210 murine leukemia cells, Cancer Res. 43:4211 (1983).
9. K. J. Scanlon, E. M. Newman, Y. Lu, and D. G. Priest, Biochemical basis for cisplatinum and 5-fluorouracil synergism in human ovarian carcinoma cells, Proc. Natl. Acad. Sci. USA 83:8923 (1986).

10. K. J. Scanlon and M. Kashani-Sabet, Elevated expression of dTMP synthase cycle genes in cisplatin-resistant A2780 cells, Proc. Natl. Acad. Sci. USA 85:650 (1988).
11. J. Chen and K. J. Scanlon, Molecular and biochemical properties of cisplatin-resistant HCT8 human colon carcinoma cells, Amer. Assoc. Cancer Res. 29:1431 (1988).
12. A. Eva, K. C. Robbins, P. R. Andersen, A. Srinivasan, S. R. Tronick, E. P. Reddy, N. W. Ellmore, A. T. Galen, J. A. Lanten-berger, T. S. Papas, E. H. Westin, F. Wong-Stall, R. C. Gallo, and S. A. Aaronson, Cellular genes analogous to retroviral onc genes are transcribed in human tumour cells, Nature, Lond. 295:116 (1982).
13. B. J. Rollins, and C. D. Stiles, Regulation of c-myc and c-fos proto-oncogene expression by animal cell growth factors, In Vitro Cellular and Developmental Biol. 24:81 (1988).
14. M. Kashani-Sabet, J. J. Rossi, Y. Lu, J. Chen, H. Miyachi, J. x. Ma, D.Blaney, L. Leong, and K. J. Scanlon, Early detection of cisplatin resistance in fresh human carcinoma cells by in vitro enzymatic amplification assay, Amer. Assoc. Cancer Res. 29:1159 (1988).
15. M. D. Sklar, Increased resistance to cis-diamminedichloroplatinum(II) in NIH 3TE cells transformed by ras oncogenes, Cancer Res. 48:793 (1988).
16. L. Vanhamme and C. Szpirer, Methionine metabolism defect in cells transfected with an activated HRAS1 oncogene, Exp. Cell Res. 169:120 (1987).
17. R. B. Gross and K. J. Scanlon, Membrane transport properties of L1210 cells resistant to cisplatin, Chemoterapia 5:37 (1986).
18. S. Shionoya, Y. Lu, and K. J. Scanlon, Properties of amino acid transport systems in K562 cells sensitive and resistant to cis-diamminedichloroplatinum(II), Cancer Res. 46:3445 (1986).

SUMMATION OF SESSION 1

John J. McGuire

Grace Cancer Drug Center
Roswell Park Memorial Institute
Buffalo, New York 14263

I would like to make a few comments about the earliest talks in the
day. The later talks in the day concentrated on TS and the effects of
dUMP, FdUMP, and various factors related to TS. What the earlier talks
point out is that there is a real need to be looking at earlier steps.
The transport of CF, for example, and the activation reaction, both have
to be considered. As Dave Duch pointed out, for example, his particular
cell line seems to be unable to be modulated because it does not activate
CF and that could potentially be a mechanism of intrinsic resistance to
this kind of modulation phenomenon and I think that should be looked at
in more detail. In terms of the transport, the pharmacokinetic data show
the 6R-isomer remains at very high levels in the plasma as the natural
isomer falls, so that ratio becomes very high. There needs to be more
work in looking at the effects of the 6R-isomer and Dr. Rustum, in fact,
is interested in doing some of those studies as are some other groups.
In terms of the activation, there were two pathways described and I think
most people seem to think that the methenyltetrahydrofolate synthetase is
the one primarily responsible for the effect of CF in these combinations,
but the other pathway has not been ruled out yet. An interesting aspect
to examine is whether both of those pathways are important or only one of
them. In terms of a basic biochemical question, at least two groups reported the normal occurrence of 5-formyltetrahydrofolate which had previously been thought to be an artifact of isolation procedures. Since we
don't have a reaction that uses 5-formyltetrahydrofolate I think it would
be interesting to determine the function of that pool. A storage role
was postulated, but the levels are very low; it seems that if you were
going to store something you'd store higher levels than the minor amount
that was reported. The transport and the activation, the steps prior to
TS, deserve more investigation.

SUMMATION OF SESSION II

Peter V. Danenberg

University of Southern California
Los Angeles, CA 90033

It has been apparent from this conference that the FUra-CF combination is of exceptional interest to investigators in all areas of cancer chemotherapy, from basic biochemistry to clinical studies. There are a number of reasons for this. First, the FUra-CF combination was proposed on the basis of rational a priori biochemical studies at the enzymological level, which revealed the role of $CH_2H_4PteGlu$ in the mechanism of interaction between FdUMP and TS. Secondly, there is a multiplicity of biochemical pathways and reactions involved in the conversion of CF to the reduced folate cofactor form. This provides the opportunity for many more biochemical studies which in turn should give rise to more ideas for drug modulation. Thirdly, the basic concept seems to hold up across the board. In contrast to many modulation ideas which seem to work basically as conceived in vitro, only to fizzle out when taken to in vivo systems, the effect of adding folates works in stabilizing the ternary complex in the test tube, it works to enhance the toxicity of the drugs in cell culture, and so far all indications are that the same biochemical mechanism is operative in human patients as well. This is encouraging in that it validates a concept of cancer drug pharmacology for which there was heretofore little precedent, namely, that finding out more about how drugs work will lead to more effective ways to use them.

In this session, the biochemistry of drug action directed at TS was explored on a wide range of levels - including x-ray crystallography of the target enzyme's active site and surrounding regions, basic enzymology, biochemical events in intact cells, and measurements of biochemical determinants of activity in tumor specimens taken from patients treated with the FUra-CF drug combination.

Houghton and coworkers reported the important observation that $H_4PteGlu$ oligoglutamates stabilized the ternary complex between TS, FdUMP and the reduced folate cofactor to a much greater extent than did the monoglutamyl cofactor. Furthermore, they showed that the stabilization of the complex increased with increasing concentration of the oligolutamyl $H_4PteGlu$ just as was found earlier with the monoglutamyl $H_4PteGlu$ (1). Their results confirm that the ordered mechanism of substrate binding to TS, where dUMP (or FdUMP) binds first to the enzyme followed obligatorily by the folate, applies also for the oligoglutamyl cofactors. This is a question that came up as a result of an earlier study on pig liver TS, in which it was proposed that the above binding sequence was reversed when $H_4PteGlu$ oligoglutamates were used as substrates (2), thereby removing much of the biochemical rationale for maintaining high intracellular reduced folate levels. We can draw the conclusion from this study that the effectiveness of the FUra-CF combination would benefit substantially from maximal oligoglutamylation of the CF.

Moran and Keyomarsi studied the effect of combining fluoropyrimidines with CF on intact cells, and reported that the presence of CF co-administered with FdUrd had two major effects compared to FdUrd alone: 1) a delayed recovery of TS activity and 2) a stabilization effect of the ternary complex in intact cells which can only be characterized as dramatic. This is a critical observation from the point of view of confirming that what goes on in the test tube also happens in the intact cell. The stabilizing effect of CF on the ternary complex in the cells is considerably more pronounced than seen with the monoglutamylfolate cofactor used previously in in vitro studies (1), and therefore is probably an effective illustration of the powerful effect of intracellular oligoglutamylation of CF.

Berger and coworkers, by studying the properties of TS in fluoropyrimidine-resistant cells, made the important connection between the presence of altered TS proteins and a lowered response of the cells to fluoropyrimidines. Even though Heidelberger in 1968 reported that an FUra resistant mouse tumor contained TS that did not bind FdUMP (3), this is a mechanism of resistance which really has not been considered very much as a factor contributing to the unresponsiveness of human cancer to fluoropyrimidines. The fact that these were innately fluoropyrimidine-resistant cells found in the same primary culture of tumor cells provides validity for investigating further the possibility of individual variation in TS genes. With modern tools of molecular biology, it should be possible to carry out these kinds of studies. Specifically relevant to the FUra-CF combination was the finding that one of the resistant cell lines was rendered sensitive to fluoropyrimidines through the co-administration of CF, suggesting that the binding of $H_4PteGlu$ to this particular altered TS was weaker than normal. Another significant result was that the TS-altered cells, selected for by resistance to FdUrd, were also cross-resistant to FUra, thereby establishing a commonality of mechanism between these two fluoropyrimidines.

The reports of both Allegra and coworkers and Spears and coworkers, besides their clinical results with the FUra-CF combination, described biochemical studies on human tumor serial biopsy specimens. These studies thereby provide a crucial link between laboratory research and the clinic. Both laboratories found a strong correlation between clincal response and TS inhibition, i.e., the amount of TS bound to FdUMP in the ternary complex. Allegra and coworkers, furthermore, saw a marked stabilization of the ternary complex when CF was present compared to FUra alone. This important result extends the cell culture observations of Moran and Keyomarsi to clinical specimens, and provides assurance that the same biochemical mechanisms are operative in human patients as in experimental in vitro and in vivo systems.

Scanlon and coworkers showed that cis-platin could enhance the activity of FUra by causing an increase in $H_4PteGlu$ pools. Beyond what was learned about the mechanism of action of cis-platin and its synergism with FUra, this paper has a broader significance, namely, that this heretofore unsuspected effect of cis-platin verifies the feasibility of biochemically modulating the amount of $H_4PteGlu$ in cells in a specific manner.

Santi reported on state-of-the-art approaches to development of unique and specific suicide inhibitors of TS. Through x-ray crystallographic pictures of the enzyme, the shape of the active site can be determined and amino acid residues that are in and around the active site of TS can be identified. With this information in hand, work can begin to design a molecule to fit precisely the shape of the active site, after which appropriate groups can be placed on this custom-designed inhibitor at the proper locations to interact with specific functional groups on the enzyme. In the past, the development of active site-directed inhibitors was done by a laborious process of establishing bulk-tolerance regions around the active site of the molecule and then placing electrophilic leaving groups at random positions into this area. It will be very interesting to see what sort of inhibitors are obtained by this ultrarational approach. There is a good likelihood that they will be folate analogs because of the numerous possibilities for structural alteration of this molecule.

REFERENCES

1. A. Lockshin and P.V. Danenberg, Biochemical Factors Affecting the Tightness of 5-Fluorodeoxyuridylate Binding to Human Thymidylate Synthetase. Biochem. Pharmacol. 30, 247-257 (1981).

2. Y.-Z. Lu, P.D. Aiello, and R.G. Matthews, Studies on the Polyglutamate Specificity of Thymidylate Synthase from Fetal Pig Liver. Biochemistry, 23, 6876-6882 (1984).

3. M. Umeda and C. Heidelberger, Comparative Studies of Fluorinated Pyrimidines with Various Cell Lines. Cancer Res., 28, 2529-2538 (1968).

THE ROSWELL PARK MEMORIAL INSTITUTE AND GASTROINTESTINAL TUMOR STUDY
GROUP PHASE III EXPERIENCE WITH THE MODULATION OF 5-FLUOROURACIL BY
LEUCOVORIN IN METASTATIC COLORECTAL ADENOCARCINOMA[1]

Nicholas J. Petrelli,[2] Youcef M. Rustum,[2] Howard
Bruckner,[3] and Donald Stablein,[4]

[2]Roswell Park Memorial Institute, Department of Surgical Oncology
 (NJP) and Grace Cancer Drug Center (YMR), Buffalo, NY
[3]Mount Sinai School of Medicine, Department of Medicine and
 Neoplastic Diseases, New York, NY
[4]The EMMES Corporation, Potomac, MD

INTRODUCTION

The therapeutic activity of 5-Fluorouracil (5-FU) in gastrointestinal (GI) malignancies may be enhanced by increasing the tumor cell
reduced folate pools in vivo[1,2,3,4]. One of the mechanisms of action
of 5-FU is its conversion into fluorodexoyuridylate (FdUMP), which
inhibits thymidylate synthetase (TS)[5]. FdUMP binds tightly to TS in
the presence of the cofactor L-5, 10-methylene tetrahydrofolate
(CH_2FH_4). This interaction of FdUMP and TS leads to the formation
of a covalent ternary complex, $TS-CH_2FH_4-FdUMP$[6]. The stability of
the ternary complex is maximal when the extracellular folate concentration is 10 umol/L in cell culture[7]. Therefore, high levels of inhibition of TS and a slow recovery of the enzyme activity can occur only in
the presence of sufficient intracellular concentrations of reduced
folates.

In a prior phase I-II trial at Roswell Park Memorial Institute, of
5-FU and leucovorin (CF) in previously treated patients with metastatic
colorectal carcinoma, partial responses were seen in nine of twenty-
three patients (38%)[3]. The recommended dose of 5-FU for a phase III
study was 600 mg/m^2 and CF 500 mg/m^2 weekly for 6 weeks followed by
a 2 week rest period.

The present report describes the results of a comparison of 5-FU
alone versus 5-FU and Methotrexate (MTX) versus 5-FU and high dose CF in
previously untreated patients with metastatic colorectal adenocarcinoma
with an update on survival. It also details the toxicity data from the
Gastrointestinal Tumor Study Group Phase III prospectively randomized
trial in metastatic colorectal adenocarcinoma (GITSG No. 6384).

[1]Supported by C21071 from the National Cancer Institute, Grant No.
 CA34184 (GITSG).

MATERIALS AND METHODS

In the Roswell Park Memorial Institute (RPMI) trial there were 74
patients previously untreated with cytostatic agents. This included 56
males and 18 females, with a median age of 60 years. All patients had
histologically confirmed colorectal adenocarcinoma and all gave written
and informed consent for entry into the study. All patients had an
Eastern Cooperative Oncology Group (ECOG) performance status 0 (normal
activity), 1 (ambulatory but symptoms), or 2 (in bed <50% of time).
All patients had normal hematologic, renal, hepatic and cardiac parameters, unless the abnormalities resulted from direct tumor invasion.
All of the patients had objectively measurable metastatic disease beyond
surgical removal diagnosed by tissue biopsy and/or radiologic or radionuclide procedures.

In the GITSG trial there were 343 patients. These patients also had
no prior chemotherapy and ECOG performance status 0, 1 or 2.

Treatment Plan

The 74 RPMI patients were randomized into one of three treatment
regimens: (1) 5-FU 450 mg/m^2 as an intravenous (IV) bolus daily for
five days of toxicity, then 200 mg/m^2 IV bolus every other day for six
doses. This was considered one course of treatment and was continued
every 4 weeks from the last day of treatment. (2) MTX 50 mg/m^2 in
normal saline by IV infusion over four hours, followed by an IV bolus of
5-FU 600 mg/m^2. This was administered weekly for 4 weeks and then
every 2 weeks. Leucovorin 500 mg/m^2 (calcium leucovorin supplied by
Lederle) in a two-hour IV infusion of normal saline with 5-FU 600
mg/m^2 as an IV bolus one hour after the leucovorin began every week
for 6 weeks, followed by a 2 week rest period.

The 343 patients in the GITSG trial[16] were randomized to one of
the following regimens: (1) 5-FU 500 mg/m^2 bolus days 1-5 every four
weeks with a 25 mg/m^2 escalation beginning at the second course of
treatment. (2) 5-FU 600 mg/m^2 IV bolus one hour after the beginning
of a two hour leucovorin infusion 500 mg/m^2 (calcium leucovorin
supplied by Burroughs Wellcome) weekly for six weeks with a two week
rest period. (3) 5-FU 600 mg/m^2 IV bolus one hour after the beginning
of a 10 minute leucovorin infusion 25 mg/m^2 weekly for six weeks
followed by a two week rest period.

Study Parameters

Before each course of therapy, every patient had a complete blood
count, serum electrolyte determination, liver function tests, serum
creatinine, blood urea nitrogen, and chest roentgenography. Radionuclide
liver scan, abdominal pelvic computer tomography (CT) scan, or ultrasound were performed where appropriate.

Response criteria for the RPMI trial used to evaluate antitumor
effect were as follows: complete response - the disappearance of all
perceptible tumor; partial response - a 50% reduction in the product of
the largest perpendicular diameters of the most clearly measurable known
malignant disease with no increase in the size of other measurable
disease and no appearance of new lesions; duration of response was
calculated from the time the response began until progression. Eight
weeks was required as a minimum response duration. Stable disease - no
change in size of the measurable lesion or a decrease in tumor size <
50% or an increase <25% with no appearance of new lesions; stable

Table 1

Platelet Nadir	Granolocyte Nadir		
	> 1500	500-1500	<500
> 100,000	Up 1*	No change	Down 1*
50,000-100,000	No change	No change	Down 1*
< 50,000	Down 1*	Down 1*	Down 2*

*One dose level is 25 mg/m^2

disease also required a minimum of 8 weeks duration; progression - the appearance of any new lesions and/or growth of any existing lesions by > 25% from the start of treatment.

Dose Reductions for Toxicity

The hematologic and gastrointestinal modifications for the RPMI phase III trial have been previously defined[8]. Table 1 defines the CITSG No. 6384 trial dose escalation/de-escalation for 5-FU loading schedule.

Table 2 defines the dose modification for hematological toxicity in the GITSG trial.

Table 3 defines gastrointestinal toxicity for the 5-FU and leuco-vorin regimens in the GITSG No. 6384 phase III trial.

Sample Preparation and HPLC Analysis

Extraction from plasma and quantitation by HPLC of FUra, dl-CF and 5-CH$_3$FH$_4$ were performed as previously described[13,14]. Briefly, FUra levels were investigated using an HPLC system equipped with a Spherisorb ODS II reverse-phase column (Alltech Assoc., Deerfield, IL) and two UV detectors set at 265 and 254 nm (Waters Assoc., Milford, MA). Elution was carried out isocratically at room temperature with a 1.5% methanol in 2.5 mM ammonium acetate buffer of pH 5. The limit of sensitivity of the assay is 2×10^{-7}M. Separation and quantitation of dl-CF and 5-CH$_3$FH$_4$ was performed using an HPLC reverse-phase ion

Table 2

WBC	Platelet Count	5-FU + Leucovorin
> 4000/mm^3	> 100,000/m^3	600 mg/m^2 + 100% CF
3000 - 3999/mm^3	75,000 - 99,000/mm^3	500 mg/m^2 + 100% CF
< 2999/mm^3	< 74,999/mm^3	No drug till recovery

Table 3

Grade	Toxicity	5-FU + Leucovorin
1	Stomatitis, mild ulcers, diarrhea vomiting 2-3 x per day	500 mg/m^2 + 100%
2	Stomatitis, moderate to severe diarrhea (4-6 x per day), intravenous hydration not required, moderate skin rash	Hold treatment until recovery, then 500 mg/m^2 of 5-FU with 100% of CF
3	GI bleeding - diarrhea 10 x per day, exfoliative dermatitis; intravenous hydration required	Hold treatment until WBC = 4000 and plts = 100,000, then 500 mg/m^2 of 5-FU with 100% of CF

pair method. The column was a μ-Bondapak C$_{18}$ (Waters Assoc., Milford, MA). Two UV detectors were set at 294 and 280 nM. Drugs were eluted from the column at room temperature with 30% methanol in 5 mM tetrabutylammonium phosphate of pH 7. The limit of sensitivity of the assay is 5×10^{-7}M for both dl-CF and 5-CH$_3$FH$_4$.

The amount of biologically active l-CF was quantitated by a microbial assay with Pediococcus cerevisiae (American Type Culture Collection 8081), a micro-organism which utilizes l-CF, but not d-CF, as a growth factor. dl-CF was collected from the HPLC (to separate from FUra), and serial dilution were made. Pediococcus cerevisiae was then incubated in the assay medium at 37°C for 18 hr. The turbidity of the culture (index of bacterial growth) was determined using a colorimeter at the end of the incubation. A standard curve was generated using known amounts of dl-CF (50% l-CF). l-CF Concentrations in samples from patients were calculated using the regression equation of the standard curve. A correction was made to account for the 85% recovery of dl-CF from HPLC. The limit of sensitivity of this microbial assay is 10^{-9}M.

Pharmacokinetic Evaluation

The elimination half-lives (T$_{1/2}$) were then evaluated by $0.693/k$ where k is the apparent first-order elimination rate constant (slope of the linear regressed terminal portion of the log concentration vs time curve). Areas under the concentration vs time curve (AUC) were calculated by the trapezoidal rule; the area from the last data point detected to infinity was estimated by first order extrapolation according to C$_z$/k, where C$_z$ was the last concentration detected. Plasma clearances (Cl) were calculated by Dose/AUC.

For the 5 days continuous infusion schedule, parameters evaluated were: steady-state plasma concentration (SSc), AUC and Cl. AUC from time zero to 120 hr were calculated by the trapezoidal rule; AUC from 120 hr to infinity were evaluated by first-order extrapolation using the mean elimination rate constant from patients treated with the 2 hr infusion schedule. Cl were calculated according to the formula: Rate of Infusion/SSc.

146

A two-tailed t test was utilized for the statistical evaluation of the data.

RESULTS

Response to Therapy

Table 4 summarizes the response to therapy in all patients on the RPMI phase III trial. In the 5-FU alone regimen 2 of 22 patients (9%) had a partial response with the duration of these responses 10 and 12 months, respectively. In the 5-FU and MTX regimen one of 22 patients (5%) underwent a partial response. The duration of this one partial responder was 19 months. In the 5-FU and high dose leucovorin regimen there were a total of 30 patients. Eleven of these patients (37%) had a partial response and there was one complete responder (3%). The median duration of response was 10 months with a range of 2 to 18 months. Comparison of the response rates for the three regimens showed a highly statistically significant difference between the three treatments (p = .009). The estimated median survival time from one study to death in the 5-FU, 5-FU and MTX and 5-FU and CF regimens was 11 months, 10 months and 12 months, respectively. However, there was no statistically significant difference between the treatment regimens with respect to survival time (p = 0.6). An update of the survival in the three regimens in April 1988 revealed a trend towards the 5-FU and Leucovorin regimen (p = 0.44).

Toxicity

Toxicity requiring a dose reduction of chemotherapy in the RPMI trial is summarized in Table 5. Emphasis is placed on the predominance of diarrhea in the 5-FU and leucovorin regimen as opposed to myelosuppression in the 5-FU and MTX regimen and 5-FU alone. As illustrated in Table 5, 13 of 30 patients (40%) on the 5-FU and leucovorin regimen required a dose reduction of 5-FU because of diarrhea. The leucovorin was maintained at 500 mg/m^2 and 8 of 13 (52%) patients who developed diarrhea not only required a dose reduction of 5-FU but also hospitalization for intravenous hydration. The remaining 5 patients required a dose reduction of 5-FU without intravenous hydration. Three patients on this regimen developed diarrhea that required further dose reductions of 5-FU to 400 mg/m^2, 400 mg/m^2 and 300 mg/m^2, respectively. Of the 13 patients with diarrhea requiring a dose reduction of 5-FU, 10 underwent a delay of treatment. The median duration of the delay was 3 weeks (range 1 to 6 weeks).

Table 4. Response to Therapy - All Patients RPMI Trial

Regimen (No. of Patients)	Partial Response (%)	Complete Response (%)
5-FU (22)	2 (11)	0
5-FU + MTX (22)	1 (5)	0
5-FU + CF (30)	11 (37)	1 (3)

Table 5.   Toxicity Requiring a Dose Reduction of Chemotherapy in the
           RPMI Trial

Regimen (No. of Patients)	Stomatitis (%)	Diarrhea (%)	Leukopenia (%)	Thrombocytopenia (%)
5-FU (22)[*]	2 (10)	5 (23)	8 (37)	0
5-FU + MTX (22)[+]	2 (10)	0	9 (40)	1 (5)
5-FU + CF (30)[+]	3 (10)	13 (40)	3 (10)	0

[*]One drug-related death secondary to leukopenia in conjunction with
hepatic failure.

[+]One drug-related death secondary to leukopenia.

There was one fatal toxicity in each of the three regimens on the
RPMI trial. All three of these patients died from sepsis secondary to
leukopenia.

Table 6 summarizes the incidence of myelosuppression in the GITSG
No. 6384 trial. The predominance of leukopenia in the 5-FU alone arm is
illustrated by the fact that 27% of the patients in this regimen
developed white blood counts below 2000/mm^3 whereas this was the case
in only 8% of the high dose leucovorin regimen and 4% of the low dose
leucovorin regimen. The median nadir white blood cell count in the 5-FU
alone arm was also significantly lower than the other two regimens.

Table 7 summarizes the incidence of diarrhea in the GITSG trial.
Mild-moderate diarrhea was defined as 4 to 6 bowel movements per day not
requiring intravenous hydration. Severe diarrhea was defined as bloody
in character and/or requiring intravenous hydration. As opposed to
leukopenia the predominant toxicity in the 5-FU and leucovorin regimens
was diarrhea.

Table 6.   Summary of Myelosuppression in GITSG No. 6484 Trial

	5-FU Alone	5-FU + High Dose CF	5-FU + Low Dose CF
Leukopenia (/mm^3)			
> 4,500	14%	52%	65%
2,000 - 4,500	59%	41%	32%
< 2,000	27%	8%	4%
Median Nadir WBC x 10^3/mm^3	2.5	4.4	5.0
Median Nadir Platelets x 10^3/mm^3	171	190	203

Table 7. Summary of Gastrointestinal (Diarrhea) Toxicity in GITSG No. 6384 Trial

	5-FU Alone	5-FU + High Dose CF	5-FU Low Dose CF
Diarrhea			
Mild, Moderate	39%	48%	51%
Severe	9%	26%	14%

Table 8 summarizes the incidence of stomatitis in the GITSG trial. This table illustrates that stomatitis was not a major toxicity in the leucovorin regimens. However, in the 5-FU alone regimen 65% of the patients developed stomatitis.

In the GITSG trial there was one treatment related death in the 5-FU alone regimen secondary to leukopenia and sepsis. In the 5-FU and leucovorin regimens there were a total of 11 deaths. Ten of these eleven deaths were in patients older than 63 years. These deaths were caused by dehydration with third space fluid loss and developing sequellae. Diarrhea occurred within the first course of treatment and death subsequently followed four to five days later.

Pharmacokinetic Studies

Plasma pharmacokinetics of d-CF, l-CF and the metabolite 5-methyl tetrahydrofolic acid ($5-CF_3FH_4$) have been reported by Straw et al. following short-term infusion (4.5 min) and oral administration of relatively low doses of dl-CF (25-100 mg) to healthy subjects[15]. The results reported by these investigators can be summarized as follows: 1) the plasma elimination half-lives of the two stereroisomers were greatly different, the l-CF half-life being 14-fold shorter than the d-CF half-life; 2) plasma clearance and renal clearance of d-CF were equal, indicating the d-CF is not significantly metabolized; 3) absorption of oral dl-CF was saturable and only partially stereo-selective. The peak concentration of l-CF in plasma after a 50 mg IV dose of dl-CF did not exceed 2.0 μM.

Table 8. Summary of Gastrointestinal (Stomatitis) Toxicity in GITSG No. Trial

	5-FU Alone	5-FU + High Dose CF	5-FU Low Dose CF
None	35%	64%	75%
Mild, Moderate	50%	32%	25%
Severe	15%	4%	0%

In the present study, plasma pharmacokinetics of high dose dl-CF (500 mg/m^2) were investigated in patients with advanced colorectal cancers treated according to the following schedules: 2 hr IV infusion of 500 mg/m^2 dl-CF and IV push of 600 mg/m^2 FUra one hour after the start of the dl-CF infusion; 5 days continuous IV infusion of 500 mg/m^2 dl-CF and 400-500 mg/m^2/d FUra and orally as divided doses of 125 mg/m^2 hx4 for a total dose of 500 mg/m^2 to patients with lung carcinoma.

The data in Table 9 indicate that although significantly higher peak plasma concentration of l-CF and 5-FH$_3$FH$_4$ was achieved by the 2h infusion of dl-CF, higher AUC were obtained by the 5 day infusion and by the hourly oral administration of CF. In addition the t 1/2 life of l-CF and 5-CH$_3$FH$_4$ were significantly longer when dl-CF was administered orally.

Pharmacokinetic studies of high dose dl-CF confirm the previously reported finding that the disposition of l-CF differs greatly from that of d-CF[13,14]. This difference of kinetic behavior may be important, since, although d-CF is believed to lack biological activity, at the very high concentrations in plasma it could compete with l-CF for its cellular uptake, metabolism and binding to thymidylate synthatase especially shortly after administration of dl-CF where the d-CF to l-CF ratio is greater than 10 at 4 h. Furthermore, it is not known whether the total systemic exposure (AUC) of l-CF or its peak plasma concentration is likely to be critical determinants in the intracellular modulations of folate pools resulting in an effective modulation of therapeutic efficacy of FUra in cancer patients. l-CF plasma levels in this study indicate that lower AUC but higher plasma peaks are achieved following the 2 hr infusion of dl-CF than during and following the 5 days infusion and p.o. treatments. The results of the 5,10 CH$_2$FH$_4$ studies seem to indicate that a high peak concentration of l-CF rather than a lower total systemic exposure (AUC) can yield a greater increase of dTMP-S folate cofactor pool and higher rate of dTMP-S inhibition[14]. The observed differences in the cellular dTMP-S folate cofactor pools may also be related to differences in the biochemical and pharmacological make-up of tumor cells obtained from patients with prior or with no prior chemotherapy. Thus, the role of dose and schedule of dl-CF administration should be more clearly defined in a well randomized clinical trial.

DISCUSSION

5-FU has been the standard therapy for the treatment of metastatic colorectal adenocarcinoma. Extensive studies on 5-FU have been previously reported[11,12,13,14].

The RPMI previous data[3] indicated that the administration of 5-FU and high dose leucovorin enhanced the antitumor activity of 5-FU in metastatic colorectal carcinoma. The dose of leucovorin for the presently reported RPMI trial was based on our clinical and pharmacokinetic data[3] and in vitro data[7], which have shown that the stability of the ternary complex is maximal when the extracellular leucovorin concentration is 10 μmol/L in cell culture. This leucovorin dose was then used in the GITSG No. 6384 trial.

In the RPMI trial of previously untreated patients, we have observed a response rate of 40% in the 5-FU and leucovorin regimen. The duration of this response was 10 months, and the estimated median survival time from on study to death for all patients was 12 months. The response

Table 9. Pharmacokinetic Parameters of 5-Formyltetrahydro Folate (CF) and Its Metabolites in Patients with Colon Carcinoma Treated with FUra (500 mg/m²) and CF (500 mg/m²) by 2h Infusion, Continuous IV Infusion per Day for 5 Days, or by Oral Route as 125 mg/m²/Hx4

	2H			5d+			P.O.		
	dL-CF	LCF	5-FH$_3$FH$_4$	dL-CF	LCF	5-CH$_3$FH$_4$	dL-CF	LCF	5-CH$_3$FH$_4$
Peak (μM)	98+38	24 +6	17 +8	51+ 17	1.2	12+ 5	4.4	< 0.5	4.6
AUC (mM.h)	71+22	2.6+1.5	14 +5	364+123	6.0	83+38	6.3	–	2.8
t1/2 (h)	8+ 1.4	0.8+0.1	7.1+1.9	8+ 1.5	0.7+1.5	7+ 1.2	16.3	–	5

+Value reported as steady state concentrations.

rate was superior to both 5-FU alone and 5-FU in combination with MTX. However, no improvement in survival time was noted and although there is a trend in the 5-FU and leucovorin regimen the updated survival is based upon a small number of patients with the p value still not significant.

The toxicity observed during the RPMI study was within acceptable limits with the exception of one therapy related death in each regimen. Our previous phase I-II trial[3] of 5-FU and high dose leucovorin demonstrated the predominance of GI toxicity, specifically diarrhea, as opposed to hematologic toxicity. In the present report, a comparison of toxicities requiring a dose reduction of chemotherapy reveals a predominance of myelosuppression in both the 5-FU alone and the 5-FU and MTX regimens. No cases of diarrhea were seen in the 5-FU and MTX regimen, but there were toxicities of stomatitis, 10%; leukopenia, 40% and thrombocytopenia, 5%. With 5-FU alone, there was a 37% incidence of leukopenia and a 23% incidence of diarrhea.

In the GITSG No. 6384 phase III trial diarrhea was also the predominant toxicity in the leucovorin regimens as opposed to leukopenia. Fifty-two percent of the patients in the high dose leucovorin regimen and 65% of patients in the low dose leucovorin regimen maintained white blood cell counts >4500/mm^3. Whereas this was the case in only 14% of the patients in the 5-FU alone regimen. In terms of stomatitis the majority of the patients on the high dose leucovorin regimen (64%) and on the low dose leucovorin regimen (75%) developed no stomatitis during the course of their treatment. However, in the 5-FU alone arm 65% of the patients developed mild-moderate or severe stomatitis. The predominant toxicity in the 5-FU leucovorin regimens was diarrhea. Seventy-four percent of the patients in the high dose leucovorin regimen developed mild-moderate or severe diarrhea and 65% of the patients in the low dose leucovorin regimen developed diarrhea. This diarrhea occurred within the first six weeks of the first course of treatment. Typically, these patients would develop four to five loose bowel movements per day either on the day of hospital discharge or at home and within one week presented with severe third space fluid loss and azotemia. If treated aggressively and immediately with intravenous hydration the diarrhea is reversible. If not, it can become fatal.

Pharmacologically, although initial evidence suggest that modulation of the intracellular folate pools requires the administration of high doses of dl-CF, especially when administered by short term infusion, the role of schedule and route of administration must be further evaluated. It is possible that selective modulation of the therapeutic efficacy of FUra may require prolonged continuous i.v. infusion of folates and/or administration of dl-CF by the oral route. Further the reasons why previously treated patients with colon carcinoma didn't respond to FUra modulation by folate remains intriguing and requires further investigation.

REFERENCES

1. D. Machover, E. Goldschmidt, P. Chollet, G. Metzger, J. Zittoun, J. Marquet, et al., Treatment of advanced colorectal and gastric adenocarcinomas with 5-fluorouracil and high dose folinic acid, J. Clin. Oncol. 4:5:685 (1986).
2. J. A. Houghton, S. J. Maroda, J. O. Phillips, et al., Biochemical determinants of responsiveness to 5-fluorouracil and its derivatives in xenografts of human colorectal adenocarcinomas in mice, Cancer Res. 41:144 (1981).

3. S. Madajewicz, N. Petrelli, Y. M. Rustum, et al., Phase I-II trial of high dose calcium leucovorin and 5-fluorouracil in advanced colorectal cancer, Cancer Res. 44:4667 (1984).

4. D. Machover, L. Schwarzenberg, E. Goldsmith, et al., Treatment of advanced colorectal and gastric adenocarcinoma with 5-FU combined with high-dose folinic acid: A pilot study, Cancer Treat. Rep. 66:1803 (1982).

5. C. Heidelberger, Fluorinated pyrimidines and their nucleosides, in: "Handbook of Experimental Pharmacology, Antineoplastic and Immuno-suppressive Agents", A. C. Sartorelli and D. G. Johns, eds., Springer Verlag, New York (1975).

6. D. V. Santi, C. S. McHenry and H. Sommer, Mechanism of interaction of thymydilate synthetase with 5-fluorodeoxyuridylate, Biochemistry 13:471 (1974).

7. R. M. Evans, J. D. Laskin and M. T. Hakala, Effect of excess folates and deoxyinosine on the activity and site of action of 5-fluoro-uracil, Cancer Res. 41:3283 (1981).

8. N. Petrelli, L. Herrera, Y. Rustum, P. Burke, P. Creaven, J. Stulc, L. Emrich and A. Mittelman, A prospective randomized trial of 5-fluorouracil versus 5-fluorouracil and high dose leucovorin versus 5-fluorouracil and methotrexate in previously untreated patients with advanced colorectal carcinoma, J. Clin. Oncol. 5:10:1559 (1987).

9. C. G. Moertel, Chemotherapy of gastrointestinal cancer, N. Engl. J. Med. 299:1049 (1978).

10. H. L. Davis, Chemotherapy of large bowel cancer, Cancer 50:2638 (1982).

11. C. A. Presant, A. E. Denes, C. Liu, et al., Prospective randomized reappraisal of 5-fluorouracil in metastatic colorectal carcinoma: A comparative trial with 6-thioguanine, Cancer 53:2610 (1984).

12. P. F. Engstrom, J. M. MacIntyre, A. Mittelman, et al., Chemotherapy of advanced colorectal carcinoma: Fluorouracil alone vs two drug combinations using fluorouracil, hydroxyurea, semustine, decar-bazine, razoxane and mitomycin: A phase III trial by the Eastern Cooperative Oncology Group, Am. J. Clin. Oncol. 7:313 (1984).

13. S. G. Arbuck, F. Trave, H. O. Douglass, Jr., H. Nava, S. Zakrzewski and Y. M. Rustum, Phase I and pharmacologic studies of intraperi-toneal leucovorin and 5-fluorouracil in patients with advanced cancer, J. Clin. Oncol. 4:1510 (1986).

14. F. Trave, Y. M. Rustum, N. J. Petrelli, L. Herrera, A. Mittelman, C. Frank and P. J. Creaven, Plasma and tumor tissue pharmacology of high dose intravenous 5-formyltetrahydrofolate inhibition with 5-fluorouracil in patients with advanced colorectal carcinoma, J. Clin. Oncol. in press (1988).

15. J. A. Straw, D. Szapary and W. T. Wynn, Pharmacokinetics of the diastereroisomers of leucovorin after intravenous oral administra-tion to normal subjects, Cancer Res. 44:3114 (1984).

16. N. Petrelli, D. Stablein, H. Bruckner, A. Megibow, R. Mayer and H. Douglass, A prospective randomized phase III trial of 5-fluorouracil (5FU) versus 5FU and high dose leucovorin (HDCF) versus 5FU and low dose leucovorin (LDCF) in patients (pts) with metastatic colorectal carcinoma: A report of the Gastrointestinal Tumor Study Group, Proc. Am. Assoc. Cancer Res. 7: p. 94 (abst. No. 357) (1988).

DISCUSSION OF DR. PETRELLI'S PRESENTATION

Dr. Hines: Did you see any lacrymal excessive secretion? One of the things we've noticed both with the PPMI/Rustum regimen with the i.v. CF and with my oral high dose is quite a bit of lacrymal excessive secretion. It's not a major toxicity but it's something that I haven't seen with FUra alone.

Dr. Petrelli: The only thing I can say is that on the GITSG trial none was reported. Now in our Phase II trial we did see, not the con-junctivitis, but the excessive tearing.

Dr. Laufman: Did you see any weakness? We've had a lot of experience with patients, especially older patients, who tolerate the regimen very poorly and take to their beds. Was that reported as a side effect?

Dr. Petrelli: You mean weakness in general or weakness secondary to the diarrhea?

Dr. Laufman:: Generalized weakness separate from the diarrhea.

Dr. Petrelli: Again, obviously very difficult to report and I would have to say no to that. Several people over the age of 65 who in general may be weak in certain aspects of daily activity anyway but none significantly here, no.

Dr. Holland: If we put your presentation together with the Mayo Clinic results, giving essentially the same low doses of CF, 25 mg/m^2, and the Mayo Clinic giving their FUra on 5 successive days instead of once a week for 6 weeks which comes up to about the same total dose, has doubled the duration of remission, 10 months instead of 5 months, and the same survival that you get in the high dose CF, which is 53% for you with the high dose CF, 55 weeks for the low CF dose, for them. This is a disease where these tight comparisons aren't really helpful except that you are advocating potentially out of your study a 25-fold increase in the cost of CF. Would you comment on the economics of this study?

Dr. Petrelli: Your point is well taken. I think if you were to look at a graphic demonstration of the cost of per mg or per 50 gm vial you would see almost the half the price of 5 years ago, but every-thing is relative. I think the cost effectiveness of this is still something to reckoned with but again, this is an investigational trial just like the Mayo Clinic's is and I still consider this modulation investigational only in controlled environments. I think it's going to take perhaps another year or so before a definitive statement can be made about this. The cost effectiveness is still a consideration today, but if the trend continues in what has happened to the price of this drug, then I think you will it become equally based with the standard drug used for this disease. But your point is well taken.

Dr. Tilchen: Would you recall if any of the diarrheas were investi-gated for bacterial causes like.

Dr. Petrelli: The problem with the diarrhea was that, in view of our own Phase II and Phase III study where we didn't see these fatal toxicities because of the aggressiveness of treatment, on the GITSG trial we were concentrating on myelosuppression. By the time these patients got diarrhea the classic story was quote in the chart "they had a little bit of diarrhea before they went home" and then they came back 5 days later with a BUN of 70 and a creatinine of 5. So in the interim it was missed. Investigation of cause was not done because these patients came in fairly morbid. Following that recognition, when it was recommended to the participants in this trial to treat this diarrhea aggressively, although it was towards the end of this trial, there were no reported fatal toxicities. These were all up front in the trial.

Audience: I'm interested in the toxicity issue and I was wondering do you have any idea of how many courses of the 6 weeks treatment had to be aborted before the 6 weeks were completed because of onset of diarrhea? That is, you have 6 weeks on, 2 weeks off, 6 weeks on how many of those courses consisted of lets say 4 weeks or 5 weeks because diarrhea seemed to be starting.

Dr. Petrelli: The diarrhea occurred usually around the 4th or 5th dose of the first course; it was all within the first 6 weeks. Once that diarrhea was noted after the fatal toxicities and treated, the median duration of delay in treatment, we were being very conservative, was 3 weeks, very similar to our in house trial. But we were using our own in house trial to tell people to wait until this completely abates. I don't know if that answers your question.

Audience: Not really. I'm not sure you have this information. Of the number of patients that were supposed to get six weeks, how many only got 4 or how many only got 5, etc.?

Dr. Petrelli: I don't have that information available at this time but it's a good point to investigate.

MOUNT SINAI CLINICAL EXPERIENCE WITH LEUCOVORIN

AND 5-FLUOROURACIL

Howard W. Bruckner

Mount Sinai School of Medicine
1 Gustave L. Levy Place, Box 1178
New York, New York 10029

INTRODUCTION

The early Mount Sinai clinical experience appears to be relevant to unresolved questions concerning both leucovorin (LV) dosage and 5-fluorouracil (FU) schedules examined in the Gastrointestinal Tumor Study Group (GITSG) and Mayo Clinic-North Central trials. In addition, recent findings in the course of evolving practice provide support for specific new applications of LV-FU for combined modality and combination chemotherapy.

Initial experience supports: re-examination of FU dose and schedule as possible variable in LV-FU clinical trials; and attempts to find novel LV-FU schedules with either atypical biologic effect or greater ease of administration. These are testable, especially promising, new applications. They include: combination chemotherapy for traditionally difficult diseases, such as gastric cancer with cisplatin (DDP) and antifolates where the LV serves for both rescue and biochemical modulation; intraperitoneal (I.P.) and intra-arterial routes of administration for refractory colon and gastric cancer; and combined modality with radiotherapy (RT) for pancreatic cancer.

METHODS

In the initial clinical experience with LV-FU, patients failing FU 5-day infusions were retreated with the identical infusion plus LV 15 mg/M^2 three times a day, first intravenously and then orally in separate patients (Table 1) (1-3). A similar oral dosage of LV was used in conjunction with hepatic artery continuous infusion of 1000 mg/M^2 of FU each day for 5 days. This was used for patients with severe symptoms due to metastases in the liver, failing systemic FU infusion, after the preceding experience had demonstrated efficacy for low-dose LV with systemic FU infusion. It was assumed these patients were in urgent need for a local response which could not be accomplished with fluorodeoxyuridine (FUDR) arterial infusion in timely fashion.

Table 1. Toxicity: LV-FU (Infusion)

Grade	WBC	PLTS	Mucositis	Median Infusion Time
1	0	0	2	88 hours (72-94)
2	1	3	3	
3	1	2	2	versus
4	0	0	1	
				106 Hours (96-120)*
	20%	50%	80%	FU without LV

Treatment consisted of: FU 1000 mg/M^2/24 hours continuous infusion to first toxicity; LV 15 mg/M^2 every 8 hours days 2,3,4 intravenously. Ten patients were treated.

*Prior treatment consisted of HexMF: Hexamethylmelamine, Mitomycin-C, and the identical FU continuous infusion.

In separate phase I trials, increasing doses of LV were next piloted with single day FU bolus and 2-day FU bolus regimens (2). Plans for testing a multiday bolus regimen were aborted because of unexpected findings: activity with the 1-day regimen, and severe toxicity with less than conventional doses of FU in the 2-day regimen (Table 2).

Based on a treatment which appeared effective during pharmacology studies of LV, a retrospective review found 20 patients, given LV over a range of dosages from 100-200 mg/M^2 and FU 1000 mg/M^2 once every 2 weeks for stage III pancreatic cancer, by several Mount Sinai physicians. Additional patients were found, given the same regimen either before or in initially lower 500 mg/M^2 FU dosage after RT, based on the highly favorable preceding experience (4). The regimens are shown in Table 3.

A new regimen has evolved, compressing 3 regimens which were found active as part of Mount Sinai and GITSG investigations: methotrexate (MTX) followed by FU (5), LV followed by FU (2), and DDP followed by FU [MLP] (6). This series has grown because of the extraordinary quality of the initial responses (7). The regimen is shown in Table 4.

Table 2. LV-FU Bolus: Dosage, Schedule & Toxicity

Daily Dosage FU	Pts. No. D1 D1-2	None D1 D1-2	Mild D1 D1-2	Moderate D1 D1-2	Severe D1 D1-2	Life-Threatening D1 D1-2
15	4^1 3	2^1 1	0 1	1 -	1 1	0 -
17.5	2 4^2	0 -	1 1	1 1	0 -	0 2^2
20	6^1 2	1 -	0 -	5^1 2	0 -	0 -
22.5	13^4 -	3^1 -	2^1 -	5^1 -	2^1 -	1 -
Total	25^6 9^2	6^2 1	3^1 2	12^2 3	3^1 1	1 2^2

Number in superscript= number treated as primary therapy.

Table 3. LV-FU Regimens

LV	FU
200 mg/M^2	1000 mg/M^2 every 2 weeks
30 min inf	bolus at 60 minutes
no change	escalate 10%

Early pancreatic cancer, 50% respond, some complete
response (CR).
Late pancreatic cancer, 30% respond, all partial
response (PR).
Following RT-FU, FU dosage is 500 mg/M^2 with escalation as tolerated. Some patients responded
(CR and PR) inside and outside RT field
(no cross-resistance).
Preceding RT, 1 of 1 complete response with
subsequent RT-FU.

The regimen was also used an I.P. versions for individuals with severe symptom-producing ascites. All day 1 drugs
were injected into the abdomen in separate full dosage in 1
liter of saline with no attempts to remove the drugs. In some
cases, the subsequent systemic (LV bolus - FU continuous infusion) followed the I.P. loading (Table 5).

RESULTS

Efficacy of Low-Dose LV

Low-dose LV, every 8 hours, significantly increased the
side effects of FU infusion (Table 1). Mucositis occurs significantly more often (80%) and also significantly earlier than
in the same patients serving as their own historical controls
(1). The incidence of leukopenia (20%) and thrombocytopenia

Table 4. MLP Schema

Hour	Drug	Dose
0	MTX	100 mg/M^2 200(2nd course); 300(3rd course)
4	FU	600 mg/M^2 bolus (2nd course)
18	LV	200 mg/M^2 *
19	FU	800 mg/M^2/24 hours x 96 hours continuous infusion
19	FU	600 mg/M^2 bolus
20	DDP	100 mg/M^2 with Mannitol

Days 1,8 prior to starting this regimen, day 15, patients
may be given MTX 100 mg/M^2 at 0 time (15 minute infusion),
FU 500 mg/M^2 at 1 hour (bolus) in order to avoid delay in
treatment required for borderline postoperative recovery.

*LV 12.5 mg every 6 hours times 4, Day 2. Double LV dosage
to 25 mg every 6 hours times 4, if complete gastrectomy
or any other high risks of side effects.

Modified from the 79th Annual Meeting of the American
Association for Cancer Research presentation, 1988.

Table 5. Intraperitoneal Regimens

Drug	mg/M^2	Time	Drug	mg/M^2	Time
MTX	200-400	0 hr	MTX	200-400	0 hr
FU	1000	2 hr	FU	1000	2 hr
LV+	100-200	3 hr			
DDP	100	4 hr	LV+	100-200	18 hr
			FU	1000	19 hr
			DDP	100	20 hr

+LV also given 10 mg/M^2 every 6 hr x 3-6 intravenously.
DDP given with full systemic hydration and mannitol
diuretics.
First time hours 2,3,4; then, if tolerated, hours
2,18,19,20; then with systemic FU continuous infusion as
in the MLP systemic regimen.

(50%) were high; the latter significantly so, compared to
prior side effects following longer administration of the same
FU infusion (with two concurrent cytotoxic drugs) (1).

FU Schedule Dependent-Toxicity

Toxicity with the 2-day bolus regimen was out of all
proportion to the total dosage of FU (2). The single dose did
not produce the same toxicity (2). Historically, 4 to 5 days
of FU in these total dosages, without LV, will not produce the
same level of toxicity (2).

Arterial Treatment

A particularly striking example of the efficacy of low-
dose oral LV was found in its ability to produce 3 of 3 rapid
objective responses of liver metastases, when FU was given as
a 1000 mg/M^2 continuous arterial infusion, days 1-5 (to first
sign of side effects). The regimen produced moderate-severe
extrahepatic toxicity, similar to the peripheral infusions,
and also more mild-moderate upper gastrointestinal toxicity
than either the peripheral infusion or arterial FU alone.
Hepatic artery LV-FU remains attractive and only appears to
require small doses of LV, but has not been pursued at Mount
Sinai, because of commitments to the development of primary
systemic therapy.

Pancreatic cancer

The LV-FU regimen produced responses of early and late
pancreatic cancer (Table 3). Some of the former responses were
complete and of 1 to 4 years in duration. Median survival will
exceed 1 year.

There were additional anecdotal partial and complete
responses after RT. There is little or no cross-resistance
between RT or FU as used in combined modality therapy and LV-
FU.

Half the patients had more than 50% improvement in tumor
markers (OC-125, CA 19-9, CEA). Toxicity was mild or moderate.

Granulocytopenia was common, conjunctivitis was frequent while diarrhea was rare.

Patients in this series tended to be atypical, because they were clinically stable (enough to come through a pro-longed referral process and to be considered for pharmacology trials). Tumors tended to involve soft tissue and often spared the liver. There was infrequent pain or ascites due to pancreatic cancer. Preliminary working definitions of early cancer have been described (4). In the `early' cases, the primary tumor was too small to evaluate for response.

Gastric Cancer Combination Chemotherapy

The MLP regimen (Table 4) commonly produces brief severe granulocytopenia and mucositis. It produced 6 complete responses, 4 partial responses, and 1 stable disease for the first 12 patients. In prior experience, complete remissions by CAT scan criteria were virtually non-existent (1-2 in 50-100 patients in different series). There was no effort to perform second surgery. These were clinical complete remissions. The patients had larger than average tumors, measurable by CAT scan, usually in soft tissues. Median survival exceeds 1 year. Both response rates and survival are significantly better than any Mount Sinai or GITSG trial for patients with stage III gastric cancer. Mild neurotoxicity almost consistently limits treatment among responders. Response appears to persist only as long as DDP can be continued. The patients are a representative group satisfying eligibility criteria for DDP therapy.

I.P. Regimen

The I.P. regimen has been used sparingly for patients with clinically massive symptomatic ascites refractory to paracentesis and sometimes to systemic chemotherapy. Three patients with gastric cancer and 2 with colon cancer had complete permanent resolution of their ascites with single treatments. Treatments were not repeated, because systemic therapy was considered more appropriate once the palliative goal had been achieved. These are clinical remissions supported by CAT scan and sonography, with no attempt at cytologic or laparoscopic evaluation. Side effects are less than those with the systemic regimen. All systemic treatment precautions were employed. Brief chemical peritonitis sometimes occurred.

DISCUSSION

The initial laboratory experiments of Santi demonstrated that low-dose $5x10^{-7}$M LV was potentially effective in the L1210 systems (8), although the majority of systems apparently demonstrate greater effect or only first demonstrate effect in the 10 to 10^{-5}M dosage range. In laboratory experiments at Mount Sinai, which were contemporary with those of Santi, LV produced a marked effect on the toxicity of FU. The degree of increased potency of FU appeared to tend to vary with FU dosage, when LV was held constant (9). The growth inhibition experiments were only a screening test and, statistically, did not serve to quantitatively discriminate between the effect of different LV or FU dosages. Moran et al. have illustrated in this symposium that these screening growth inhibition tests only measured the tip of the iceberg (10). Clinicians had to consider that this LV-FU combination might represent a new drug with different patterns of toxicity. At the time of first clinical application, its selectivity or any measure of impact on normal tissue had not been examined in the laboratory.

There was concern about the safety of LV. At Mount Sinai, it was considered mandatory to begin with the smallest dosage pharmacologically effective for 'rescue'. The FU infusion was selected because its dose-limiting side effects were the least likely to be fatal. It was also least likely to produce profound bone marrow toxicity, although this did not prove the case in practice.

Mount Sinai phase I LV for dose finding trials, with a toxicity endpoint, screening evidence of biologic activity, appear to find that multiple exposures to LV at low-doses have more profound effect than single applications of 2-3 times more cumulative LV or even a ten times larger single dose of LV (2,3,11). This was the basis for the early advocacy of a low-dose LV arm in controlled trails, as tested by both the GITSG and the Mayo Clinic-North Central Group.

The relative contribution of multiple exposures to LV or protracted multiple exposures to FU are unknown. Single hit enzyme kinetics did not predict that the dose or schedule of FU would affect the LV-FU interaction with biologic effects may be the complex sum of interactions in a dynamic biochemical meleu, dependent on more than the enzyme hit alone. Formation of the complex is only a first step toward cell death. This is compatible with the still unexplained profound diverse impact of scheduling on FU and FUDR as single agents. FU schedule differences may offer a unifying hypothesis for the Mayo Clinic-North Central Group and GITSG phase III trials. Low-dose LV is effective in a multiday schedule, but has little impact on the weekly intermittent schedule. These findings are identical to the earlier Mount Sinai experience with analogous schedules (1,2,11).

Increased FU toxicity is possibly an important indicator of LV activity. Since the qualitative and quantitative toxicities of different regimens are not the same, it would be dangerous to assume that laboratory (LV dosage) cytotoxicity tests can predict the selectivity, severity, or form of side effects in clinical trials of LV-FU. The Mount Sinai experience, now apparently supported by 2 phase III trials, illustrates that it may not be enough to find the minimum effective dose of LV. Investigators may perhaps profit from examining the diversity of LV dose-FU schedule effects. Multiday LV-FU regimens produce far more and different toxicity than single day regimens (2). Multiday regimens may be effective with low-dose LV. With single intermittent doses, even 100 mg/M^2 of LV fails to have greater impact than 15 mg/M^2 (11). Intermittent regimens may require very large (500 mg/M^2) doses of LV to provide high rates of objective response. They also produce a pattern of gastrointestinal toxicity, unlike the low-dose regimens suggesting different therapeutic targeting.

The implications of widely different effect, due to either LV or FU schedule change, have been relatively neglected, and can be recommended for renewed interest. It may be possible to find novel schedules with atypical biologic effects, perhaps broadening the spectrum of LV-FU application. Critical changes in FU dosage schedule may produce a window of activity, not only in toxicity, but in therapeutic effect. The concept of serially testing low-dose and high-dose regimens remains attractive.

The GITSG trial may not demonstrate a failure of efficacy for low-dose LV. LV appears to have some effect with intermittent dose schedules. It probably produces an improvement in therapeutic index compared to the more dose-intensive 'control' FU loading regimen (12). It is not an optimum application of LV in conjunction with the once weekly FU regimens, as Petrelli et al. have shown in an update of the GITSG phase III trial (13).

A high order and quality of benefit was observed when the every 2-week regimen was applied to patients with pancreatic cancer as part of pharmacology trials. This trial produced a broad preliminary phase II experience as one of its by-product; bile duct tumors may also respond (4). Since then, several oncologists familiar with the results have used it as treatment for patients who requested novel, but not extraordinary treatment (by toxicology or complexity criteria). LV-FU produces a 35% cumulative rate of response, an additional 15% have marked fall in tumor assays (OC-125, CA 19-9, and CEA). Median survival exceeds a year. One patient is a 4-year complete responder, without disease at second-look surgery.

This experience with pancreatic cancer is, in theory, confounded by the absence of prospective registration and the use of an otherwise untested high-dose FU regimen. Nevertheless, the order and quality of activity, and the physicians practical choice to use it over and over again, provides strong evidence that some LV-FU regimen can be developed as a new best treatment for pancreatic cancer. The alternatives are nihilism and markedly toxic experimental regimens which do not easily lend themselves to integration with other therapy.

Anecdotally, this LV-FU regimen is well tolerated and active after RT-FU fails. In addition, it can be integrated with combined modality RT. Integration of LV-FU with 'proven' effective therapies (such as GITSG combined modality and adjuvant therapies) may have much greater impact then pursuing a single drug treatment to its limit. There is substantial potential for combined modality therapy of pancreatic cancer, because RT in combination with FU infusion, high-dose DDP and other drugs (without adding LV as yet) already produce 25% complete response and 50% partial durable response of simultaneously irradiated stage II pancreatic cancer (Bruckner unpublished). As noted in this symposium, LV has possible synergistic interaction with both FU infusion and DDP.

Gastric cancer may represent an example of a disease in which LV-FU can be applied to combination chemotherapy. In theory, breast cancer and head and neck cancer should be even better subjects for such application, because the standard combinations are more well characterized, and may have greater impact, even as adjuvant therapy. Striking initial clinical success has led to repeated use of a clinical regimen, compressing proven components of earlier work (5-7). This MLP biochemical modulation of FU regimen, which was first used for patients with urgent need of response (in clinical circumstances where prior regimens were individually consistently ineffective) has produced the highest complete response rates to date. Experience with MTX-FU-adriamycin and etoposide-adriamycin-DDP suggest that components of the new combination improve rates of complete response (14,15). It is impossible for a phase II experience to prove the contribution of the LV, because of the complexity of this MLP regimen, which contains 6 potentially synergistic drug combinations (7). The level of activity, the availability of tissue with endoscopy, and the theoretical rationale for LV-FU-DDP, make this regimen ideal for study of clinical laboratory correlates. Preliminary findings by Preusser et al. and Arbuck et al., presented as part of this symposium, also strongly support directing investigational efforts to adding LV to combination chemotherapy for gastric cancer.

The Mount Sinai experience strongly supports and provides new clinical models for testing several of the major options for development of LV-FU. It identifies the schedule of FU as a possible variable affecting optimum dose and schedule of LV. It identifies LV-FU as a clinical adjunct to combined modality RT and combination chemotherapy.

REFERENCES

1. H. W. Bruckner, J. A. Storch, and J. F. Holland, Leucovorin increases the toxicity of 5-fluorouracil: phase I clinical pharmacological trials, Proc Am Assoc Cancer Res, 22:192 (1981).

2. H. W. Bruckner, J. Roboz, M. Spigelman, E. Ambinder, R. Hart, and J. F. Holland, An efficient leucovorin-5-fluorouracil sequence: dosage escalation and pharmacologic monitoring, in: "Advances in cancer chemotherapy. The current status of 5-fluorouracil-leucovorin calcium combination," H. W. Bruckner, J. Rustum, eds., Park Row Publishers, New York (1984)

3. H. W. Bruckner and M. K. Spigelman. Leucovorin as a clinical potentiator of 5-fluorouracil. Toxicity and anticancer efficacy, Mount Sinai J Med (1988). In Press

4. H. W. Bruckner, J. Crown, A. McKenna, and R. Hart, Leucovorin and 5-fluorouracil as a treatment for disseminated cancer of the pancreas and unknown primary tumors, Cancer Res (1988). In Press

5. H. W. Bruckner, J. Cohen, MTX/5-FU trials in gastrointestinal and other cancers, Sem Oncol, 10:32 (1983).

6. H. W. Bruckner, and D. M. Stablein for the Gastrointestinal Tumor Study Group, A randomized study of 5-
   fluorouracil and doxorubicin with semustine, cis-platin,
   or triazinate for treatment of advanced gastric cancer.
   Proc Am Soc Clin Oncol, 5:90 (1986).

7. H. W. Bruckner, Gastric cancer trials: implications of the
   gastrointestinal tumor study group and the Mount Sinai
   Medical Center experience, in: Gastric Carcinoma
   Workshop, Utopia Medical Publications, Inc., New
   Isenburg, (1988), In Press

8. D. V. Santi, A biochemical rationale for the use of 5-FU
   in combination with leucovorin, In: Advances in cancer
   chemotherapy: the current status of 5-FU-leucovorin
   calcium combination, H. W. Bruckner and Y. M. Rustum,
   eds., Park Row Publishers, Inc., New York (1984)

9. H. W. Bruckner, M. Rubinoff, and S. Waxman, Limited effectiveness of in vitro high-dose methotrexate and
   leucovorin to overcome resistance in L1210 leukemia
   cells with elevations of dihydrofolate reductase, Europ
   J Cancer, 16:1057 (1980).

10. R. G. Moran, P. V. Danenberg, and C. Heidelberger C,
    Therapeutic response of leukemic mice treated with fluo-
    rinated pyrimidines and inhibitors of deoxyuridylate
    synthesis, Bioch Pharmacol, 31:2929 (1982)

11. H. W. Bruckner, R. Hart, M. Spigelman, E. Feuer, J. F. and
    Holland, An intermittent leucovorin-5-fluorouracil
    regimen for advanced adenocarcinoma of the colon, Proc
    Am Assoc Cancer Res, 28:202 (1987)

12. H. W. Bruckner, N. J. Petrelli, D. Stablein, R. Mayer, J.
    Novak, and the Gastrointestinal Tumor Study Group,
    Comparison of unique leucovorin and "maximum" dosage
    strategies. Natl Cancer Inst Monqr, 5:179 (1987)

13. N. Petrelli, D. Stablein, H. Bruckner, A. Megibow, R.
    Mayer and H. Douglass, A prospective randomized phase
    III trial of 5-fluorouracil (5FU) versus 5FU + high-dose
    leucovorin versus 5-FU + low-dose leucovorin in patients
    with metastatic colorectal adenocarcinomas. Proc Am Soc
    Clin Oncol, 7:94 (1988).

14. P. Preusser, H. Wilke, W. Achterrath, U. Fink, J. Meyer,
    U. Schmitz-Hubner, and H. Bunte, Advanced gastric carci-
    noma: a phase II study with etoposide, adriamycin and
    split course cisplatin (EAP), Proc Am Soc Clin Oncol
    6:75 (1987)

15. J. Wils, H. Bleiberg, O. Dalesio, G. Blijham, N. Mulder,
    A. Planting, T. Splinter, and N. Duez, An EORTC gastro-
    intestinal group evaluation of the combination of
    sequential methotrexate and 5-fluorouracil, combined
    with adriamycin in advanced measurable gastric cancer, J
    Clin Oncol, 4:1799 (1986).

DISCUSSION OF DR. BRUCKNER'S PRESENTATION

Dr. O'Connell: Those are really impressive numbers for both the
   gastric and pancreatic cancer. I was wondering, are these all
   advanced metastatic patients with pancreatic and gastric cancer or
   did you include locally advanced patients?

Dr. Bruckner: These are big tumors and metastatic. Obviously this
   is something that needs to be confirmed as a first step. Numbers
   are small but the quality of some of these responses is unlike what
   we've seen before and that just mirrors what other people told you
   earlier today. We have complete responses and that deserves attention.

HIGH-DOSE WEEKLY ORAL LEUCOVORIN AND 5-FLUOROURACIL IN PREVIOUSLY UNTREATED PATIENTS WITH ADVANCED COLORECTAL CARCINOMA: A PHASE I STUDY

John D. Hines, David J. Adelstein, Jeffrey L.
Spiess, Susan Gear Carter, and Joan E. Trey

Cleveland Metropolitan General Hospital
3395 Scranton Road
Cleveland, Ohio 44109

INTRODUCTION

Chemotherapy has remained the major treatment modality for patients with metastatic or recurrent colorectal carcinoma. The chemotherapeutic agent, 5-fluorouracil (FUra), has been the "standard" therapy for a number of years. The objective response rate for this single agent has been disappointing with most series reporting response rates between 12 and 20%. Recent studies involving intracellular pharmacokinetics of FUra have provided information concerning mechanisms which lead to cellular resistance to the active metabolite, FdUMP, which binds to intracellular thymidylate synthetase (TS). A number of recent studies have now been performed which suggest that increased levels of intracellular reduced folate analogs can overcome intracellular drug resistance to FdUMP.

A number of Phase I-II trials of different schedules of FUra and leucovorin have now been published (1). Hines, et al (2) employed the R.P.M.I. dosage schedule using 500 mg/m^2 IV leucovorin and 600 mg/m^2 of IV FUra weekly for six weeks in 27 refractory and 4 previously untreated patients with advanced colorectal cancer. The combined CR-PR rate for this patient cohort was 45% with acceptable toxicity (2).

One potential disadvantage of IV administration of leucovorin is the rapid increase in the concentration of the d-isomer. Oral administration of leucovorin offers the advantage that little of the d-isomer is absorbed, with a selective preferential absorption of the "active" l-isomer. An additional advantage of administration of oral leucovorin is that the l-isomer is rapidly converted to $5-CH_3H_4PteGlu$, the predominant reduced folate analog in cells. Bioavailability of oral leucovorin is nearly 100% at doses of 25-30 mg (3). At higher doses, bioavailability decreases to 80% for 40 mg, 60% for 60 mg, but appears to reach a plateau of 30% for higher oral doses. Although bioavailability decreases, the area under the curve (AUC) for total reduced folate continues to increase in serum as a function of higher oral doses. Hines, et al (4) recently reported on the bioavailability of high dose oral leucovorin at doses from 400 mg to 1600 mg administered at equally split doses from 0 to 3 hours. Based on the serum levels and the AUC data, we initiated the following Phase I clinical trial employing 500 mg/m^2 of oral leucovorin administered in equal split dose regimens of FUra. The first was FUra at 450 mg/m^2 and the second was 600 mg/m^2 administered as an IV bolus at the 5th hour following the start of oral leucovorin ingestion. This schedule was repeated weekly x 6 with a two week rest period and was then reinstituted.

MATERIALS AND METHODS

From February 1, 1986 through November 1, 1987 a total of 34 patients were entered on this study. The first six patients entering this study received FUra at a dose of 450 mg/m²/week and the remainder of the patients received 600 mg/m²/week. All patients received leucovorin at the 500 mg/m² dosage schedule. A total of thirty evaluable patients comprise this report. The patient characteristics are summarized in Table 1. Serial serum levels were prepared for analysis of 5-CHO-H₄PteGlu and total reduced folate, but these results are not yet complete and will not be discussed in this report. None of these patients had received prior chemotherapy although 8 had received prior radiation therapy. All patients had objectively measurable disease that included precisely defined palpable tumor or parenchymal lesions that could be defined by imaging procedures (chest x-ray, endoscopy, computerized tomography [CT], ultrasongraphy, or radionuclide scan). Neither serosal effusions nor abnormal accessory laboratory tests (including CEA) were considered measurable disease. All 30 patients had a blood CEA determination prior to and after each six week treatment cycle. Prior to each weekly treatment, all patients had a complete physical examination and a complete blood count. Biochemical monitoring of hepatic and renal function were performed every two weeks. Response was determined quantitatively after each treatment cycle using all of the appropriate imaging and radionuclide procedures. Response was graded as a CR when all measurable disease had been eradicated, PR when there was a reduction in the sum of the products of the largest perpendicular diameters of all measurable lesions by >50% of the pretreatment value, and stable disease when a <50% reduction occurred or no further disease progression could be detected for 2 or more cycles of therapy.

Table 1. Patient Characteristics
Evaluable N = 30

1. 17 Male   13 Female
2. Median age 60. 5 yr (24-76)
3. All previously untreated (FUra)
4. 8 prior R.T.
5. Site of Metastatic Disease
     Liver only   12
     Lung only   4
     Liver and other   11
     Other sites   3

RESULTS

All 30 patients were evaluable for response. Five (17%) achieved a CR. Four of the five had documented pulmonary metastases. One patient achieved a CR after one 6 week cycle of therapy whereas 4 achieved a CR after two full cycles of therapy. Eight (27%) achieved a PR, 3 after one cycle and 5 after 2 cycles of therapy. Seven (23%) achieved stable disease after one cycle of therapy. Disease progression was documented in 10 patients during or after one cycle of therapy. The overall response rate for this regimen was 44%.

Thus far, the median disease-free survival for the CR patients is 19.8 months (9-28.5) and for the PR patients 11.5 months (5.5-16.5). The median time to progression for those patients with stable disease was 8.7 months (5.5-11.7). The median survival for the CR patients is 26.7+ months and for the PR patients 16.5 months (7.5-22). The median survival for those patients with stable disease was 9.5 months and in patients with disease progression 5.5 months.

The toxicity was graded according to the Eastern Cooperative Oncology Group and is summarized in Table 2. The predominant toxicity occurring with this regimen was diarrhea which ranged from grade I (43%), and grade II (20%) to grade III (7%). Two patients with grade III toxicity required hospitalization for IV hydration. However, no treatment related deaths occurred. All 30 patients completed the first six week cycle of therapy without any dose reduction of the FUra.

Table 2. Toxicity – E.C.O.G. Grade No. and (Percent)

Type	0	I	II	III	IV
GI:					
Nausea & Vomiting	19(63)	3(10)	8(26)	–	–
Diarrhea	9(30)	13(43)	6(20)	2(7)	–
Lacrymal	14(47)	16(53)	–	–	–
Cutaneous	20(67)	6(20)	4(13)	–	–
Mucositis	19(63)	8(27)	3(10)	–	–
Myelosuppression	27(90)	3(10)	–	–	–

Other toxicities included a mild degree of nausea and vomiting (36%), excess lacrymal secretion (53%), cutaneous erythemia (33%), mucositis (37%), and minimal myelosuppression (10%). Aside from the two patients requiring hospitalization, no patients encountered any weight loss exceeding 5% of pretreatment weight.

Pretreatment CEA levels exceeded 60 units in all 30 patients. The serum CEA levels returned to normal in all 5 CR patients and to either normal or significantly lower levels in the 8 PR patients. In those 7 patients with stable disease, the serum CEA decreased significantly in 5, with 2 patients exhibiting no change. The serum CEA was an excellent predictor of disease progression, increasing significantly in all but one patient at or prior to disease progression. The CEA levels continued to increase in all the patients exhibiting disease progression.

DISCUSSION

In most large clinical trials which have been conducted employing FUra as a single agent for treatment of advanced colorectal carcinoma, the overall response rate has been less than 20%.

Initial clinical trials that used FUra combined with leucovorin in treatment of advanced colorectal cancer were performed by Bruckner et al (5,6). These early trials provided evidence indicating that administration of low dose leucovorin resulted in increased therapeutic utility of FUra. Machover, et al (7) published an update of 86 patients with advanced colorectal carcinoma where the leucovorin was administered at 200 mg/m^2 IV bolus for 5 consecutive days in combination with IV FUra (340–400 mg/m^2). Grem, et al (1) have recently published an excellent review of all of the current Phase I-II and III clinical trials that have been published or are still ongoing. The majority of these trials have demonstrated that low or high doses of leucovorin potentiate the clinical effectiveness of FUra in the treatment of advanced colorectal carcinoma.

At the present time the major unanswered questions are: 1) what is the optimal dosage of leucovorin and FUra and, 2) what is the optimal schedule and route of administration of leucovorin when co-administered with FUra.

The results of our Phase I trial demonstrate that oral high-dose leucovorin with weekly bolus FUra yields results that are comparable to our previous published study employing IV high dose leucovorin (500 mg/m^2/ week) with bolus FUra at the same dosage (2). Two potential advantages can be realized with this high-dose oral leucovorin schedule. The first is that the l-isomer ("natural" isomer) is preferentially absorbed over the d-isomer. The second is the prolonged elevation of total reduced folate concentrations that are observed in serial serum samples (3).

It is our opinion that these treatment results warrant a randomized Phase III trial of high-dose oral leucovorin vs. high-dose IV leucovorin coadministered with FUra in the treatment of advanced colorectal carcinoma.

ACKNOWLEDGEMENT

The authors wish to thank Mr. Paul Giroski for his expert technical assistance and Ms. Anne Lagania for secretarial assistance.

REFERENCES

1. J. Grem, D. Hoth, J.M. Hamilton, Overview of current status and future directions of clinical trials with 5-fluorouracil in combination with folinic acid, Cancer Treat. Rep. 12:1249-1264 (1987).

2. J.D. Hines, M. Zakem, D.J. Adelstein, et al, Treatment of advanced stage colorectal adenocarcinoma with fluorouracil and high-dose leucovorin calcium: A Pilot Study, J. Clin Oncol. 6:142-146 (1988).

3. J.A. Straw, D. Szapary, W.T. Wynn, Pharmacokinetcis of the diastereo isomers of leucovorin after intravenous and oral administration to normal subjects, Cancer Res. 44:3114-3119 (1984).

4. J.D. Hines, M. Zakem, D.J. Adelstein, et al, Bioavailability of high-dose oral leucovorin, Development of folates and folate antagonists in cancer chemotherapy, N.C.I. Monographs 5:57-60 (1987).

5. H.W. Bruckner, T. Ohnuma, R. Hart, et al, Leucovorin potentiation of 5-fluorouracil, efficacy and potency, Proc. Assoc. Cancer Res. 23:434 (1982).

6. H.W. Bruckner, J. Roboz, M. Spiegelman, et al, An efficient leucovorin and 5-fluorouracil sequence dosage escalation and pharmacologic monitoring, Proc. Am. Assoc. Cancer Res. 24:547 (1982).

7. D. Machover, E. Goldschmidt, P. Chollet, et al, Treatment of advanced colorectal and gastric adenocarcinoma with 5-fluorouracil and high-dose folinic acid. J. Clin. Oncol. 4:685-696 (1986).

DISCUSSION OF DR. HINE'S PRESENTATION

Dr. O'Connell: It was very interesting that you have 5 patients that had complete responses. Certainly in our series of patients we had some 111 patients and only had a handful of patients that had complete regression of indicator lesions. How did you stage these patients? Was it just that the indicator lesion went away completely?

Dr. Hines: Four of the 5 were patients with pulmonary metstases with rectal cancer and I think Dr. Madajewicz might want to refer to this in his data. We did MRI, CT scan and needle biopsy on 2 patients where we thought there was residual disease. Interestingly only 1 of the 5 has had an overt relapse; the rest, as far as we're aware, are still in remission. We check them every 2 months now. We used MRI's for all abdomen and chest lesions in addition to CT scanning. The one patient with a hepatic metastasis which we felt was a partial, we called the patient a partial, and we went ahead because he developed some adhesions which had to be operated on. The surgeon went in and rebiopsied extensively where we felt we had a lesion and there was no lesion. That patient's out about 36 months.

Dr. O'Connell: So there are 5 patients, 4 had pulmonary disease and 1 was hepatic?

Dr. Hines: Four were lung and 1 was liver.

Dr. Arbuck: While we all hope that the data that you showed in the patients who had failed on FUra alone holds up, I want to point out that there was a lot of delight initially with the Roswell Park study where 6 of 12 previously treated patients responded and we thought that this was a great salvage regimen. In reviewing the data about a year ago, predominantly in the Phase II trials, there was about a 12% response rate so I just issue that caution.

Dr. Hines: I quite agree, Susan. I just thought that since I had the data I'd give it.

Dr. Pinedo: It was nice to see that you had some responses in previously treated patients. We have done a phase II study in previously treated patients, but we used the lower 200 mg/m^2 CF and we observed no responses. Perhaps the dose of CF for pretreated patients may be quite important and may be different for non-pretreated patients.

Dr. Moran: Just to restate some of the obvious facets of the advantages of your oral technique. You're not going to have much in the way of 6R-CF getting across, maybe 5-10% at maximum. The way you are giving this, allowing the curve to come back down again then giving another oral dose, you are simulating an i.v. infusion that is going to keep the levels up for a substantial period of time. I just think it is a super idea.

Dr. Hines: Exactly. I mentioned that we have actually done a prospective study of six patients where we have loaded them with that
same oral dose the night before their primary colorectal surgery.
The total reduced folate pool, that we have analyzed in the 6,
ranges from 0.96 to almost 3.2 ?M at 12 or 14 hr following the
administeration of the oral dose. Dr. Rustum currently has that
tissue in his freezer and he will analyze the TS value for us some
time.

Dr. P. Houghton: My colleague Siebold Graff has been working with
intravenous infusions of 5-methyltetrahydrofolate which is
predominently what you are going to have in the plasma. In mice it
causes lachrymal symptoms whereas CF doesn't.

A CONTROLLED CLINICAL TRIAL INCLUDING FOLINIC ACID AT TWO DISTINCT DOSE
LEVELS IN COMBINATION WITH 5-FLUOROURACIL (5FU) FOR THE TREATMENT OF
ADVANCED COLORECTAL CANCER: EXPERIENCE OF THE MAYO CLINIC AND NORTH
CENTRAL CANCER TREATMENT GROUP*

Michael J. O'Connell

Mayo Clinic, Rochester, MN

ABSTRACT

A prospectively randomized clinical trial was conducted to determine
the therapeutic effect of five individual combination chemotherapy regimens
compared to single agent FUra for the treatment of advanced colorectal
cancer. For the purposes of this symposium, the detailed results of
therapy will be presented only for PTS treated with FUra alone or FUra +
LV* in a high dose (200 mg/m^2) or a low dose (20 mg/m^2) daily for five
days. Two hundred twelve PTS were randomized to one these three regimens,
and 208 PTS (98%) were available for analysis. Median time from
randomization is 18 months and approximately 70% of PTS have died. Both
LV* + FUra regimens are associated with significantly improved survival
compared to single agent FUra (p $\leq$ 0.03). In addition,
interval-to-tumor-progression, measurable tumor response rates, and
measures of quality of life (performance status, weight gain, symptomatic
relief) were also significantly improved with the addition of LV*. The
most favorable regimen in the trial is low dose LV* + FUra based on
considerations of both therapeutic results and cost. A national intergroup
trial will examine the efficacy of the low dose LV* + FUra regimen in the
surgical adjuvant setting.

INTRODUCTION

Past experience with the chemotherapy of advanced colorectal carcinoma
has met with limited success. The most widely studied agent, FUra, has
produced objective tumor responses in only 15%-20% of PTS. Furthermore,
there has been no evidence of improved PT survival. Any increase in tumor
response rates with a variety of combination chemotherapy regimens has
frequently been overshadowed by an increase in toxicity.

There is a great deal of current interest in exploiting the scientific
principles of biochemical modulation in the design of chemotherapy regimens
for the treatment of colorectal cancer. This report will focus on the use
of LV* to enhance the activity of FUra. Previous papers presented at this
symposium have outlined the laboratory rationale for the use of these two
agents in combination: enhancement of the ability of FUra to inhibit TS by
increasing the amount of covalent ternary complex formed as a result of

---

*Statistical Analysis Performed by Harry S. Wieand, Ph.D.

increasing the intracellular levels of reduced folates. The optimal amount of LV* to enhance FUra cytotoxicity is not clearly known since some laboratory investigations suggest a concentration of 1 μM is sufficient (1) whereas other studies have suggested optimal FUra cytotoxicity with total LV* concentrations of 20 μM (2). These studies, therefore, provide a preclinical rationale for the use of LV* doses ranging from as low as 10-20 mg/m^2 to as high as 150-600 mg/m^2.

We have conducted a controlled clinical trial designed in part to determine whether the addition of LV* at two distinct dose levels (20 mg/m^2 and 200 mg/m^2 respectively) can enhance the therapeutic activity of FUra compared to the use of FUra as a single agent. Three other chemotherapy regimens were also studied in this trial (FUra + cisplatin, FUra + high dose MTX with LV* rescue, and FUra + low dose MTX). The full details of our overall trial have been submitted for publication (3). This paper will review our controlled experience with LV*/FUra as part of this symposium on the expanding role of folates and fluoropyrimidines in cancer chemotherapy.

MATERIALS AND METHODS

PT Eligibility

All PTS were required to have histological or cytological confirmation of unresectable metastatic colorectal cancer, with the site of origin confirmed radiologically or surgically to be in the large bowel. The single exception to the requirement for tissue proof was in the PT with previous histologic confirmation of a primary colorectal cancer and a radiographic diagnosis of pulmonary metastasis with no other tumor area accessible to biopsy. Under these circumstances two or more nodular lesions on chest x-ray which had either newly appeared or increased in size at least 25% were required. PTS who were classified as having measurable disease had a known tumor mass that could be clearly measured on physical examination or x-ray. Malignant hepatomegaly was employed as a measurable lesion if the liver edge extended at least 5 cm below the costal margin on quiet respiration, or if there was a defect on CT scan or radionuclide liver scan measuring at least 5 cm in greatest diameter. All PTS were ambulatory and maintaining an oral intake of $\geq$ 1200 calories per day. PTS with any of the following conditions were excluded from study: white blood count < 4,000 cells/mm^3, platelet count < 130,000 cells/mm^3, any elevation of serum creatinine (unless creatinine clearance was documented to be greater than 75 cc/minute), any prior chemotherapy, recent major surgery, radiation to the axial skeleton in the previous four weeks, signifiant third space fluid accumulation, congestive heart failure or medical condition which would preclude IV hydration as stipulated by protocol, or other concurrent cancers.

Randomization Procedures

PTS were stratified according to performance status using the ECOG scale (0, fully active to 4, totally disabled), anatomic sites of metastatic disease, and institution. PTS were then randomized to one of the six chemotherapy regimens. The chemotherapy administration schedules for the FUra alone control and the two LV*/FUra regimens are indicated below:

1. FUra alone - FUra is given by rapid IV push at 500 mg/m^2 for five consecutive days with courses repeated every five weeks.

2. FUra + high dose LV* - LV*† was given at 200 mg/m^2 immediately
    followed by FUra at 370 mg/m^2. Both drugs were given by rapid IV
    injection daily for five consecutive days. Courses were repeated at
    four weeks, eight weeks, and every five weeks thereafter.

3. FUra + low dose LV* - LV*† was given at 20 mg/m^2/day immediately
    followed by FUra at 370 mg/m^2/day. Both drugs were given by rapid IV
    injection daily for five consecutive days. Courses were repeated at
    four weeks, eight weeks, and every five weeks thereafter.

When toxicity patterns were analyzed following treatment of the first
100 PTS on the overall protocol, the starting FUra dose was increased to
425 mg/m^2/day for five consecutive days in the low dose LV*/ FUra regimen.
Throughout the duration of the study, escalations of FUra by 10% were
allowed in the event that no myelosuppression nor significant
nonhematologic toxicity was documented on the preceding cycle of
chemotherapy. The intent was to escalate the FUra dose to produce definite
but clinically tolerable and essentially comparable toxicity for each of
the chemotherapy regimens.

Response Criteria for PTS with Measurable Disease

Complete response required total disappearance of all tumor initially
observed with no evidence of new areas of malignant disease. PR required >
50% reduction in the sum of the products of the longest perpendicular
diameters of all measurable indicator lesions or > 30% decrease in the sum
of liver measurements below the costal margin with no new lesions
appearing. Transient tumor regressions lasting less than eight weeks were
excluded.

Criteria for Evaluation of Palliative Effect

PTS were evaluable for assessment of improvement in performance status
if the pretreatment performance status was impaired to some degree (i.e.,
ECOG performance status 1, 2, or 3). Likewise, PTS were evaluable for
symptomatic improvement if there were definite pretreatment symptoms
attributable to malignant disease.

Statistical Considerations

The Pearson's chi-square statistic was used for toxicity and response
comparisons. The survival curves were generated using the Kaplan-Meier
method. When p - values are shown for survival comparisons of treatment
arms, the p values were obtained using the log-rank statistic. When
survival, response, or palliative effect comparisons are presented for the
FUra regimen vs. a combined therapy regimen, the p values are one-sided.
Two-sided values are given for toxicity comparisons.

RESULTS

Administrative Data

Seventy PTS were randomized to FUra alone, 69 PTS to FUra + high dose
LV*, and 73 PTS to FUra + low dose LV*. Two hundred and eight of these 212
PTS (98%) were properly entered, eligible, and received chemotherapy
according to protocol, and were therefore included in the analysis.

---

† Supplied by Lederle Laboratories, Division of American Cyanamid

TABLE 1

Patient Characteristics According to Treatment Arm

% of Patients

Characteristics	5FU Alone (N=70)	5FU + High LV (N=68)	5FU + Low LV (N=70)
Male	54	66	53
Age, yr			
< 50	19	13	·17
50-69	64	65	64
≥ 70	17	22	19
Performance Score*			
0	34	31	33
1	50	56	51
2-3	16	13	16
Symptomatic	54	51	54
Measurable Disease			
Liver	24	26	27
Lung	26	18	17
Other	6	9	9
Total Measurable	56	53	53
Grade of Anaplasia†			
1-2	71	79	75
3-4	29	21	25

*   ECOG Score, 0 fully ambulatory to 4, totally disabled

†   Broder's classification 1, well-differentiated, to 4, poorly-differentiated

Pretreatment PT Characteristics

PT characteristics are displayed in Table 1. The variables listed are distributed without significant differences between these three treatment arms. Slightly more than half of the PTS had definite symptoms attributed to malignant disease. A similar proportion had measurable malignant disease.

Interval to Tumor Progression

The interval to tumor progression according to treatment regimen is illustrated in Figure 1. Both the high and the low dose LV* + FUra regimens (p = 0.03 and 0.01 respectively) are superior to single agent FUra. None of the other regimens in the overall trial showed superiority to FUra alone.

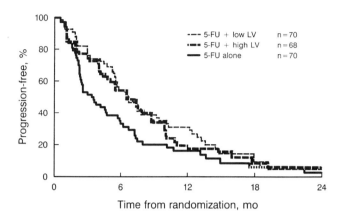

Figure 1

PT Survival

Approximately 70% of PTS have died. The median follow-up for PTS still alive is 11 months. There is a significant superiority for each of the LV* + FUra arms (p ≤ 0.03) compared to single agent FUra (see Figure 2). The high dose MTX with LV* rescue + FUra arm (not illustrated) showed borderline improvement (p < 0.06). The remaining treatment regimens did not show a significant survival advantage compared to FUra alone. Note that there is no significant survival difference between FUra + high dose LV* and FUra + low dose LV*.

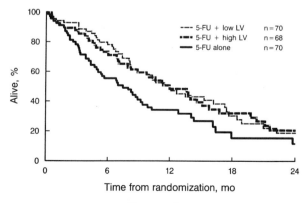

Figure 2

Objective Tumor Response

Figure 3 illustrates the objective tumor responses among the 111 PTS with measurable disease who were treated with FUra alone or FUra + LV*. FUra + low dose LV* was associated with the highest objective response rate (43%) and was significantly superior to FUra alone (p = 0.001). The FUra + high dose LV* regimen was also associated with an improved response rate compared to single agent FUra (p = 0.04). Of the other regimens tested, only FUra + low dose MTX showed an improved response rate compared to single agent FUra (26%, p = 0.04). The median time-to-progression among responding PTS was ten months, with no significant differences between treatment regimens.

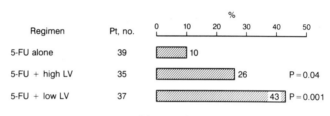

Figure 3

Palliative Effects

The impact of treatment on three measures of quality of life are summarized in Table 2. Of all regimens tested, only the FUra + low dose LV* regimen was associated with a significant improvement in each of the parameters of quality of life compared to FUra alone (p < 0.05).

Toxicity

As documented in Table 3, hematologic toxicity associated with LV* + FUra was significantly less than observed with FUra given alone. There was only one treatment-related death among PTS treated with FUra alone or in combination with LV*, and that PT received FUra + high dose LV*.

TABLE 2

Comparative Palliative Effect

	5FU Alone	5FU + High LV	5FU + Low LV
Improvement in Performance Status			
No. evaluable	46	44	48
% improved	13%	34%*	33%*
Weight Gain of 5% or More			
No. evaluable	70	68	70
% improved	14%	25%*	31%*
Improvement in Symptoms			
No. evaluable	38	42	36
% improved	34%	40%	69%*

* Significant improvement compared to 5-FU alone $P < 0.05$

TABLE 3

Hematologic Toxicity

	% of Patients		
	5FU Alone	5FU + High LV	5FU + Low LV
Leukopenia			
< 4,000/cu mm	93	71**	83
< 2,000/cu mm	48	19**	21**
Thrombocytopenia			
< 130,000/cu mm	32	19	28
< 50,000/cu mm	3	5	0

** Less frequent than with 5FU alone $p < 0.01$

TABLE 4

Non-Hematologic Toxicity

	% of Patients		
	5FU Alone	5FU + High LV	5FU + Low LV
Nausea			
Any	60	60	76
Severe	6	8	10
Vomiting			
Any	40	34	46
Severe	7	6	9
Diarrhea			
Any	43	61	64**
Severe	11	9	14
Stomatitis			
Any	58	76*	80*
Severe	16	30**	26**
Alopecia	37	40	34

More frequent than with 5FU alone   **p $<$ 0.05   *p $<$ 0.01

Table 4 displays nonhematologic toxicity. The dose-limiting effect associated with the LV* + FUra regimens was ulcerative stomatitis which was severe in 26%-30% of PTS. Severe diarrhea was not seen more frequently with the FUra + LV* compared to FUra alone. There were no deaths attributed to nonhematologic toxicity.

DISCUSSION

Our study demonstrates a definite therapeutic advantage for the LV* + FUra regimens compared to single agent FUra in the management of advanced colorectal cancer. The superiority of the LV*/FUra combinations is reflected consistently in this PT population by multiple parameters as indicated above. This benefit was observed to the greatest degree and most consistency with our low dose LV* + FUra regimen. We did not demonstrate any advantage for the use of LV* at a dose level ten times higher on this treatment schedule. From a practical standpoint, the issue of LV* dose is of more than academic concern in view of the high cost of this agent.

Although not illustrated in this paper, it is possible that our high dose MTX with LV* rescue + FUra regimen may also improve survival, but this advantage was not statistically significant and was not as great as that observed with either of the LV* + FUra regimens. Neither low dose MTX + FUra nor FUra + cisplatin provided any substantial advantage to the use of single agent FUra. The full details of these comparisons are given elsewhere (3). In conclusion, available data from our study and those of others reviewed elsewhere at this symposium indicate that therapy with combined LV*/FUra represents an authentic improvement in the treatment of advanced colorectal cancer. It should be recognized that the magnitude of this improvement in PTS with advanced disease is only moderate. These results do, however, provide a strong scientific rationale for controlled studies of LV*/FUra combination regimens as adjuvant therapy following surgical resection of primary colorectal cancer where such treatments may have the potential to produce a much more substantial effect on long-term survival or cure. Based upon considerations of cost, toxicity, and advanced disease survival benefit, our low dose LV* + FUra regimen would seem to be the most attractive for such studies.

REFERENCES

1. K. Keyomarsi and R. G. Moran: Folinic acid augmentation of the effects of fluoropyrimidines on murine and human leukemic cells. Cancer Res 46:5229-5235, 1986.

2. Y. M. Rustum, F. Trave, and S. F. Zakrzewski, et al: Biochemical and pharmacologic basis for potentiation of 5-fluorouracil action by leucovorin. NCI Monograph 5:165-170, 1987.

3. M. A. Poon, M. J. O'Connell, C. G. Moertel, et al: Biochemical modulation of fluorouracil: Evidence of significant improvement of survival and quality of life in advanced colorectal carcinoma. Submitted for publication April 1988.

DISCUSSION OF DR. O'CONNELL'S PRESENTATION

Dr. Rustum: Have you made the calculation of the total dose of FUra given to the patient per arm and the total dose of CF you were able to administer to these patients? The high dose versus low dose versus FUra alone.

Dr. O'Connell: We haven't done that specific analysis. We did allow a 10% escalation of FUra dose in any of the arms of the trial in the absence of toxicity. It turns out that most patients treated with the 500 mg/m^2 dose level of FUra alone had stomatitis, diarrhea, or leucopenia; a few of those patients were able to have a substantial escalation. The CF doses were kept constant regardless of toxicity and so, for example, if a patient developed severe stomatitis, we would continue CF at the 200 mg/m^2 dose level but simply reduce the FUra dose.

Dr. Rustum: Was there a difference in each arm in the number of courses the patients received?

Dr. O'Connell: I haven't specifically analyzed number of courses. I would suspect that the answer is yes because patients treated with FUra progressed at an early stage compared to those with FUra/CF. I didn't mention that the overall median survival for patients treated with FUra alone was 6 months and for FUra/CF was 13 months. I am sure that if we were to do the analysis you asked about we would find that there were fewer courses on the average of FUra administered.

Dr. Erlichman: I believe in the low-dose arm you used a higher dose of FUra than in the high-dose arm, is that correct?

Dr. O'Connell: We started with the same dose, 370/m^2 of FUra but found that we were seeing minimal toxicity when we gave the 20 mg/m^2 CF dose with it. So after the accrual of the first 100 patients in the study, we analyzed toxicity patterns; at that point we found we could escalate to 425 mg/m^2 of FUra and found at that dose, that that was an equitoxic regimen compared to 370 of FUra combined with 200 of CF.

Dr. Erlichman: Do you think that, and this is obviously speculation, that that may be a factor in terms of equalizing the effects that you have seen in the 2 arms, that is a somewhat higher dose of FUra with a lower dose of CF, may be as good as a higher dose of CF with a slightly lower dose of FUra?

Dr. O'Connell: That would be my interpretation, yes.

Dr. Houghton: Can you tell us something about the plasma levels of L-leucovorin that are achieved in each arm?

Dr. O'Connell: We have not yet performed the pharmacokinetic assays but have sampled a group of 12 patients, 6 receiving high dose CF, 6 receiving a low dose and those analyses are being conducted at the present time. I'm sorry that I cannot share those with you right now.

Dr. Wittes: The point that Chuck Ehrlichman just made is really a key
point. When you make the conclusion that there is no evidence that
200 mg of CF, is any better than 20 mg of CF, it would be important
to include the proviso that there was a dose difference of FUra in
the 2 arms.

Dr. O'Connell: Agree.

Dr. Wittes: Can you tell us about how many patients had grade 3 or
worse toxicity of any kind, by arm? It's obviously difficult when
you're comparing toxicities if the toxicities are qualitatively
different as they are here between the arms.

Dr. O'Connell: Yes. Again, I have to give you this sort of off the
cuff. For the CF regimens, about 30% of patients that had severe
stomatitis. Approximately 15% of patients had severe diarrhea but
some of those in that subset may have had both nonhematologic
toxicities so that we're probably dealing with a 35-40% overall
severe nonhematologic toxicity rate. The incidence of leucopenia
with white counts below 2000 was also in the 15% range. So my
estimate would be that in the range of 40-50% of patients treated
with a high dose CF or low dose CF and FUra combinations had grade 3
or higher toxicity.

Dr. Wittes: And for the FUra alone?

Dr. O'Connell: For FUra alone, 50% of patients had a white count
nadir below 2000 to start out with, so half of that group had what
we would consider grade 3 or higher hematologic toxicity. Only
10-15% had significant diarrhea or stomatitis. I would say though
that there would be a slightly higher proportion of patients with
grade 3 or higher toxicity in the FUra alone group, probably in the
range of 60%. The control was at least as toxic if not somewhat
more toxic than the FUra/CF combinations.

Dr. Budd: In the toxicity slide you showed us for the low dose CF arm,
is that all the patients or were those the patients entered after
100?

Dr. O'Connell: That was all patients combined and therefore the
patients treated with 425 mg/m^2 of FUra plus CF had a higher rate
of ulcerative stomatitis than those in the cohort from the initial
group of patients. So those were combined statistics.

184

5-FLUOROURACIL (FUra) AND FOLINIC ACID (FA) THERAPY IN PATIENTS WITH
COLORECTAL CANCER

Charles Erlichman

Department of Medicine, Princess Margaret Hospital
Associate Professor of Medicine and Pharmacology
University of Toronto
NCI of Canada Colorectal Subcommittee

INTRODUCTION

Colorectal cancer is the third most common cancer in North America today
(1). Whereas surgery is the mainstay of primary therapy for this disease,
it cures on average only 50% of all patients who develop this disease(2).
The impact of surgery is greatest at the early stages of this cancer. When
the tumour has penetrated to serosa or metastasized to local or distant sites
the probability of cure with surgery alone is decreased markedly. In
attempts to improve the prognosis for patients in this latter category, new
therapies are constantly tested in the metastatic setting(3) and some are investigated in the adjuvant setting(4). We have performed a randomized trial
comparing FUra to FUra and FA in patients with previously untreated metastatic colorectal cancer(5). I will describe this study and an ongoing trial
of this combination in the adjuvant treatment of patients who have undergone
curative resection of the colon.

MATERIALS AND METHODS

Patients referred to the Princess Margaret Hospital and the Tom Baker
Cancer Centre with the diagnosis of metastatic colorectal cancer from March
1984 to March 1986 were considered for the trial. The study design is shown
in figure 1.

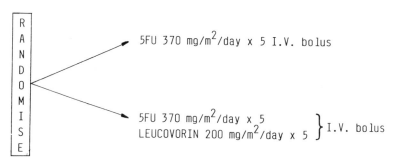

TREATMENT REPEATED EVERY 28 DAYS

FIGURE 1

Patients who met the eligibility criteria (table 1) were randomized to
receive FUra or FUra and FA at the starting doses shown in figure 1.
The dose of FUra was adjusted in subsequent courses to achieve equitoxicity
in both arms. The study outcomes were response rates, survival and toxicity.
Response was defined as partial or complete response using the standard
criteria and had to be of 8 weeks duration. Minor responses were considered
no response for the purposes of the study analysis. All radiological
responses were determined by one of two radiologists who were blinded to
treatment arm allocation of the patient entered. Survival status was
determined as status at last follow-up in March 1987. Toxicity endpoints
were mucositis, diarrhea and myelosuppression. The scales for mucositis
grade and diarrhea are shown in table 2. Myelosuppression was defined by
neutrophil and platelet nadir. The chi-square test was used to compare
response rates and the Fisher exact test was used to compare toxicity
between the two arms. Survival and time to disease progression curves
were constructed according to the method of Kaplan and Meier. Log rank
analysis was used to compare survival times and time to progression curves
for the two therapies.

Table 1. PATIENT ELIGIBILITY CRITERIA

1. Biopsy proven colorectal cancer
2. Measurable metastatic or recurrent disease
3. ECOG status 0, 1, 2
4. Life expectancy > 8 weeks
5. Serum bilirubin < 2 mg%
6. No cerebral metastases or CNS disorders
7. No prior chemotherapy

Table 2. TOXICITY SCALES

STOMATITIS

0 - No oral pain or mouth ulcers
1+ - Pain present with no ulceration
2+ - Ulceration present but able to eat
3+ - Any degree of ulceration where patient is unable to eat

GASTROINTESTINAL

0 - No nausea, vomiting, diarrhea or change of appetite
1+ - Mild nausea, 4 bowel movements per day, mild anorexia
2+ - Nausea and vomiting requiring antiemetics, 4 bowel
     movements per day, nocturnal diarrhea
3+ - Any above with guaiac positive stools

CO.3 is a National Cancer Institute of Canada Clinical Trials Group study
designed to determine whether adjuvant therapy with FUra and FA is effective
in increasing survivorship and prolonging the disease-free interval in
patients undergoing curative resection of colonic adenocarcinoma. The
definition of a colon tumour is any tumour of the large bowel in which the
tumour does not extend below the peritoneal reflection. The study design
is shown in figure 2.

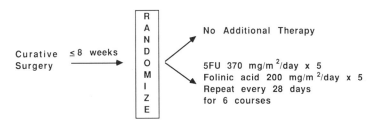

FIGURE 2

Patients who meet the eligibility criteria are randomized to no further therapy or 6 cycles of FUra 370 mg/m^2/day x 5 and FA 200 mg/m^2/day x 5. Patients who are randomized to therapy receive a mouthwash consisting of allopurinol 1 mg/ml with which to rinse and cover their lips at time 0, 1, 2 and 3 hours after the FUra is given on each treatment day. Eligibility criteria are as follows: 1) complete resection of primary tumour; 2) patient consent; 3) WBC $>$4 x 10^9/L and platelets $>$100 x 10^9/L; 4) serum creatinine $<$ 150 umol/L and bilirubin $<$35 umol/L; 5) performance status 0, 1, 2, (ECOG scale); 6) tumour stage $T_1N_{1,2}$, $T_2N_{1,2}$, T_3N_{0-2}; 7) randomization within 8 weeks of surgery. T_1 lesions invade the submucosa, T_2 lesions invade the muscularis propria, and T_3 lesions invade through the muscularis propria penetrating the subserosa or into nonperitonealized pericolic tissues. N_0 means no nodal involvement, N_1 indicates 1 to 4 positive nodes and N_2 signifies 5 or more positive nodes. Patients who present with intestinal obstruction treated with a prior or concomitant colostomy are eligible as are patients whose tumours involved adjacent stuctures by direct extension pro-vided an en bloc resection could be effected for cure. Study endpoints are survival, disease-free interval and toxicity. WHO criteria are used to grade toxicities.

RESULTS

One hundred and thirty patients with metastatic recurrent colorectal carcinoma and measureable lesions were randomized on the trial of patients with metastatic disease. Five were inevaluable, 61 received FUra and 64 received FUra and FA. The patients were balanced for 11 clinical character-istics including age, sex, performance status, weight loss, time to first recurrence, serum albumin, serum alkaline phosphatase, serum SGOT, serum LDH and site of disease (5).

The mean dose of FUra in the control arm was 425 mg/m^2/day and was 370 mg/m^2/day in the combination arm. The dose-limiting toxicity was oral mucositis and diarrhea. These were significantly greater on the first course of therapy in the FUra and FA arm as compared to the control but became equivalent as the doses of FUra were adjusted on subsequent courses. The frequency of grade 2 and 3 stomatitis was 18.2% and 0.06% of 325 courses of the combination administered. The frequency of grade 2 and 3 diarrhea was 22.8% and 0.02%. Neutropenia $<$1 x 10^9/L occurred in 22% of 262 cycles of FUra and FA. Platelet nadirs $<$100 x 10^9/L occurred in 3% of 264 cycles of the combination. Two episodes of febrile neutropenia requiring hospitaliza-tion occurred and one patient died during a period of thrombocytopenia. This death was secondary to an intra-abdominal hemorrhage which could not be controlled surgically. Alopecia, nausea and vomiting were minor toxicities and no neurotoxicity was observed. Four of 61 patients receiving FUra responded for a response rate of 7% (0-13%, 95% confidence limits) and 21 of 65 patients treated with FUra and FA achieved a response - response rate = 33% (22-45%, 95% confidence limits). The difference in response rate of 26% is significant at p 0.005. The median time to progression was 2.9 months for the control arm and 5.1 months for the combination. This was significant (p= 0.023). The median survival for FUra therapy was 9.6 months and was 12.6 for FUra plus FA. The survival of patients receiving FUra plus FA was significantly greater than that of those receiving FUra alone (p= 0.05).

CO.3 has been open for 10 months and is currently accruing patients from participating centres across Canada. The study will continue to its accrual target of 400 evaluable patients. Two hundred patients per study arm are required to identify a 15% difference in survival between the two arms (α= 0.05, β= 0.01).

DISCUSSION

Our results indicate that FUra plus FA is superior to FU alone in causing tumour regression, increasing time to tumour progression and duration of survival. The development of the FUra plus FA combination is the first important advance in the management of patients with metastatic colorectal cancer since the introduction of FUra. The results of the study we have performed demonstrates that this treatment is superior to FUra alone. Although the incidence of stomatitis and diarrhea are increased when FUra and FA are combined, survival has been increased significantly also. This would indicate that the combination is a good first line therapy at this stage of the disease. Our study does not indicate whether the combination is useful in the management of patients who have had prior chemotherapy as all patients entered on the trial had not received prior chemotherapy. Since no complete responses were observed in the combination arm, we must consider this an initial step. These positive results do not eliminate the need for further improvements in therapy which may be in the form of changes in drug doses, different drug schedules or addition of other drugs or therapies to this combination.

The positive results which FUra and FA have achieved in the metastatic setting make this combination an attractive one to explore in the adjuvant setting. The National Cancer Institute of Canada Clinical Trials Group study - CO.3, is designed to determine its role in the setting of colon cancer. We have incorporated use of allopurinol mouthwash to minimize stomatitis. This technique was suggested by the results of previous studies of biochemical modulation(6) and one report of a small series of patients who received FUra alone(7). The results of this ongoing study will be important in defining FUra plus FA's role in early stage disease.

The development of a new therapy can be considered an important advance. But, the improvement raises many questions also. The reasons for resistance to the combination in patients with colorectal cancer must be sought. This may open new therapeutic leads to be explored in well designed and conducted clinical trials.

ACKNOWLEDGEMENT

Supported in part by the National Cancer Institute of Canada and Lederle Cyanamid, Canada.

REFERENCES

1. Silverberg, E., Lubera, J.A., 1968, Cancer Statistics 1988, Ca- A
    Cancer Journal for Clinicians, 38:5.

2. Surgarbaker, P., Gunderson, L.L., Wittes, R.E., 1985, Colorectal Cancer,
    in: Cancer Principles and Practices of Oncology, DeVita, V.T., Helleman,
    S., Rosenberg, S.A. ed. Lippincott Co., Toronto, 795-884.

3. Buroker, T.R., Moertel, C.G., Fleming, T.R. et al, 1985, A Controlled
    Evaluation of Recent Approaches to Biochemical Modulation or Enhancement
    of 5-fluorouracil therapy in Colorectal Carcinoma, J. Clin. Oncol. 3:1624.

4. Wolmark, N., Fisher, B., Rockette, H. et al, 1988, Post-operative adjuvant
    chemotherapy or BCG for colon cancer: results of NSABP protocol C-01, J.
    Natl. Cancer Inst., 80:30.

5. Erlichman, C., Fine, S., Wong, A., Elhakim, T., 1988, A Randomized Trial
    of Fluorouracil and Folinic Acid in Patients with Metastatic Colorectal
    Cancer, J. Clin. Oncol., 6:469.

6. Kroener, J.F., Saleh, F., Howell, S.B., 1982, 5-FU and Allopurinol:
    Toxicity Modulation and Phase II Results in Colon Cancer, Cancer Treat.
    Rep., 66:1133.

7. Clark, P.I., Slevin, M.L., 1985, Allopurinol mouthwashes and 5-fluoro-
    uracil induced oral toxicity, Europ. J. Surg. Oncol., 11:267.

DISCUSSION OF DR. ERLICHMAN'S PRESENTATION

Dr. Hudlen: The response rate of 7% for FUra is a little low by most oncology standards. Any comment on that?

Dr. Erlichman: I agree with you, but there are several points to be made. First of all, for studies done at our institution, 7% is the standard response rate for any chemotherapy for colon cancer, so it is not out of line with our previous experience. Secondly, response criteria were extremely strict and perhaps stricter than some centers might use. Thirdly, if you look at the confidence limits, the response rate could have been up to 13%. In fact, we have gone through another mathematical analysis in which we doubled the FUra response rate to 14%. Is the difference still significant? The answer is yes. The P-value obviously drops but it is still significant.

Dr. Hudlen: Regarding your FUra at dose escalation. You mentioned in the FUra-alone arm you escalated a number of patients. In the second arm was the FUra de-escalated when your CF was used?

Dr. Erlichman: I can't give you the exact number of patients that were escalated, but the majority of them were on the second course. For the FUra/CF arm very few, I think it was on the order of 3 patients, were escalated and they had to be de-escalated again so, in fact, we really couldn't get much above 370 with the combination. Some patients were de-escalated. The median dose of FUra over 10 courses for all patients, and of course patients are dropping out over that period of time, stayed at 370 mg/m^2.

Dr. Marsh: It is customary to include primaries from both colon and rectum in advanced disease and yet to separate them in adjuvant trials. Did you observe any difference in response rate between primaries originating in the rectum or the colon?

Dr. Erlichman: That is certainly an important question which we wanted to ask of our data. Unfortunately, if we separated the rectals and colons into the 2 arms, the numbers were so small that the statistician told me that doing the analysis would give us no difference just because of numbers.

Dr. Frei: Another point with respect to dose. The 370 mg/m^2 for the FUra, I take it, tended to remain the same through the study or get escalated whereas the FUra with CF tended to go down. Could you tell us at equilibrium what the proportionate difference in FUra-dose delivery was?

Dr. Erlichman: Just to clarify one point. In the FUra-alone arm it was actually increased, it did not stay the same. Then getting to your question, the mean dose for the FUra alone was 425 mg/m^2 and the mean dose for or median dose for FUra with CF was 370 mg/m^2.

Dr. Frei: So it is about a 4 to 3 or 5 to 4 ratio?

Dr. Erlichman: Yes, those are mean, some of the FUra patients got higher than 425.

Dr. Frei: The other question relates to time to response. If response kicked in after 1 or 2 courses, and there was a big difference in toxicity with the first course only, you do have the possibility that there is a correlation between toxicity and response.

Dr. Erlichman: Since this data have come up, we've tried to look at determinants or predictors of toxicity on this study putting all patients into the pool. In fact, response and toxicity did not correlate. We looked at quite a few parameters and it just didn't correlate.

Dr. Frei: What was the median time to response?

Dr. Erlichman: I can't give you median time to the response. What I can say is 1/3 of the patients responded after 2 courses, 2/3 after 4 courses and 95% responded after 6 courses.

Dr. Arbuck: You are predicting a response rate in your control arm of above 40% and yet you are including Bs. Obviously this is a difficult area, but I feel compelled to point out that the GITSG results in B2s of untreated patients approaches 70% survival.

Dr. Erlichman I accept that. I think that when we chose that number it was not just the Bs it was also the Cs in there and we are assuming that there will be a reasonable distribution such that it will bring it down to approximately 40%.

Dr. Wittes: Just to ask the dose question in a somewhat different way. Would you like to speculate about the possible effect of the need to escalate in the FUra-alone arm over the first course versus the results? In other words do you think the results would have been different if you had started at the dose that was most nearly the maximum tolerated dose in the absence of CF?

Dr. Erlichman: No, I don't believe so. Metastatic colon cancer does not grow that rapidly, so we're not talking about 1 course changing things that rapidly. So I don't believe it would make difference. As I said, one can go through various maneuvers to determine if increasing the response rate might make a difference. You can keep increasing it and saying what response rate would I have needed in FUra not to see a difference. We've done those sort of numbers.

Dr. Gullo: In a recently completed trial through the Mid Atlanta Oncology Program using infusion of FUra continuously, 24 hr/day, for approximately 8 out of 10 wk, the group was able to demonstrate a response of approximately 30% in a multi-institution multi-practice trial. That group was also able to demonstrate that 7% was a reproducible figure for FUra given by the bolus technique daily x5. I think your 7% response rate is quite accurate. In terms of an adjuvant study I was wondering if you would comment on your feelings about using infusion of FUra at a much lesser cost than using FUra by bolus along with CF.

Dr. Erlichman: That is a good question. In Canada we are doing a study basically repeating that study. We should be finishing in about 9 months and we will, first of all have, hopefully, confirmative information. Then I think it will be most interesting to look at, assuming that the infusion arm is better in that study also, a comparison of infusion FUra vs bolus FUra plus CF. Then we should get our medical economists in and let them tell us which costs more and what is a quality of life index that is most appropriate in terms of using these treatments in the adjuvant setting.

A NORTHERN CALIFORNIA ONCOLOGY GROUP RANDOMIZED TRIAL OF
SINGLE AGENT 5-FU VS. HIGH-DOSE FOLINIC ACID + 5-FU VS.
METHOTREXATE + 5-FU + FOLINIC ACID IN PATIENTS WITH
DISSEMINATED MEASURABLE LARGE BOWEL CANCER

Frank H. Valone, Peter S. Wittlinger, Marshall S.
Flam, Tom Drakes, Peter D. Eisenberg and John
Hannigan

UC San Francisco, San Joaquin Valley CCOP, UC
Davis, Marin County Oncology Program and the
Northern California Oncology Group, Belmont, CA.

INTRODUCTION

Numerous Phase II and Phase III trials have demonstrated
that combinations of folinic acid plus 5-FU or sequential
methotrexate, 5-FU, folinic acid are effective treatments for
patients with advanced carcinoma of the colon or rectum
(1-10). In many of these studies the objective response rates
in previously untreated patients were greater than 30%. These
rates are in excess of those expected for treatment with 5-FU
alone (11) suggesting that these combinations are more
effective than 5-FU for treatment of patients with advanced
colorectal carcinomas.

In 1983, the Northern California Oncology Group (NCOG)
began a randomized trial to compare the effectiveness of
standard treatment with 5-FU to experimental treatment with
folinic acid plus 5-FU or with sequential methotrexate, 5-FU
and folinic acid. In order to compare optimally active
treatment regimens, the drug schedules, dosages and dose
escalations were chosen to reach the maximally tolerated dose
on each treatment arm. The specific objectives of the study
were to evaluate and compare the objective response rates for
the three chemotherapy regimens; to evaluate the durations of
response; to compare the survival of patients receiving each
treatment; and, to study the toxicity of the three regimens.
A separate two-arm trial examined cross-resistance between
5-FU and the two experimental treatments. In that trial,
patients who failed treatment with 5-FU were randomized to
treatment with folinic acid plus 5-FU or to sequential
methotrexate, folinic acid, 5-FU. The results of the two-arm
trial were reported previously (12). This report presents an
update of the results of the three-arm trial for treatment of
patients who had not received prior 5-FU.

METHODS

Patient selection. Patients with measurable, locally
recurrent or metastatic cancer of the colon or rectum who had
not received prior chemotherapy and who provided signed
informed consent were eligible for this study. All patients
had adequate hepatic, renal and hematologic function as
defined previously (10,12). Patients were stratified by
Karnofsky performance status and history of prior
radiotherapy.

Treatment. Eligible patients were randomized to one of three
treatment regimens. An unbalanced 1:2:2 (A:B:C)
randomization scheme was used. Arm A, the control arm, was
5-FU 12 mg/kg/day intravenously for 5 days followed by 5-FU
15 mg/kg intravenously every week. The dosage of 5-FU was
increased by 10% if a blood count on the day of treatment
showed WBC $\geq$ 3,500 and platelets $\geq$ 150,000 and the patient
had only mild non-hematological toxicity. Patients who
failed treatment on Arm A and who continued to meet study
entry criteria were eligible for re-randomization to one of
the experimental treatments in the two arm study (12). Arm B
was the regimen described by Machover (1) namely folinic acid
200 mg/m^2 intravenously followed immediately by 5-FU 400
mg/m^2 as a 15 min infusion on days 1-5 of a 28 day cycle.
The dosage of 5-FU was increased by 10% if only mild systemic
toxicity occurred and a blood count on day 15 showed WBC $\geq$
3,000 and platelets $\geq$ 100,000 or WBC $\geq$2,000 and platelets $\geq$
150,000. Arm C was methotrexate 50 mg/m^2 orally every 6
hours for 5 doses plus 5-FU 500 mg/m^2 intravenously 24
hours after starting methotrexate plus folinic acid 10
mg/m^2 orally every 6 hours for 6 doses starting 6 hours
after 5-FU. Initially Arm C was administered weekly. After 6
months of accrual, treatment was changed to every other week
because of severe toxicity.

Evaluation of treatment toxicity. All patients who received
treatment were evaluable for toxicity. Toxicity was graded
using standard NCOG criteria (10). Criteria for hematologic
toxicity were: leukopenia grade 1, 3,000-4,400; grade 2,
2,000-2,900; grade 3, 1,000-1,900; grade 4, <1,000;
thrombocytopenia grade 1, 90,000-129,000; grade 2,
50,000-89,000; grade 3, 25,000-49,000; grade 4, <25,000.
Patients were evaluable for response following completion of
the first four weeks of therapy unless disease progression
occurred earlier.

RESULTS

Patients. A total of 265 patients were entered in the study
(55 on Arm A, 107 on Arm B and 103 on Arm C). The patient
characteristics were equally distributed on each arm. The
median age was 62.3 years with a range of 19-85 years. The
male: female ratio was 1.7:1. The mean Karnofsky performance
status was 87.4%

Analysis of toxicity. Non-hematologic toxicity accounted for
the bulk of the grade 3 or greater toxicity observed on each
treatment arm (Table 1). Gastrointestinal toxicity

TABLE 1

ANALYSIS OF TREATMENT TOXICITY

NUMBER OF PATIENTS

	GRADE	ARM A 5-FU	ARM B FA+5-FU	ARM C MTX,5-FU,FA
PATIENTS RADOMIZED		55	107	103
PATIENTS EVALUABLE		52	103	98
HEMATOLOGIC TOXICITY	3	7	6	4
	4	3	4	0
	5	1	2	0
NON-HEMATOLOGIC	3	18	21	13
TOXICITY	4	4	2	1
	5	0	2	0

(mucositis and diarrhea) accounted for most of the non-hematologic toxicity. Treatment with 5-FU alone was substantially more toxic than treatment with either of the experimental regimens. Grade 3 or greater non-hematologic toxicity was observed in 22 of 52 evaluable patients treated with 5-FU alone (42.3%), 25 of 103 evaluable patients treated with folinic acid plus 5-FU (24.3%) and 14 of 98 evaluable patients treated with sequential methotrexate, 5-FU, folinic acid (14.3%). Similarly, the control arm had substantially greater hematologic toxicity. Grade 3 or greater toxicity was observed in 11 of 52 evaluable patients treated with 5-FU alone (21.2%), 12 of 103 evaluable patients treated with folinic acid plus 5-FU (11.7%) and 4 of 98 evaluable patients treated with sequential methotrexate, 5-FU, folinic acid (4.1%). Leukopenia (WBC<2,000) was the dominant hematologic toxicity. Only one episode of grade 3 thrombocytopenia was observed. Five patients were hospitalized with leukopenia: (three on Arm A and two on Arm B). There were 5 treatment-related deaths: one on Arm A (infection) and four on Arm B (three infection and one entercolitis).

DISCUSSION

This study compared three regimens for treatment of advanced colorectal cancer: 5-FU alone (Arm A), folinic acid + 5-FU (Arm B) and sequential methotrexate, 5-FU, folinic acid (Arm C). The treatment schedules were different on each of the three arms so this study did not rigorously examine the effects of folinic acid and methotrexate on 5-FU's activity. Rather this study compared three different treatment regimens each given in a maximally active fashion. Intensity of chemotherapy drug dosage may be an important determinant of tumor response to treatment (13). This study was designed to escalate 5-FU doses in order to treat each patient with the maximally tolerated dose of 5-FU thereby achieving maximal dose intensity. In spite of this goal, standard treatment with 5-FU was substantially more toxic than either of the two experimental treatments. Arm C was only minimally toxic and much of the toxicity occurred during the first 6 months of the study when patients were treated weekly instead every other week. Thus most patients on Arm C were not treated at the maximally tolerated dose.

This study has been closed to further patient accrual. Preliminary analysis suggests that the three treatment arms are equally effective in terms of objective response rates and overall survival. If these preliminary observations are substantiated after further follow up then the choice of which treatment to offer patients with colorectal carcinomas would be based on the relative toxicity of each regimen. In that setting treatment with sequential methotrexate, 5-FU, folinic acid may be the regimen of choice because of its minimal toxicity with apparently equal effectiveness to that of more toxic treatments

REFERENCES

1. D. Machover, E. Goldschmit, P. Chollet, et al: Treatment of advanced colorectal and gastric adenocarcinomas with 5-fluorouracil and high-dose folinic acid, J. Clin. Oncol. 4:685-698, (1986).
2. P. Bryne, F. Smith, M.W. Treat, et al: 5-Fluorouracil and higher dose folinic acid treatment of colorectal carcinoma patients, Proc. ASCO 2:121, (1983).
3. G.T. Budd, T.R. Fleming, J.D. Bukowski, et al., 5-Fluorouracil and folinic acid in the treatment of metastatic colorectal cancer: A randomized comparison, J. Clin. Oncol. 5:272-277, (1987).
4. J.D. Hines, M.H. Zakem, D.J. Adelstein, et al., Treatment of advanced-stage colorectal adenocarcinoma with fluorouracil and high-dose leucovorin calcium: A pilot study, J. Clin. Oncol. 6:142-146, (1988).
5. C. Erlichman, S. Fine, A. Wong, et al., A randomized trial of fluorouracil and folinic acid in patients with metastatic colorectal carcinoma, J. Clin. Oncol. 6:469-475, (1988).
6. J.H. Doroshow, M. Bertrand, E. Newman, et al., Preliminary analysis of a randomized comparison of 5-fluorouracil vs 5-fluorouracil and high-dose continuous-infusion folinic acid in disseminated colorectal cancer, NCI Monographs 5:171-174, (1987).
7. R. Hermann, J. Spehn, J.H. Beyer, et al: Sequential methotrexate and 5-fluorouracil: Improved response rate in metastatic colorectal cancer, J. Clin. Oncol. 2:591-594, (1984).
8. N.E. Kemeny, T. Ahmed, R.A. Michaelson, et al., Activity of sequential low-dose methotrexate and fluorouracil in advanced colorectal carcinoma: Attempt at correlation with tissue and blood levels of phosphoribosylpyro-phosphate, J. Clin. Oncol., 2:311-315, (1984).
9. B.A. Leone, A. Romero, M.G. Rabinovich, et al., Sequential therapy with methotrexate and 5-fluorouracil in the treatment of advanced colorectal carcinoma, J. Clin. Oncol., 4:23-27, (1986).

10. R.J. Ignoffo, M.A. Friedman, M. Gribble, et al., Phase II study of sequential methotrexate and 5-FU plus mitomycin and leucovorin in patients with disseminated large bowel cancer: Northern California Oncology Group Study, Cancer Treat. Rep. 68:983-988, (1984).
11. C.G. Moertel, Chemotherapy of gastrointestinal cancer. New Engl. J. Med. 299:1049, (1978).
12. F.H. Valone, M. Kohler, K. Fisher, et al, A Northern California Oncology Group randomized trial of leucovorin plus 5-fluorouracil versus sequential methotrexate, 5-fluorouracil, and leucovorin in patients with advanced colorectal cancer who failed treatment with 5-fluorouracil or 5-fluorodeoxyuridine alone, NCI Monographs 5:175-177, (1987).
13. W. Hryiuk, The impact of dose intensity on the design of clinical trials, Seminars Oncol. 14:65-74, (1987).

DISCUSSION OF DR. VALONE'S PRESENTATION

Dr. O'Connell: Frank, it was interesting that the time to progression distributions were significantly different showing an advantage for the experimental treatments over the FUra alone control but there was no difference in survival. I note in your abstract that there were a certain percentage of patients who crossed over from FUra to one of the experimental regimens at the time of progression. I wonder what percentage of patients actually crossed over and how valid do you think the survival comparisons are in the presence of that cross over?

Dr. Valone: I can answer that for you. 18 patients out of the 52 that were randomized to FUra alone were then re-randomized to either arm B or arm C in this study. We had a separate salvage study going on at the same time. We had one responder out of those 18 to the methotrexate/FUra. We then ran survival curves on the 18 who were crossed over compared to the other patients and found they were superimposable; we couldn't distinguish that subset from the other patients. So although you are right, the crossover potentially muddies the survival data, we can't find anything about that group that suggests that we selected out a subset and helped them do better.

Dr. O'Connell: Was there any other factor that might explain the disparate results between time to progression and survival? If it is not the crossover effect?

Dr. Valone: No, I don't have one. The clinicians who were doing this called me up saying, "I've got these patients who've had a PR that has lasted for months, I just had never seen that before". But, eventually the patients relapsed and died quite abruptly.

Audience: In your FUra single arm study, you administered FUra more optimally perhaps than other studies mentioned here because you've seen toxicities, but it differs from other institutions presenting today. Can you make comments on that? In case of response and were the responses similar

Valone: Responses were similar. My mind raises the question about whether what FUra/CF does is simply allow you to give FUra at a relatively well tolerated dose; if you really wanted to push FUra up to this type of toxicity where 1/3 of your patients are in the hospital, you may do just as well. So here we are probably finding an advantage in terms of therapeutic ratio rather than absolute benefit in terms of response.

Audience: Your FUra/CF arm is very similar to the Mayo Clinic FUra/CF arm at the high dose folinic acid; both your response rates are very similar, too. I wonder if anybody wants to make a comment about why we are seeing such different response rates when the dose of CF is dropped and FUra is raised just a tiny bit.

Dr. Valone: Basically we all leaned on Machover's regimen, Erlichman also used it and came up with a response rate of 33%. I don't know whether we're simply looking at the lowering of response rates due to cooperative groups or whether indeed the high CF is somehow giving us a lower response rate. I don't think we can answer that based on the studies we have done.

Dr. Marsh: You mentioned a very high number of complete responders. Was there anything unusual about the location. For example, were they lung as in John Hines' patients.

Dr. Valone: They were lung and liver. We had 16 CRs and 31 PRs in the study. I insisted on seeing all the X-rays myself for those CRs. There were several very well documented CRs in livers as well as in the lungs.

CLINICAL EXPERIENCE WITH CF-FUra

Leslie R. Laufman, Wayne D. Brenckman, Jr., Kathy A.
Stydnicki, E.D. Morgan, Mary Collier, Victoria B. Knick,
David S. Duch, Robert Mullin and Robert Ferone

Columbus CCOP, Columbus, OH 43215, Duke University Medical
Center, Durham, NC 27710, Burroughs Wellcome Co., Research
Triangle Park, NC 27709

ABSTRACT

Two trials of CF-FUra in patients with metastatic colorectal cancer
were performed, both using a 3 day loading dose and then weekly maintenance doses to minimize toxicity. The first trial used CF by IV
infusion with constant dose of FUra 400 mg/m^2, and the second trial
used oral CF with escalating doses of FUra.

In the first trial, 45 eligible patients (20 with and 25 without
prior therapy) were treated. Toxicity usually consisted of diarrhea or
weakness and was controlled by delaying or decreasing 5FU dose. Subjective responses occurred in 75% of patients but did not correlate with
antineoplastic effect. Objective responses were seen in 36% and
stabilization of disease in 31% of patients, and correlated with prolonged survival. Median survival was 8 months for patients with prior
treatment and 10 for those without, and 12 month survival was 32% and
40%, respectively. There was no correlation between the development of
toxicity and response or survival.

The second trial was recently conducted in cooperation with Duke
University to determine toxicity and efficacy of oral CF with IV FUra
prior to a randomized trial of this combination versus placebo with IV
FUra. Eighteen patients were treated and serum levels of folates were
obtained on 10. First toxicity occurred at FUra doses ranging from 375
to 850 mg/m^2, and consisted of diarrhea in 9, lethargy in 7, nausea/
vomiting in 4, dermatitis in 4, conjunctivitis in 2, hypersalivation in
2, stomatitis in 1, and profound granulocytopenia in 1. Response rate
was 35% and stabilization was 35% with median survival of 14 months and
12 month survival of 56%.

INTRODUCTION

Improved antineoplastic effect of FUra may be accomplished by modulation of its metabolism and effect on the target enzyme TS.
Theoretical models have suggested several biochemical alterations which
might allow enhanced growth inhibition of malignant cells by FUra[1].

201

Evidence from tissue culture and animal models has suggested an advantage for these new methods of FUra administration, but the ultimate test of these principles is in patients with malignancy.

Thus far, the only biochemical modulation of FUra which has yielded improved response rates and survival of cancer patients has been CF pretreatment[2]. Clinical trials were performed initially in patients with colon cancer because FUra has been the only effective chemotherapy for that disease, but with a substantial margin for improvement[3]. Trials by Machover[4] and Bruckner[5] showed an improved response rate for patients with colon cancer, a finding confirmed by subsequent trials[6]. Recent controlled studies of CF-FUra versus FUra alone demonstrate the superiority of CF-FUra [7,8,9]. Because toxicity is also increased by CF pretreatment, it is unclear whether therapeutic index is improved.

Previous trials have described the absorption of oral CF to be excellent if given to fasting subjects[10]. There is a selective absorption of the active l- isomer, which could theoretically be advantageous for cellular uptake and metabolism of CF[11]. Hines has reported clinical effectiveness of oral CF and IV FUra in colon cancer patients[12].

The experience of the Columbus Community Clinical Oncology Program with CF-FUra is reported herein. Our observations of patients treated informally with Machover's regimen and patients enrolled on a Southwest Oncology Group protocol using a similar 5 day schedule, impressed us not only with the antineoplastic but also the toxic potential of CF-FUra. The toxicities of diarrhea and profound weakness occur late, resolve slowly, and must be comletely resolved before additional therapy can be given. During this recovery period, which may last several weeks, the antineoplastic effect may be lost, and tumor regrowth occur. Therefore, a less intense, more frequent schedule (once weekly) was attempted, and found to have similar antineoplastic effect with milder toxicity, greater safety, and better patient acceptance.

Two formal clinical trials of CF-FUra have been done. The first, hereafter designated the IV trial[6], used a schedule suggested by Aaron Sholnick and others of the Michigan State University Cancer Treatment Consortium, with a 3 day loading dose of both CF 80 mg/m^2 IV infusion and FUra 400 mg/m^2 IV bolus, followed by weekly maintenance doses of both drugs. The second trial, the PO trial, was performed in conjunction with Duke University as a pilot study leading to a randomized double-blind placebo-controlled trial, now underway. This PO trial was designed using 3 day loading dose of large dose oral CF before IV FUra treatment. After the loading dose, oral CF and IV FUra are given weekly, but with FUra dose escalations, until the development of toxicity, after which each patient is maintained on his maximal nontoxic dose. The therapeutic effects and toxicity of both regimens are reported herein. Serum CF levels were obtained on 3 patients treated according to the IV trial protocol, and on 10 patients in the PO trial.

METHODS

Patient Population

Nonpregnant patients at least 18 years old with histologically confirmed colorectal adenocarcinoma were included if they had no prior malignancy, except in situ cervical carcinoma, or completely excised basal or squamous skin cancer. All patients had measurable metastatic

Table 1. Definition of Measurable Disease

- Bidimensional lung lesions on x-ray
- Palpable, quantifiable lymph nodes >2x2 cm
- Palpable abdominal mass >2x2 cm
- Pidimensional liver or abdominal mass on CT or MRI scan
- Palpable hepatomegaly >5 cm below costal margin or xiphoid process with CT or nuclear scan confirmation

---

disease as defined in Table 1, expected survival of at least 6 months, minimum granulocyte count of 2000/mm^3, platelet count of 150,000/mm^3, and bilirubin <2.0 mg%, BUN <30 mg%, and creatinine <1.5. Patients with brain metastases were excluded. Patients with prior chemotherapy or radiotherapy were excluded from the PO trial but represent 20 of the 45 patients in the IV trial. Pretreatment characteristics of all patients are shown in Table 2. Patients in the PO trial have better PS (Karnofsky 80-100%), whereas those in the IV trial had SWOG PS 0-2 (Karnofsky 50-100%). Patients in the PO trial also have a lower incidence of multiorgan metastases, and lower incidence of documented disease progression prior to therapy.

Table 2. Pretreatment Characteristics

	IV		PO
	Prior Rx	No Prior Rx	PO
Total	20	25	18
Male	10 (50)	14 (56)	10 (56)
Age range	46-77	37-78	40-79
Sites of metastases			
Liver only	1 (5)	8 (32)	9 (50)
Lung only	5 (25)	0 (0)	2 (11)
Abd-Pelvic Mass	3 (15)	5 (20)	1 (6)
Multiple	11 (55)	12 (48)	6 (33)
Performance Status			
Karnofsky SWOG			
100% 1	8 (40)	12 (48)	6 (55)
90%			4
80% 2	5 (20)	12 (48)	8 (44)
70%			-
50% 3	7 (35)	1 (4)	- (0)
CEA > 10	13 (65)	19 (76)	14 (78)

(Percent of total in parentheses)

Treatment

Both trials used a 3 day loading dose followed by weekly maintenance doses.

In the IV trial, a <u>loading dose</u> of CF 80 mg/m^2 was infused over 20h followed by FUra 400 mg/m^2 IV bolus, with both drugs given daily for 3 days. The once weekly <u>maintenance dose</u> consisted of CF 80 mg/m^2 infused over 1h followed by FUra 400 mg/m^2 IV bolus. No dose escalations occurred. Doses were delayed until toxicity resolved. FUra doses were decreased if 400/m^2 reproducibility caused toxicity lasting more than one week, a rare occurrence.

In the PO trial, a <u>loading dose</u> of CF 100 mg orally was given to fasting patients each hour for 4 doses, and then every 4h for 3 days. FUra 375 mg/m^2 was given IV bolus at the time of the fourth CF dose and then repeated on day 2 and day 3. The once weekly <u>maintenance dose</u> consisted of CF 100 mg orally given to fasting patients each hour for 4 doses and then every 4h for 1 day with FUra 375 mg/m^2 IV bolus at the time of the fourth CF dose. FUra dose was escalated to 400 mg/m^2 on the second weekly maintenance dose, and then increased by 50 mg/m^2 per week until toxicity occurred. After resolution of toxicity patients subsequently received the highest nontoxic dose weekly. CF doses remained the same throughout.

Serum Folate Determinations

Serum folates were analyzed by <u>L</u>. <u>casei</u>[13] and by HPLC[14]. Samples were prepared for analysis by extraction of folates and precipitation of protein material with a 5 min incubation with 4 ml of 1% sodium ascorbate containing 1% mercaptoethanol. Samples were concentrated, following cooling and centrifugation at 20,000 g for 20 min, by use of C18 cartridges[15,16]. Results were quantitated based upon recovery of standards added to control sera. 5-Formyl tetrahydrofolate pools from serum samples were collected following C18 HPLC and subjected to chiral analysis after concentration of C18 cartridges and reconstitution in chiral HPLC mobile phase[17].

Study Parameters

Complete blood count and toxicity assessment were performed weekly, and tumor measurements and CEA were performed at least every 3 months. Eligibility and response were determined by second party review.

Definitions

<u>Response</u>. Tumor area was defined as the product of the peripendicular diameters of the measurable lesion or the sum of the products of all measurable lesions in a given patient. Complete response (CR) was defined as the disappearance of all clinical evidence of tumor for at least 4 weeks; partial response (PR) as at least 50% decrease in tumor area, lasting at least 4 weeks, without increase in any site of malignant disease and without the appearance of any new site of malignant disease; and stable disease (SD) as no change or <50% decrease in tumor area lasting at least 3 months, without increase in any site of malignant disease, and without the appearance of any new site of malignant disease. Progression (PD) was defined as a >25% increase in tumor area or the appearance of new sites of malignant disease known not to be present at the start of therapy, occurring within the first 3 months of therapy. Relapse was defined as a >25% increase in tumor area in a

patient previously classified as having a response or stable disease, or the appearance of new sites of malignant disease in previously responding or stable patients.

Survival. Time in months from initiation of therapy to death.

RESULTS

Clinical

Both treatment regimens were well tolerated. In the IV trial, toxicity was generally mild, with the exception of 2 patients. One died of neutropenic urosepsis, having had prior pelvic irradiation and chronic bacteriuria related to an ileal bladder. Another patient experienced reversible cerebellar ataxia and discontinued therapy. The commonest toxicities were weakness (62%), nausea, vomiting (53%), and diarrhea (47%). Diarrhea required dose delays or reductions in 21 patients (47%), and could be severely exacerbated if additional therapy was given before complete recovery. A severe exacerbation can mimic a bowel obstruction, clinically and radiologically, and should be managed conservatively. Gastrointestinal bleeding, occult or overt, was seen in some patients with CF-FUra diarrhea. Patients treated on the PO trial had a similar pattern of toxicity, but because of the trial design, all patients eventually experienced some toxicity, though at widely variable doses (Table 3). There was no correlation between any pretreatment characteristic and maximal dose tolerated. First toxicity was most often diarrhea, though weakness or conjunctivitis also occurred frequently, and were often associated with diarrhea. Milder symptoms of stomatitis, nausea, vomiting, and skin changes (rash, hyperpigmentation) were seen frequently. One 70 year old man experienced life threatening toxicity following the loading dose and first maintenance dose. His past history included heart disease, with pacemaker insertion, glaucoma, and mild diabetes mellitus, and was enrolled for treatment of liver metastases with a PS of 90%.

On the third day of the loading dose he received trimethoprimsulfamethoxazole for a urinary infection, and the first weekly maintenance dose was given on day 7, despite his complaint of a dry mouth. On day 10 he developed severe ulcerative stomatitis due to herpes simplex and

Table 3. FUra Dose That Caused First Toxicity

Dose mg/m^2	No. of Patients
375	3
400	1
450	1
500	1
550	0
600	6
650	2
700	–
750	1
800	2
850	1

candida, and required hospitalization for dehydration. On day 18 his
WBC was 1200/mm^3 with 0% granolocytes, and platelets were 76,000/
mm^3. Antibiotic therapy for beta streptococcal sepsis resulted in a
complete recovery. Subsequently, he received 4 consecutive weekly doses
of CF-FUra at 375 mg/m^2 without stomatitis or hematologic toxicity,
but declined further treatment because of diarrhea and weakness.

The efficacy of these two regimens in terms of response and survival
is shown in Table 4. Roughly one third of patients develop a response,
one third exhibit disease stabilization, and one third have progression. All patients with response or stabilization have biochemical
improvement (liver function and CEA), whereas those with PD have worsen-
ing of these parameters. The time required to achieve a response was
similar in both IV and PO trials, ranging from 2 to 9 months, with a
median of 3 months. Duration of disease stabilization was 3 to 16+
months with a median of 12 months. Median survival is better for
patients in the PO trial versus IV trial (14 versus 8 months). In the
IV trial, previously untreated patients survive longer than treated (10
vs 8 months). The proportion of patients surviving 1 year (56% vs 40%
vs 32%) reflects the same pattern, though small sample size and differences in populations could account for this finding. In both trials,
patients who achieved a response or disease stabilization had markedly
improved survival compared to those with progressive disease.

In patients with a pretreatment CEA > 10, a CEA decline which occurs
in the first 2 months predicts development of either a response or
disease stabilization. The amount of CEA decline also predicts survival.

In neither IV nor PO trial is there a correlation between patient
outcome, measured by response or survival, and FUra dose or toxicity.

Table 4. Response and Survival

	IV Trial		PO Trial
	Prior Rx	No Prior Rx	
Total Patients	20	25	18
Inevaluable	1	1	1
Evaluable	19	24	17
CR/PR	6 (32)	10 (42)	6 (35)
SD	7 (37)	7 (29)	6 (35)
PD	6 (32)	7 (29)	5 (28)
Median Survival	8 mo	10 mo	14 mo
12 mo survival	32%	40%	56%
18 mo survival	21%	33%	> 16%

206

Table 5. Serum Folate Levels (μM) in 3 Patients Following IV Infusion
80 mg/m^2

Time (hr)	Total LV	%1-LV	MeTHF
	E.K. (1-hr inf)		
Pre	0	0	0
0	12.35	20.0%	6.37
2	1.25	6.2%	4.33
	A.R. (20-hr inf)		
Pre	0	0	0
0	5.20	39.2%	5.06
2	4.19	19%	5.05
	G.D. (20-hr inf)		
Pre	0	0	0
0	8.13	30.2%	6.86
2	3.70	5.2%	2.48

Serum Levels

Serum folate levels for 3 patients treated according to the IV trial protocol are shown in Table 5. Levels were drawn before (pre), immediately after (T-0) and 2h after completion of either a 1h or a 20h infusion of CF.

The serum folate levels obtained on 10 patients in the PO trial using reverse phase and chiral HPLC and L. casei methods are shown in Table 6. Analysis of 5-formyltetrahydrofolate by chiral HPLC indicates that it is present almost exclusively as the d-isomer at all time points. If one assumes that the L. casei is measuring 5-methyltetrahydrofolate (as d-5-formyltetrahydrofolate does not support growth), the two methods, L. casei and HPLC, give equivalent results for 5-methyltetrahydrofolate levels.

DISCUSSION

While many authors have described CF enhancement of FUra antitumor activity, most have used either the 5 day schedule[4] or a high CF dose once weekly[7]. The 2 studies reported herein combine the advantages of the traditional FUra loading dose and the more easily regulated toxicity of the once weekly schedule. The antineoplastic effect of this treatment compares favorably to other schedules, and the incidence of severe toxicity is lower. Both effects are more closely related to the dose and schedule of FUra, as opposed to CF. An unexpected finding in the PO trial was the wide range of maximally tolerated FUra doses, suggesting that future protocols should be more flexible in FUra dosing.

Table 6. Mean Serum Folate Concentration (μM)
(N=9)

	Total HPLC (d-+l-)	5-Formyl TNF (d-)	5-Methyl THF (l-)	Total L. Casei
Day 1 Pre LV	ND	ND	ND	< .1
2 h	1.6 $\pm$ .5	0.9 $\pm$ .3	0.8 $\pm$ .2	0.7 $\pm$ .2
4 h	2.6 $\pm$ 1.0	1.4 $\pm$ .6	1.2 $\pm$ .4	1.1 $\pm$ .4
6 h	2.8 $\pm$ .8	1.5 $\pm$ .4	1.3 $\pm$ .5	1.2 $\pm$ .4
8 h	2.9 $\pm$ .9	1.7 $\pm$ .5	1.2 $\pm$ .4	1.2 $\pm$ .4
Day 2	4.0 $\pm$ 1.0	2.5 $\pm$ .8	1.5 $\pm$ .4	1.3 $\pm$ .4
Day 3	5.1 $\pm$ 1.5	3.2 $\pm$ 1.1	1.9 $\pm$ .5	1.7 $\pm$ .5

A major issue is that of CF dose. While some in vitro studies suggest that 10 μM levels of CF are necessary for maximal FUra binding and inhibition of TS[18], other studies suggest that 1 μM levels are adequate to produce this effect[19,20]. Our two clinical studies show that modest serum folate levels can accomplish antineoplastic and toxic effects very similar to those achieved with higher serum folate levels. It is likely that extrapolation of serum folate levels to events which occur intracellularly is misleading. Malignant cells are folate depleted, compared to normal cells, for reasons that are poorly understood. Probably, FUra inhibition of malignant growth occurs only if intracellular folates exceed a threshold level, adequate to form the stable ternary CF-FUra-TS complex. Available data is consistent with this threshold replacement concept rather than a traditional dose response association for folates, but either simplistic concept will be modified as the many additional factors regulating folate metabolism and TS inhibition are understood.

ACKNOWLEDGEMENTS

Dr. Richard Schilsky performed CF serum assays for patients treated with IV CF infusions, Beverly Sullivan, Albert Guaspari, Dr. Diane Wald, and Dr. Neil Cledennin assisted in data management and interpretation, and Lisa Kerstein assisted in manuscript preparation.

REFERENCES

1. S. G. Arbuck, 5-FU/Leucovorin: Biochemical modulation that works?, Oncology 1:61 (1987).

2. T. R. Buroker, C. G. Moertel, T. R. Fleming, et al., A controlled
    evaluation of recent approaches to biochemical modulation or
    enhancement of 5-fluorouracil therapy in colorectal carcinoma, J.
    Clin. Oncol. 3:1624 (1985).
3. S. K. Carter, Large bowel cancer: The current status of treatment,
    JNCI 56:3 (1976).
4. D. Machover, G. Schwarzenberg, E. Goldschmidt, et al., Treatment of
    advanced colorectal and gastric adenocarcinomas with 5FU combined
    with high dose folinic acid: A pilot study, Cancer Treat. Rep.
    66:1803 (1982).
5. H. W. Bruckner, T. Ohnuma, R. Hart, et al., Leucovorin (LV) poten-
    tiation of 5-fluorouracil (FU) efficiency and potency, Proc. Am.
    Assoc. Cancer Res. 23:111 (1982).
6. L. R. Laufman, K. A. Krzeczowski, R. Roach, et al., Leucovorin-5-
    fluorouracil: An effective treatment for metastatic colon cancer, J.
    Clin. Oncol. 5:1394 (1987).
7. N. Petrelli, L. Herrera, Y. Rustum, et al., A prospective randomized
    trial of 5-fluorouracil versus 5-flurouracil and high-dose
    leucovorin versus 5-fluorouracil and methotrexate in previously
    untreated patients with advanced colorectal carcinoma, J. Clin.
    Oncol. 5:1559 (1987).
8. C. Erlichman, S. Fine, A. Wong, et al., A randomized trial of
    fluorouracil and folinic acid in patients with metastatic colorectal
    carcinoma, J. Clin. Oncol. 6:469 (1988).
9. M. J. O'Connell and H. S. Wieand, A controlled clinical trial
    including folinic acid at two distinct dose levels in combination
    with 5-fluorouracil (5FU) for the treatment of advanced colorectal
    cancer: Experience of the Mayo Clinic and North Central Cancer
    Treatment Group, This Volume.
10. B. W. McGuire, L. L. Sia, J. D. Hayes, et al., Absorption kinetics
    of orally administered leucovorin calcium: Development of folates
    and folic acid antagonists in cancer chemotherapy, NCI Monograph
    5:47 (1987).
11. J. A. Straw, D. Szapary and W. T. Wynn, Pharmacokinetics of the
    diastereoisomers of leucovorin after intravenous and oral adminis-
    tration to normal subjects, Cancer Res. 44:3114 (1984).
12. J. D. Hines, D. J. Adelstein, J. Bast, et al., High-dose oral (PO)
    leucovorin (CF) and intravenous 5-fluorouracil (5FU) in advanced
    metastatic colorectal carcinoma: Results of a pilot-phase I study,
    Proc. Am. Soc. Clin. Oncol. 7:110 (1988).
13. E. M. Newman and J. F. Tsai, Microbiological analysis of 5 formyl
    THF and other folates using an automatic 96 well plate reader,
    Analyt. Biochem. 154:509 (1986).
14. D. S. Duch, S. W. Bowers and C. A. Nichol, Analysis of cofactor
    levels in tissues using high performance liquid chromatography,
    Anal. Biochem. 130:385 (1983).
15. R. J. Mullin, B. R. Kieth and D. S. Duch, Distribution and metabo-
    lism of calcium leucovorin in normal and tumor tissue, This Volume.
16. E. E. Vokes, K E. Choi, R. L. Schilsky, et al, Cisplatin, fluoro-
    uracil, and high-dose leucovorin for recurrent or metastatic head
    and neck cancer, J. Clin. Oncol. 6:618 (1988).
17. K. E. Choi and R. L. Schilsky, Resolution of the stereosiomers of LV
    and 5MTHF by chiral high performance liquid chromatography,
    Analytical Biochem. 168:398 (1988).
18. R. M. Evans, J. D. Laskin and M. T. Hakala, Effects of excess
    folates and deoxyinosine on the activity and site of action of
    5-fluorouracil, Cancer Res. 41:3288 (1981).

19. B. Ullman, M. Lee, D. W. Martin Jr., et al., Cytotoxicity of
    5-fluoro-2'-deoxyuridine: Requirement for reduced folate cofactors
    and antagonism by methotrexate, Proc. Natl. Acad. Sci. USA 75:980
    (1978).
20. K. Keyomarsi and R. G. Moran, Folinic acid augmentation of the
    effects of fluoropyrimidines on murine and human leukemic cells,
    Cancer Res. 46:5229 (1986).

DISCUSSION OF DR. LAUFMAN'S PRESENTATION

Dr. Hines: L.casei does not measure CF, it measures total reduced folates. P. cerevisiae is the micro-organism that measures 6S-CF. Secondly, I think both Dr. Rustum's group and my own group in the past used i.v. CF at much higher doses. When we got up to 750 mg/m^2/wk at 500 mg CF, I didn't see one patient that didn't get severe toxicity. I don't know of anybody who can get up to those doses with our schedule. Now your schedule obviously differs but a lot of us feel the higher doses of CF may contribute to toxicity so I would be hesistant if you are using a higher dose schedule to get any higher than 600/meter/week. We didn't see any additional benefit when we tried that.

Dr. Laufman: I think the point is that you have to individualize for each patient, not that everybody should be treated at the higher dose.

Audience: I was wondering whether any of your patients who tolerated these higher doses received allopurinol at the same time?

Dr. Laufman: No.

Dr. Berken: I'm an oncologist in private practice cooperating with a group of oncologists in Paris and Quebec in a FUra/CF program that uses CF 200 mg/m^2 day 1, day 2, and FUra in a range, but most of my patients have been getting 800 mg/m^2, day 1, day 2, divided half i.v. bolus, half over a 24 hr period by infusion, repeated every 2 weeks. From what I can see, it is a substantial dose of FUra compared to those which have been talked about this morning, and somewhat less CF. Toxicities I think have been less, certainly no more than the least that have been reported this morning. The diarrhea has not been much of a problem but has been the reason most people have not had higher doses of FUra given. I, too, have seen in the patients I've treated a lot of tearing which has been a problem for the patients, and an occasional case of conjunctivitis. One of the things I have seen which has not been reported this morning, which is very troublesome to my patients and to me is sclerosis of the veins. Now I think this may be more related to the fact that we are using prolonged infusions of FUra because I've seen it in patients which have not gotten CF but have gotten prolonged infusions of FUra. That has led to my suggesting for many of my patients that we use the Infusaport rather than peripheral veins. One other point about cost. In general, I'm really very concerned as a practicing physician, about the attention now being given to cost. I feel like I'm being pushed into a corner; I have the American College of Physicians telling me what tests I should not order because they lead to other tests which are expensive. I resent that kind of treatment, I'm not being treated as a professional who is supposedly able to make decisions like that on the basis on what is best for his patients. I must say also that I spoke to the Lederle man outside. Leucovorin is now down to $15 per 15 mg vial which is a lot less I think in total cost than some of the foolish antibiotic programs that are being used. I think perhaps cost is not as great an issue as it has been made out to be. I would appeal to my fellow practitioners to resist being pushed into the corner that some of our so called advocates are placing us in.

A RANDOMIZED TRIAL OF 5-FLUOROURACIL ALONE VERSUS 5-FLUOROURACIL AND HIGH DOSE LEUCOVORIN IN UNTREATED ADVANCED COLORECTAL CANCER PATIENTS

M.T. Nobile[+], L. Canobbio[+], A. Sobrero[+], E. Galligioni[°], M.G. Vidili[+], T. Fassio[°], G.Lo Re[°], A. Rubagotti[+], M.R. Sertoli[+], and R. Rosso[°]

[+]Istituto Nazionale per la Ricerca sul Cancro, Genova and
[°]Centro di riferimento Oncologico, Aviano, Pordenone, Italy

It has been experimentally proven that high doses of the reduced folate leucovorin (LV) enhance the therapeutic efficacy of 5-fluorouracil (5FU) by increasing the FdUMP-TS binding. This rationale prompted various phase II clinical trials whose results apparently showed enhancement of the 5FU antitumor activity.

The only way to prove clinically that LV enhances the efficacy of 5FU is to compare the maximum tolerated dose (MTD) for a certain schedule with the same 5FU dose and schedule plus LV. Since the known MTD for weekly bolus 5FU is 600 mg/m^2, we compared 5FU 600 mg/m^2 I.V. weekly bolus versus LV 500 mg/m^2 infused i.v. over 2 hours and 5FU 600 mg/m^2 I.V. bolus given 1 hour after the beginning of the LV infusion, weekly, until progression.

Patients with histologically proven adenocarcinoma of the colon-rectum with locally advanced or metastatic disease were considered eligible. All patients had measurable disease and were previously untreated. Further requirements included a PS   3, age   75 and no RT on measurable lesions.

Ninety-five patients have entered the study so far and the 2 groups are comparable for age, sex, site of disease (Table 1).

Analysis of dose intensity is crucial to determine whether or not LV alters the MTD of 5FU. Table 2 shows that the median dose intensity of LV+5FU actually delivered during the first 2 months of treatment was approximately 20% lower than that of 5FU alone. This is consistent with the higher toxicity observed in the combination arm (Table 3).

The hematologic toxicity was mild in both treatment groups, but patients treated with the combination of LV+5FU experienced more frequent and severe stomatitis and diarrhea.

Thirty nine patients in the 5FU group and 43 pts. in the LV+5FU group are evaluable for response. Thirteen pts. are not evaluable: 4 just entered the study and 9 represent major protocol deviations. Table 4 shows the objective response rates (WHO criteria).

Table 1. Patient Characteristics

	5FU	5FU + LV
N° of entered pts	45	50
Median age	63 (43-75)	62 (49-75)
Median ECOG PS	0 (0-3)	1 (0-3)
Sex		
Male	20	27
Female	25	23
Site of primary tumor		
Colon	24	24
Rectum	21	26
Site of disease		
Liver	34	31
Lung	8	11
Bone	2	2
Lymph nodes	1	5
Other	7	6

Table 2. Dose Intensity

	5FU		5FU + LV	
	Mean (SD)	Median (range)	Mean (SD)	Median (range)
DOSE INTENSITY DURING THE FIRST 4 TREATMENTS (mg/sq.m/wk)	587.0 (41.59)	600 (450-672)	540.4 (91.4)	600 (222-600)
DOSE INTENSITY DURING THE FIRST 8 TREATMENTS (mg/sq.m/wk)	532.9 (108.8)	600 (225-634)	443.0 (143.9)	494 (150-600)

The response rate was not significantly different in the 2 groups (p = 0.1). Median duration of response was 4[+] and 5.5[+] months for 5FU and LV+5FU respectively and the median survival was 10 and 9 months, respectively. Despite a good dose intensity, the response rates in our study are much lower than that reported by several other groups. Therefore we investigated the possibility that stricter criteria for response were used in this trial, and conducted another analysis, including minor responses (MR), in the calculation of the p value. Table 5 indicates that the advantage in response rate for the LV-5FU arm is highly significant (p=0.01) when calculated in this way.

Table 3. Toxicity

Evaluable pts	5FU (N° of pts=45)				5FU + LV (N° of pts=50)			
Grade WHO	I	II	III	IV	I	II	III	IV
Nausea and vomiting	12	8	1	–	13	5	2	1
Leucopenia	7	2	–	–	9	4	–	–
Thrombocytopenia	2	–	–	–	1	–	–	–
Stomatitis	4	1	1	–	7	4	3	–
Diarrhea	5	6	3	–	4	6	7	4

These data mandate extreme caution in drawing conclusions about the efficacy of LV+5FU. In this connection, we plan to randomize another 30 patients before terminating the study. In the meantime we can pre-liminarily conclude that 1) LV+5FU is more toxic than 5FU alone 2) LV+5FU results in lower dose intensity, nevertheless the combination may be more effective than 5FU alone 3) LV+5FU adds nor survival advantage (at lower dose intensity).

Table 4. Responses

	5FU °pts (%)	5FU + LV °pts (%)
Total	39 (100)	43 (100)
CR	0 (0)	2 (4.7)
	(5.1)	(16.3)
PR	2 (5.1)	5 (11.6)
SD	23 (59)	19 (44.2)
P	14 (35.9)	17 (39.5)

Table 5. Responses, Including MR's

	5FU °pts (%)	5FU + LV °pts (%)
Total	39 (100)	43 (100)
CR	0	2 (4.7)
PR	2 (5.1) → (5.1)	5 (11.6) → (30.2)
MR	0	6 (14)
SD	23 (59)	13 (30.2)
P	14 (35.9)	17 (39.5)

DISCUSSION OF DR. CANNOBIO'S PRESENTATION

Dr. Rustum: Just to clarify one point on your protocol for the FUra
vs high dose FUra/CF. You had weekly for 6 weeks, do you have 2
weeks rest?

Dr. Canobbio: No.

Dr. Rustum: No rest?

Dr. Canobbio: No. The treatment has been given weekly, a delay of
the treatment has been planned according to toxicity observed. The
plan for the treatment was for 12 weeks administration of the drug.

Laufman: I'm wondering if you have any explanation or any thought as
to why you are not seeing a difference between the folate treated
group and the FUra alone group. I'm wondering if there might be an
explanation on the basis of the diet of northern Italians compared
to those from Ohio and non-San Francisco parts of the US.

Dr. Canobbio: It makes a difference in terms of survival and in
time to progression, I think, because in our experience there is a
difference in terms of remission rate also if the group of patients
treated with FUra alone achieved a very low remission rate, 4.5% I
think, that is one of the lowest remission rates reported in the
literature. However, this difference in terms of objective initial
rate did not reflect any difference in terms of survival and time to
progression. I don't think that diet can be an explanation also
because I know that the American people are shifting their diet from
the American diet to a Mediterranean diet so in these terms a group
of patients should be more comparable.

Dr. Arbuck: I didn't appreciate the differences in schedule that Dr.
Rustum just brought out. In your FUra/CF and your FUra arms in the
several studies you presented there is no break. I'm talking about
the weekly regimen?

Dr. Canobbio: No breaks were planned.

Dr. Arbuck: Is it possible then that perhaps you saw a significant
toxicity such that you ended up having longer delays and a lower
dose intensity.

Dr. Canobbio: Yes. We looked at the percent of patients who delay
or who needed a reduction of treatment. There is a slight difference but not a significant within the 2 groups of patient because
95% of patients on FUra alone had a reduction or a delay in the
treatment versus 40% of patients in the combination. It is really
not significant.

Dr. Arbuck: Well, I don't know about that. I think it might be very
significant and I would suggest that it would be worth looking at
the dose intensity of both regimens in both studies.

Audience: I find difficulty supporting your conclusions because of
the relatively small number of patients that you have in your
study.   But perhaps more so is the fact that stable disease seems to
be a major portion of your patients and perhaps you can explain or
amplify on what you call stable disease since there was no
difference in survival in either one of your groups.   What does that
mean to you?

Dr. Canobbio: I define a stable disease according to <u>WHO</u> criteria,
we follow these criteria strictly and so I don't think that there is
any significant difference according to the response assessment
because the response assessment is being strictly according to this
criteria so it should be quite similar to the criteria that have
been following those and all the other trials that have been
presented.

PHARMACODYNAMICS OF 5-FLUOROURACIL AND LEUCOVORIN

Bengt G. Gustavsson, Göran Carlsson, Roland Frösing, and
C. Paul Spears

Östra sjukhuset, The University of Gothenburg, Sweden and
The University of Southern California, Comprehensive Cancer
Center, Los Angeles, CA 90033

INTRODUCTION

Fluoropyrimidine therapy is a corner-stone of chemotherapeutic
management of metastatic cancer. Although only about 15% of patients
respond to initial single-agent FUra therapy, a greater number may have
disease stabilization with comparatively mild toxicity[1,2]. Fifteen
years ago, we reported that continuous intraportal infusion of FUra in
a significant prolonged survival compared to historical controls[3]. Since
then, significant discoveries of the mechanisms of action of FUra and
attempts at rational approaches in its application have been made.

We have developed ultrasensitive [3H]FdUMP ligand-binding assays for
TS and FdUMP and reported the feasibility of using these assays for
clinical pharmacodynamic analyses of parameters of TS inhibition[4,5].
Ultrasensitive methods have also been developed for $CH_2-H_4PteGlu$ determination in animal tumors as well as in human carcinomas.[6]

MATERIAL AND METHODS

Patients

Fifty patients received a test dose of IV bolus FUra and were then
submitted to laparotomy. The primary site of origin of tumor was large
bowel or rectum in 33; gastric cancer in 5; and pancreatic carcinoma in
4 patients. In a separate group of 10 patients with gastrointestinal
carcinoma LV, 30mg/m^2 was given as an IV bolus. Serial tumor biopsies
up to 90 min. were taken after the LV injection.

Tissue Handling

Specimens paired of fat and necrotic tissue were immediately frozen
in liquid nitrogen or dry ice. Homogenization was done by groud-glass
grinding followed by sonication. Nucleotides were extracted from homogenate with acetic acid. The nucleotide extracts were diluted with water
to conductivities 1 mmho or less prior to DEAE column chromatography.

Assays

FdUMP assay by isotope-dilution of $[^3H]$FdUMP binding to L.Casei TS, and dUMP assay by L.Casei TS synthesis of $[^{14}C]$dTMP were done essentially as previously described[6]. The assay for CH_2-H_4PteGlu levels in tissues is based on using TS-$[^3H]$FdUMP trapping of folate as charcoal-isolable ternary complex[7].

Animal Tumor Model

A cell suspension of a transplantable nitrosoguanidine induced colonic adenocarcinoma is inoculated directly into the central liver lobe of inbread Wistar rats. The liver is explored during ether anaesthezia through a midline incision[8]. The induced tumor growth is solitary and the tumor volume can be calculated by measuring the greatest (a) and smallest (b) perpendicular diameters according to the formula:

$$V = \frac{a \cdot b^2}{2} \quad [8]$$

The tumor model has been used for testing different therapeutic modalities both concerning treatment of macroscopic tumors and microscopic tumors i.e. adjuvant treatment.

The effect of FUra (30 mg/kg) alone and in combination with LV (15 mg/kg) has been used as adjuvant treatment using this tumor model. During three consequtive days following tumor cell inoculation one group of animal was given saline, one group FUra alone, and one group FUra and LV. All drugs were given as intraperitoneal bolus injections. Fourteen days following inoculation of the tumor cells relaparotomy was performed and the tumor take i.e. existence of palpable and measurable tumor growth was registered. Results are expressed as mean ± standard error of mean (SEM). Students t-test and chi-square analyses were used for statistical calculations.

RESULTS

No mortality was observed during the first 14 days. Tumor take on day 14 was lower in animals given FUra in combination with LV 9/20 (45%), compared with untreated animals 20/20 (100%) ($p < 0.01$) (fig. 1). The tumor volume on day 14, including animals with measureable tumors, was significantly smaller in animals given FUra alone or FUra in combination with LV compared with untreated animals ($p < 0.001$. LV added to FUra retarded the tumor growth compared with FUra alone ($p < 0.01$) (fig. 2).

Single Biopsy Data in Patients with Gastrointestinal Carcinomas

500 mg/m^2 of FUra has been given as IV push injection and biopsies have been taken from the gastrointestinal tumor during laparotomy. The total number of patients receiving fluoropyrimidines who had tissue material assayed for TS related parameters is now more than 120. The average time interval between intra- or pre-operative FUra and tumor biopsy was similar in all groups, with an overall average of 100 min. (15-400). In all tissues, maximal TS inhibition appears to be reached by 90-120 min. with the majority of specimens, however, studied prior to this.

FdUMP levels varied enormously, showing two orders of magnitude difference among colorectal specimens at the apparent peak of 30-60 min. Only a few specimens failed to show FdUMP in significant excess of total TS levels.

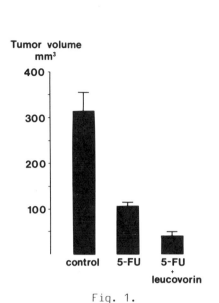

Tumor volume
mm³

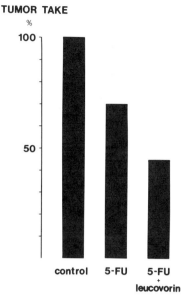

TUMOR TAKE
%

Fig. 1.

Measurable tumor in per cent on day
14 in the different groups.

Fig. 2.

Tumor volume on day 14 in the
different groups.

Correlation of FUra Pharmacodynamics with Response

An analysis at this time of 54 patients who received FUra chemotherapy
subsequent to pharmacodynamic tumor testing of metastatic disease, (using
IV bolus FUra) showed highly significant difference in free TS; per cent
TS inhibition and dUMP levels between patients benefitting from FUra and
those who progressed.

TS Inhibition in Normal Tissues

Normal hepatic tissue and colonic mucosa are highly resistant to toxic
effects of IV bolus FUra. Moreover, in our patient studies we have found
a very low percentage of inhibition of TS, low FdUMP levels, and very low
FdUMP/dUMP ratios in these tissues (Table I). These findings are consistent
with the postulate that TS inhibition is an important correlate of FUra
cytotoxicity. A comparison of surgically normal liver and hepatic tumors
obtained simultaneously in 15 patients has shown that TS inhibition is
highly significant greater in malignant tissue compared to normal liver.
Average FdUMP values is fourfold higher in tumor than in liver. Levels of
dUMP show no difference.

Serial tumor biopsies up to 90 min. after bolus IV injection of low
dose LV (30 mg/m^2) showed inconsistent increases in CH_2-H_4PteGlu levels,
on average 50% increase by 40 min. In intraoperative liver biopsies taken
before and after IV injection of low dose LV, we found that prefolinic
acid levels rose 1.9-fold at 10 min. after drug administration.

DISCUSSION

Our pharmacodynamic TS studies of tumors from patients receiving FUra
without LV are strongly supportive of the importance of low post-FUra free
TS levels for achieving response. It has also been shown that total TS is

Table I

PARAMETERS OF TS IN SINGLE POST-5-FUra BIOPSIES
OF NORMAL TISSUES OF PATIENTS GIVEN BOLUS IV 5-FUra, 500 MG/SQM

	Time min	TS, pmole/g			Nucleotides		
		free	total	inhib[c] %	FdUMP pmole/g	dUMP nmole/g	FdUMP/dUMP[d] ratio x 100
NORMAL TISSUES:							
Normal Liver (19)[a]	102[b] ±105	1.98 ±1.81	3.56 ±3.63	36.1 ±22.0	58 ±107	27.2 ±13.9	0.201 ±0.398
Normal Mucosa (3)	363 ±569	2.23 ±0.91	3.59 ±1.56	37 ±17	13 ±14	27.8 ±20.0	0.050 ±0.053
Bone Marrow (5)	78 ±40	0.88 ±0.54	2.65 ±1.39	64.8 ±17.2	123 ±126	246.5 ±209	0.060 ±0.060

[a]Numbers in parentheses, number of patients.

[b]Average values, ±S.D.

[c]Percentage inhibition of TS = [(Total TS - Free TS)/Total TS]x100.
Values corrected for isotope dilution by cytosolic FdUMP and for 13%
ternary complex dissociation during 20-min [^{3}H]FdUMP labeling.

[d]Gives FdUMP as a percentage of dUMP molecules present.

a predictor of survival. Thus among 54 patients with TS more than 2.5
pmole/g, the survival time was significantly less than those patients with
low TS levels. LV addition to FUra therapy of carcinomas has been shown to
result in significant increased response rates. Based on our biochemical
studies of single post-FUra biopsies from over 50 patients, most of them
should benefit from LV administration due to low FdUMP formation, low
folates, or high dUMP levels. The levels of CH_2-H_4PteGlu after IV bolus
administration of low dose folinic acid increased rapidly but transiently
in our study. In biopsies of metastatic colon carcinoma the levels of
CH_2H_4PteGlu are generally about one-tenth the levels found in normal liver.
Determination of pharmacodynamic events relevant to TS inhibition in biopsies of metastatic tumors after FUra and LV administration can provide vital
information regarding dose and schedule of these drugs used in combination.

ACKNOWLEDGEMENT

The study was supported by grants from Swedish Medical Research
Council, Assar Gabrielsson Foundation, and the University of Göteborg.

REFERENCES

1.   B. Gustavsson and L. O. Hafström, Adjuvant and palliative treatment
        of colo-rectal cancer with fluorinated pyrimidines - a pharmaco-
        logical and clinical review, Acta Chir Scand Suppl 504 (1981).

2. F. Ansfield, J. Klotz, T. Nealon, G. Ramirez, J. Minton, G. Hill, W. Wilson, H. Davis, and G. Cornell, A phase III study comparing the clinical utility of four regimens of 5-fluoruracil, Cancer 39:34 (1977).

3. O. Almersjö, L. O. Hafström, and B. Gustavsson, Results of regional portal infusion of 5-fluorouracil to patients with primary and secondary liver cancer, Acta Chir Gyn Fenn 65:27 (1976).

4. C. P. Spears, B. G. Gustavsson, M. S. Mitchell, D. Spicer, M. Berne, L. Bernstein, and P. V. Danenberg, Thymidylate synthetase inhibition in malignant tumors and normal liver of patients given intravenous 5-fluorouracil, Cancer Res 44:4144 (1984).

5. C. P. Spears, B. G. Gustavsson, and R. Frösing, Folinic acid modulation of fluorouracil: kinetics of bolus administration, Invest New Drugs 6: in press (1988).

6. C. P. Spears, A. H. Shahinian, R. G. Moran, C. Heidelberger, and T. H. Corbett, In vivo kinetics of thymidylate synthetase inhibition in 5-fluorouracil-sensitive and -resistant murine colon adenocarcinomas, Cancer Res 42:450 (1982).

7. C. P. Spears and B. G. Gustavsson, Methods for thymidylate synthase pharmacodynamics: serial biopsy, free and total TS, FdUMP and dUMP, and H_4PteGlu and CH_2-H_4PteGlu assays, in: "The Expanding Role of Folates and Fluoropyrimidines in Cancer Chemotherapy", Y. Rustum and J. McGuire eds., Plenum Publ Corp, N.Y. (1988).

8. G. Carlsson, L. Hafström, and B. Gullberg, Estimation of liver tumor volume using different formulas. An experimental study in rats, J Cancer Res Clin Oncol 105:20 (1983).

DISCUSSION OF DR. GUSTAVSSON'S PRESENTATION

Dr. Frei: Your analysis for TS would indicate that the lower the level the better the responsiveness.

Dr. Gustavsson: Yes.

Dr. Frei: One would suspect since that's a DNA synthesis determining enzyme, that might also reflect the cytokinetics of the tumor. Was there evidence of a positive correlation between the level of TS and tumor agressiveness as measured by volume doubling time or what have you?

Dr. Gustavsson: We have looked at TS level compared to tumor grading according to Duke's grade classification and that has been difficult to show actually; also, if you look at poorly differentiated or highly differentiated tumors we haven't found a significant difference but there is a tendency toward's it. I think it could be that we have too small numbers.

Dr. Frei: Also, the difference in TS levels in your responders vs nonresponders was 5-10-fold; lower in the responders.

Dr. Gustavsson: Yes.

Dr. Frei: To the extent that that would reflect tumor cytokinetics, it might be that response and duration of response and survival is intrinsic to the biochemistry of the tumor as well as being a function of response to chemotherapy. It's something we have to keep in mind in terms of interpreting this kind of data.

Dr. Gustavsson: Yes. I think so.

Dr. J. Houghton: Could you tell me what the optimal time is after treating with FUra for making your correlations between the different parameters that you have been measuring and sensitivity?

Dr. Gustavsson: Yes. If you're just looking at peak values, which we started with, it is around 30-60 minutes. What we have learned is that there is no correlation between FdUMP levels and what's happening to the patient. It is more a question of total TS and greater inhibition. Some time between 30 or 180 minutes is adequate because there you have a steady-state more or less and if you have 90% TS inhibition and you take several biopsies you will be still be at that level.

Dr. Rustum: Just a short comment to agree with you. Our experience here at Roswell Park indicates somewhere around 2 hours.

5-FLUOROURACIL AND 5-FORMYLTETRAHYDROFOLATE

IN ADVANCED MALIGNANCIES

Reinhard Becher[1], Erhard Kurschel[1], Ursula Wandl[1],
Otto Kloke[1], Max Scheulen[1], Olivia Weinhardt[1], Klaus
Höffken[1], Norbert Niederle[1], Hakeem Khan[1], Stefan
Bergner[2], Wolfgang Sauerwein[3], Ursula Rüther[4] and
Carl G. Schmidt[1]

Innere Universitätsklinik (Tumorforschung)[1], Urolo-
gische Klinik[2], Strahlenklinik[3], Westdeutsches Tumor-
zentrum, Universitätsklinikum Essen, Katharinenhospi-
tal Stuttgart[4], FRG

INTRODUCTION

As conventional FUra monochemotherapy with remission rates
of about 20% remained disappointing, the addition of CF to FUra
heralded an important step towards an improved therapy of advanced colorectal cancer (1). In a broad phase II study we evaluated response, toxicity and survival of patients receiving combination treatment of FUra and CF, primarily in colorectal cancer. In addition we treated pts with prostatic cancer, breast
cancer, gastric cancer and various other poor risk malignancies
with this combination. We used two different schedules of FUra
and CF. Our data indicate improved response in colorectal cancer
as compared to FUra alone and are promising in breast cancer and
adenocarcinoma of unknown primary.

PATIENTS

121 pts with histologically proven advanced and progressive
metastatic cancer entered in this study since June 1986. 100 pts
are evaluable so far. Bidimensionally measurable tumors were a
prerequisite, as well as a Karnofsky index at or above 60%.
Patients data, diagnosis, the number of cases, age, pretreatment
and sex are shown in Table 1. Local treatment modalities had already been exhausted.
The pts with colorectal cancer were mostly untreated except for
2 of 17 pts in study I(1 pt FUra, 1 pt FUra plus Vincristin) and
8 of 28 pts from study II (5 pts FUra, 2 pts schedule I, 1 pt
FUra plus MTX). The metastatic sites of pts with colorectal
cancer are shown in Table 2.
All 15 pts with prostatic cancer had been pretreated with addi-
tiv and/or ablative hormonal modalities, and had received estramustine until progression. The 12 pts with breast cancer had
already had extensive combination chemotherapy prior to this

Table 1.   Characteristics of patients

Diagnosis	No.pts	Age range (median)	Pretreat-ment	Sex male/female
Colorectal (I)	17	28-75 (53)	2	10 / 7
Colorectal (II)	28	29-79 (56)	6	20 / 8
Prostate	15	47-79 (66)	14	15 / 0
Breast	12	28-60 (45)	12	0 /12
Gastric	8	42-71 (51)	2	6 / 2
NSLC	4	47-72 (48.5)	2	3 / 1
Kidney	3	56-62 (58)	2	2 / 1
Pancreatic	3	40-51 (50)	0	2 / 1
Unknown Primary	3	53-68 (64)	1	2 / 1
Biliary tract	2	53-66 (59.5)	0	1 / 1
Liver	1	60	0	1 / 0
Head & Neck	1	46	1	1 / 0
Adrenal	1	53	0	0 / 1
Carcinoid	1	59	0	0 / 1

Table 2.   Metastatic site of pts with colorectal cancer

	Liver	Lung	Abdominal mass	Nodes	1 site	More sites
Group I (n=17)	13	7	3	5	6	11
Group II (n=28)	22	8	3	2	18	10

study, usually with at least 2 different modalities including anthracyclins and various hormonal treatments.

TREATMENT

Two different schedules were employed. Schedule I consited of a 5 day course of continuous infusion of FUra in a dose of 600 mg/m² and CF in a dose of 200 mg/m² as a rapid infusion repeated at day 22. Schedule II, also a 5 day course, consisted of a push infusion of 400 mg/m² FUra after an infusion of CF (200 mg/m²) during a time period of exactly 2 hours. This schedule was also repeated at day 22. In cases of grade III toxicity or 2 or more grade II toxicities the dose of FUra was reduced to 70% or less if necessary. The dose of CF remained unchanged. Most pts were treated on an out patient basis.

TOXICITY

The toxicity was assessed according to the WHO score and documented at the start of every treatment.

Table 3.   Treatment results

Diagnosis	CR	PR	NC	PD
Colorectal Ca. Schedule I	0/17	3/17 (18%)	11/17 (64%)	3/17 (18%)
Colorectal Ca. Schedule II	1/28 (4%)	6/28 (21%)	10/28 (36%)	11/28 (39%)
Prostate	0/15	0/15	2/15	13/15
Breast	0/12	2/12	6/12	4/12
Gastric	0/ 8	1/ 8	5/ 8	2/ 8
Kidney	0/ 4	0/ 4	0/ 4	4/ 4
NSLC	0/ 4	0/ 4	1/ 4	3/ 4
Pancreatic	0/ 3	0/ 3	0/ 3	3/ 3
Unkn. Primary	0/ 3	1/ 3	2/ 3	0/ 3
Biliary tract	0/ 2	0/ 2	1/ 2	1/ 2
Liver	0/ 1	0/ 1	0/ 1	1/ 1
Head & Neck	0/ 1	0/ 1	0/ 1	1/ 1
Adrenal	0/ 1	0/ 1	0/ 1	1/ 1
Carcinoid	0/ 1	0/ 1	1/ 1	0/ 1

EVALUATION

Only bidimensionally measurable lesions were utilized for the evaluation of response which was classified according to generally accepted standards as CR, PR, no change (NC) and PD. The evaluation as NC required the absence of progression for at least 3 months.

RESULTS

Schedule I.   17 pts with advanced colon cancer were trea-ted with this schedule. Treatment results were 3 (18%) PR (all not pretreated pts) and 11 (64%) NC (2 pretreated pts), while 3 pts were progressive. The median time to progression after PR was 6 months (range 5-8 months) and after NC 7 months (range 3-15 months). The toxicity was tolerable. A dose reduction was neces-sary in 1 case with PD because of severe mucositis.

Schedule II. 28 pts with advanced colorectal cancer were evaluable. A CR was achieved in 1 pt with disseminated hepatic lesions and documented by ultrasound and CT-scan. Six pts achie-ved a PR. The metastatic sites of these pts were: liver 2 cases, abdominal mass 2 cases, liver and abdominal mass one case, and liver and lung one case. Ten previously progressive pts exhibi-ted stable disease (Metastatic sites: liver 5 cases, lung and liver 2 cases, lung 1 case, abdominal mass 1 case, liver, lung and lymphnodes 1 case). The median time to progression after an objective response was 10 months (range 3-12 months) and after NC 5 months (range 4 to 9 months). One of 7 pts with an objec-tive response and 2/10 pts who achieved stable disease had been pretreated. In 2 pts who responded with NC for 4 months and PR for 8 months, a switch to schedule II resulted in a second NC

Table 4. Maximum Toxicity

A) Schedule I   colorectal cancer (n=17)

WHO	0	1	2	3	4
Mucositis	6	6	5	0	0
Diarrhea	13	2	2	0	0
Nausea/Vomiting	17	0	0	0	0
Leucopenia	16	0	1	0	0

B) Schedule II   colorectal cancer (n=28)

WHO	0	1	2	3	4
Mucositis	11	11	6	0	0
Diarrhea	15	5	7	1	0
Nausea/Vomiting	24	3	1	0	0
Leucopenia	27	1	0	0	0

C) Schedule II   breast cancer (n=12)

WHO	0	1	2	3	4
Mucositis	6	3	2	1	0
Diarrhea	9	1	1	1	0
Nausea/Vomiting	11	1	0	0	0
Leucopenia	10	1	1	0	0

D) Schedule II   prostatic cancer (n=15)

WHO	0	1	2	3	4
Mucositis	12	2	1	0	0
Diarrhea	13	1	0	1	0
Nausea/Vomiting	14	1	0	0	0
Leucopenia	12	1	2	0	0

for 6 months, and a second PR for 10 months. For the analysis of survival of pts as related to response (CR, PR vs NC vs PD) the pts who received schedule I and/or II were summarized. As shown in figure 1, the median survival had not yet been reached in pts with objective response. The median survival for pts with NC and PD was 8 months. There is a clearcut trend to longer survival in pts with an objective response (p=0.28).
Dose reductions in order to reduce toxicity were made in 10 of 43 pts with colorectal cancer. These were subsequently evaluated as CR (1 pt), PR (2 pts), NC (5 pts) and PD (2 pts). Three pts who objectively responded (1 CR and 2 PR) had been pretreated.
In 15 pts with prostatic cancer no case of objective remission

was observed. Two pts achieved a NC status for 4 and 5 months
which was associated with pain relief and an improvement of
laboratory findings. In 8 pts with gastric cancer 1 PR (time to
progression 4 months) and 5 NC (median time to progression 3
months, range 3-8 months) could be induced.
Two of 12 pts with advanced and heavily pretreated breast cancer
achieved PR (time to progression 9 months and 5+ months) and
6 pts responded with NC (median time to progression 3.5 months,
range 3-8 months). The metastatic sites of objective responders
were lung and lymph nodes in one pt and extensive inflammatory
cutaneous spread and lymph nodes in the second. Treatment results of single pts with other malignancies are summarized in
Table 3. Remarkable to us seems the achievment of one PR and
2 NC in 3 pts with adenocarcinoma of unknown origin.

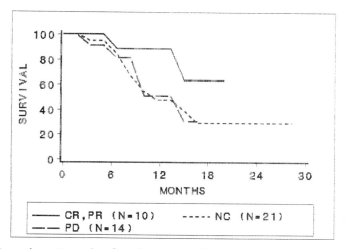

Fig. 1. Survival of pts with colorectal cancer

TOXICITY

Hematologic side effects were generaly mild and showed no
subsequent evidence of cumultative myelosuppression. Mucositis
and diarrhea were more frequent, however, and could easily be
managed by dose reduction in subsequent courses. Toxicity seemed
only slightly increased in the 12 pts with breast cancer
(Table 4 C) who had been intensively pretreated and was still
tolerable in the relatively older patients with prostatic cancer
(median age 66 years). In one responding pt with colorectal cancer a severe dermatitis (WHO grade 3) was observed after the
first course but did not reappear after dose reduction. The
maximum toxicity observed in each patient is shown in table 4 A
and B for colorectal cancer (schedule I and II respectively),
table 4 C for breast cancer and table 4 D for prostatic cancer.

DISCUSSION

Earlier studies have shown that a continuous infusion of
FUra is less toxic than push injections of equal doses. Therefore our initial study was begun with continuous infusion of
FUra. This study, however, yieled only 17% objective remissions.
As schedule I showed a mild level of toxicity, our findings indicated the possibility for dose escalation or push infusions of
FUra. Since continuous infusion requires hospitalization or the
use of portable infusion systems, we switched to short term FUra
infusions in patients who were unresponsive or progressive to
schedule I at tolerable toxicity. A further consideration which
led us to use short term infusion was that high FUra doses should
be given in the presence of excess CF. However, after push application of FUra in the dose of (600 mg/m²) after CF (200 mg/m²)
we observed an intolerable level of toxicity. Therefore we had
to reduce FUra to 400 mg/m² (push) given directly after CF in a
dose of 200 mg/m² (period of infusion 2 hours). Using this
schedule it was observed that 2 pts achieved a second PR (10
months) and NC (6 months) after switching to schedule II and as
a result, we terminated schedule I and continued with schedule
II. This study has resulted in 21% objective remissions (CR+PR)
and 38% NC, so far.

Schedule II is almost identical to that published by Machover et al.(1) except for a shorter time interval in our protocol. In spite of a higher dose intensity, however, our response
rates were clearly lower, even if the pretreated pts were excluded. Our results are more similar to those reported in a prospective study published by Budd et al.(2). One explanation for
our less encouraging findings, may be the selection of pts with
poor prognoses. We started treatment only in the presence of
measurable and progressive tumor lesions. On the other hand the
median time to progression of 10 months in the responding pts
of our study is similar or even better than that reported by
others (3, 4, 5). There was also improved survival in responders in our study.

FUra and CF in advanced prostatic cancer produced no objective remissions and the duration of disease stabilization
was very short. This discouraging result could be due to prior
hormonchemotherapy with estramustine which may have induced
secondary resistance.

In breast cancer, however, even after intensive cytotoxic
pretreatment, objective remissions and disease stabilizations
were achieved at a low level of toxicity.

Results in gastric carcinoma are still limited. They are,
however, similar to those shown by Arbuck et al.(6), which indicate that FUra and CF are active in this disease. Regarding
the other malignancies, the results in carcinoma of unknown
origin seem encouraging. These require further evaluation as
the number of cases was small.

Toxicity was mild in schedule I for pts with colorectal
cancer. Only one pt required dose reduction for mucositis and
diarrhea. We observed no case of limiting hematologic toxicity.
In pts receiving schedule II the dominant kind of toxicity was
diarrhea (Figure 4B). About one third of pts needed dose reductions. In pts with breast and prostatic cancer myelosuppression

230

(leucopenia) was more frequent, related to the extensive cytotoxic pretreatment in the first and the higher age of pts in
the first and the higher age of pts in the latter group.

In conclusion, FUra and CF are effective in advanced colorectal cancer, however, remission rates were somewhat low in
our study. Results were disappointing in prostatic cancer, but
encouraging in breast cancer and cancer of unknown origin, where
further investigation is warranted.

REFERENCES

1. D. Machover, F. Goldschmidt, P. Chollet, G. Metzger, J.
   Zittoun, J. Marquet, J.-M. Vandenbulcke, J.-L. Misset, L.
   Schwarzenberg, J.B. Fourtillan, H. Gaget, and G. Mathe:
   Treatment of advanced colorectal and gastric adenocarcinomas
   with 5-fluorouracil and high-dose folinic acid. J. Clin.
   Oncol 4:685 (1986).
2. G.T. Budd, T.R. Fleming, R.M. Bukowski, J.D. McCracken, S.F.
   Rivkin, R.M. O'Bryan, S.P. Balcerzak, and J.S. Macdonald:
   5-fluorouracil and folinic acid in the treatment of
   metastatic cancer: a randomized comparison. A southwest
   oncology group study, J. Clin. Oncol. 5:272 (1987).
3. D. Machover, M. Timus, L. Schwarzenberg, J.-M. Vandenbulcke,
   J.-L. Misset, G. Mathe, D. Baume, E. Goldschmidt, and P.
   Chollet: Treatment of advanced colorectal and gastric adenocarcinomas with 5-fluorouracil combined with high-dose
   leucovorin: an update, in: The current status of 5-fluor-
   ouracil-leucovorin calcium combination, H.W. Bruckner, and
   Y.M. Rustum, eds., John Wiley & Sons Inc. (1984).
4. P.J. Byrne, J. Treat, M. McFadden, P.S. Schein, P.V. Woolley,
   T.B. Huinink, and G. McVie: Therapeutic efficacy of the
   combination of 5-fluorouracil and high-dose leucovorin in
   patients with advanced colorectal carcinoma; single daily
   intravenous dose for five days, in: The current status of 5-
   fluorouracil-leucovorin calcium combination, H.W. Bruckner,
   and Y.M. Rustum, eds., J. Wiley & Sons Inc. (1984).
5. J.L. Misset, M. Timus, J.M. Vandenbulcke, J. Zittoun, and
   G. Mathe: Treatment of advanced colorectal (CRC) and gastric
   adenocarcinomas (GC) with 5-FU and high dose folinic acid
   (FA), 3rd European Conference on Clinical Oncology and Cancer
   Nursing, June 16-20, abstract 412, Stockholm (1985).
6. S.G. Arbuck, H.O. Douglass, F. Trave, S. Milliron, M. Baroni,
   H. Nava, L.J. Emrich and Y.M. Rustum: A phase II trial of
   5-fluorouracil and high-dose intravenous leucovorins in
   gastric carcinoma, J. Clin. Oncol. 5:1150 (1987).

DISCUSSION OF DR. BECHER'S PRESENTATION

<u>Audience</u>: May I ask you the same question. How long do you treat
your patients?

<u>Dr. Becher</u>: We treated patients with a minimum of 3 courses and in
case of stable disease or operative remissions we continued to treat
patients according to treatment success. So, in the patient in
which we achieved a complete remission we continue 2 more courses
and those with partial remission we continued until we saw improvement. If we saw no improvement, we stopped treatment. I think that
is an important point. It's very difficult for the clinician to
stay to a fixed schedule so I think it's possible also in randomized
studies to adapt treatment according to the biological features of
the specific case.

FOLINIC ACID (CF)/5-FLUOROURACIL (FUra) COMBINATIONS IN ADVANCED GASTROINTESTINAL CARCINOMAS

Hansjochen Wilke, H.-J. Schmoll, P. Preusser, U. Fink, M. Stahl, C. Schöber, H. Link, M. Freund, A. Hanauske, H.-J. Meyer, W. Achterrath, and H. Poliwoda

Hannover University,Medical School,3 Hannover, FRG

Colorectal cancer

The introduction of CF promises to be an important step towards a more successful treatment of colorectal cancer. CF (CH_2-H_4Pte Glu) is a biochemical modulator of fluoropyrimidine action and enhances cytotoxicity of FUra and FUDR in vitro and in vivo. CF/FUra combinations have been investigated in a number of clinical trials. Objective response rates of 30% - 40% were reproducibly achieved indicating a superiority of CF/FUra over FUra alone (1-7). However, inspite of these promising results the benefit of chemotherapy in colorectal cancer remains undetermined with respect to patient survival which is influenced by factors leading to a wide range of spontaneous survival time of patients with advanced colorectal cancer, e.g. stage of disease , tumor load, and particularly rate of tumor growth at time of diagnosis. If tumor growth rates are not determined prior to therapy treatment outcome might be biased by slowly or rapidly proliferating tumors and not necessarily reflect drug activity. Also, lack of tumor growth during observation period might be misinterpreted as antineoplastic effect ("no change","stabilisation").

Our group has initiated the following two sequential phase II trials with CF/FUra in advanced and progressive colorectal cancer since 1982. In both trials, a documented increase of >25% of measurable tumor parameters, as determined by two investigations 6 to 8 weeks apart or the manifestation of new metastases, were included into eligibility criteria. Other eligibility criteria were measurable disease, age $\leq$ 75 years, WHO performance status $\leq$ 2, and no prior chemotherapy.

Staging and evaluation of tumor response during chemotherapy were done by chest x-ray, abdominal CT, abdominal sonography, bone scan, and physical examination. Complete peripheral blood cell count, LDH, SGOT, SGPT, alkaline phosphatase, γGT, serum bilirubine, serum creatinine, CEA, CA 19-9, as well as measurable +/- evaluable tumor parameters were determined prior to each chemotherapy cycle. Blood counts were performed weekly. Evaluation of tumor response, toxicity, and median remission duration was done according to WHO criteria. Survival was calculated from the first day of treatment.

Table 1. Pat. characteristics (n = 93)		Table 2. Results (n = 93)	
Age	54 years (26 - 74)	CR + PR	11(12%)
Male/female	49/44	MR/NC	39(42%)
WHO performance status		P	43(46%)
0	21	CR + PR	
1	54	synchr. met.	3/30(10%)
2	18	metachr. met.	8/61(13%)
Locally recurrent dis.	2	MR/NC	
synchroneous metast.	30	synchr. met.	14/30(47%)
metachroneous metast.	61	metachr. met.	25/61(41%)

Study 1

Treatment plan: CF 200 mg/m² 10 min. inf., followed 50 min.
later by FUra 30-40 mg/kg body weight i.v. bolus injection,
once every 3 weeks until progression or intolerable toxicity
occurred.
Hundred patients have been entered in this trial. Ninety-three
are evaluable for response and toxicity. Four patients were excluded from analysis because of major protocol violations and
3 patients are lost to follow up. Patient characteristics are
summarized in table 1.
A mean of 7,5(1 -23) cycles were administered per patient. The
objective response rate (CR/PR) was 12%(11/93) including one
CR. Thirty-nine patients had MR/NC (42%) and 43 patients (46%)
had progressive disease. There was no difference in response
rate and tumor control rate (MR/NC) of patients with synchroneous and metachroneous metastases. Treatment results concerning responses are summarized in table 2.
Median remission duration was 12 months (3-17). Patients with
MR/NC progressed after a median duration of 6 months (2-17).
Overall survival time was 10 months (2-34), 19 months (6-30)

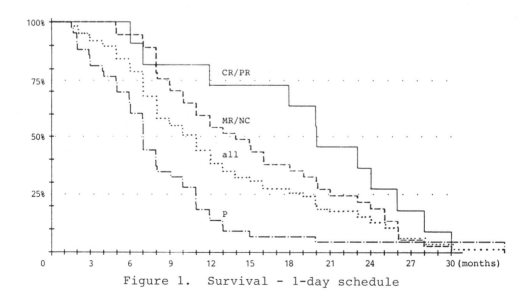

Figure 1. Survival - 1-day schedule

Table 3. Toxicity - WHO grade (n = 93)

	1	2	3	4
Leukocytes	16 (17%)	29 (31%)	22 (24%)	∅
Thrombocytes	15 (16%)	3 (3%)	∅	∅
Nausea/vomiting	21 (23%)	13 (14%)	2 (2%)	∅
Mucositis/stomat.	21 (23%)	11 (12%)	6 (6%)	∅
Diarrhea	8 (9%)	5 (5%)	∅	∅
CNS-toxicity	19 (20%)	20 (22%)	6 (6%)	∅
Infection	∅	7 (8%)	∅	∅
Skin	14 (15%)	10 (11%)	7 (8%)	∅
Alopezia	28 (30%)	21 (23%)	19 (20%)	∅

for CR/PR, 14 months (5-30) for MR/NC, and 7 months for progressive disease (Figure 1).
Myelosuppression was moderate. Leukopenia of WHO grade 2 and 3 were seen in 31% and 24% of patients, respectively. Thrombocytopenia of WHO grade 3 occurred in 3%, only.Seven patients had severe but manageable infections. Mean leukocyte nadir was 2,8 x 10^9/l (1,0 - 5,9), and the mean platelet nadir was 171 x 10^9/l (70 - 394). Peripheral blood cell counts recovered on day 20 (16 - 24). Mucositis/stomatitis of WHO grade 2 and 3 were observed in 12% and 6% of patients, respectively. A high incidence of CNS-toxicity was observed with this schedule of CF/FUra. Twenty-two percent and 6% of patients experienced confusion, vertigo, and ataxia of WHO grade 2 and 3. No other severe side effects were seen. Toxicity data are listed in table 3.

Study 2

Treatment plan: CF 300 mg/m² 10 min. inf., followed 50 min. later by FUra 600 mg/m² i.v. bolus injection, given on day 1,2, 3. Cycles were repeated on day 22 (-28). After induction of a complete remission two additional cycles for consolidation were administered. Patients without progressive disease (PR/MR/NC) recieved a total of six cycles. Patient characteristics are listed in table 4.
One hundred and fourty-four cycles (median 4 (1-8)) were administered to 37 patients. Thirty-six patients were evaluable for response (≧ 2 cycles). One patient refused further treatment after the first cycle. Thirty-seven patients were evaluable for

Table 4. Pat. characteristics (n = 37)

Age	57 years (35 - 75)
Male female	21/16
WHO performance status	
0	4
1	20
2	13
Synchroneous metastases	15
Metachroneous metastases	22

Table 5. Results (n = 36)

CR	2(6%)
CR + PR	14(39%)
MR/NC	13(36%)
CR/PR/MR/NC	27(75%)
P	8(22%)
Toxic death	1
CR + PR	
synchron. met.	1/15(20%)
metachron. met.	10/20(50%)

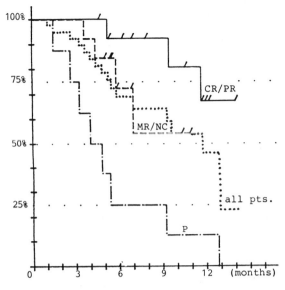

Figure 2. Survival - 3-day schedule

toxicity (≥1 cycle). The objective response rate (CR/PR) was
39% (14/36) including 2 CR's. Thirteen patients had MR/NC (36%)
resulting in an overall tumor control (CR/PR/MR/NC) of 75%
(27/36) in patients with progressive disease. Eight patients
showed tumor progression. There was one treatment related death
of a patient with concurrent irradiation of the small pelvis.
CR/PR in patients with synchroneous and metachroneous metastases were 20% and 50%, respectively. Treatment results concerning response rates are summarized in table 5.
Median remission duration of CR/PR was 7,5 months (4,5 - 13).
Patients with MR/NC progressed after a median duration of 5,5
months (2 - 7). Overall survival time is 12 months (1,5 - 14+),
14+ months (5,5 - 14+) for CR/PR, 11+ months (4 - 11+) for MR/
NC, and 4 months (1,5 - 13) for progressive disease (Figure 2).
Major toxicities of this regimen included myelosuppression
and gastrointestinal side effects. Leukopenia of WHO grade 3
and 4 were seen in 14% and 11% of patients, respectively. One
patient developed thrombocytopenia of WHO grade 4. There were

Table 6. Toxicity - WHO grade (n = 37)

	1	2	3	4
Leukocytes	5 (14%)	10 (27%)	5 (14%)	4 (11%)
Thrombocytes	4 (11%)	1 (3 %)	Ø	1 (3%)
Nausea/vomiting	5 (14%)	5 (14%)	Ø	Ø
Mucositis/stomat.	6 (16%)	12 (32%)	6 (16%)	Ø
Diarrhea	6 (16%)	4 (11%)	6 (16%)	Ø
Alopezia	7 (18%)	4 (11%)	3 (8%)	Ø
Infection	1 (3%)	1 (3%)	1 (3%)	3 (8%)
Skin	3 (8%)	5 (14%)	Ø	Ø
CNS-toxicity	3 (8%)	Ø	Ø	Ø

three severe infections in leukopenic patients including one septic death. Mean leukocyte nadir was $3,5 \times 10^9/l$ $(0,5 -6,5)$ and the mean platelet nadir was $180 \times 10^9/l$ $(14 - 487)$. Peripheral blood cell counts recovered on day 21 /17 - 28). Mucositis/stomatitis of WHO grade 2 and 3 occurred in 32% and 16% of patients, and diarrhea grade 2 and 3 in 11% and 16%, respectively. One patient developed severe angina pectoris after CF/FUra during the first cycle, which occurred again after re-exposition to CF/FUra. Three other patients with dose escalation up to 700 mg/m² of FUra showed cardiotoxic side effects (one arrhythmia, one angina pectoris gravis, one cardiac infarction). No other severe toxicities were observed. Toxicity data are summarized in table 6.

Discussion

During the past 25 years, FUra has been the mainstay of colon cancer chemotherapy despite the drawback that it produces short-lived responses in 20% of patients (8,9). With CF/FUra-combinations, higher response rates and possibly a prolongation of survival appears to be a realistic goal. Nevertheless, the benefit of chemotherapy in colorectal cancer still remains unproven. Patient subpopulations which might benefit from cytostatic treatment are not properly defined. One way to improve the impact of chemotherapy on survival and palliation might be to treat only patients with documented tumor progression. Tumor progression is a poor prognostic sign with a median expected survival of 6 - 8 months, depending on tumor load and site of metastatic spread at time of diagnosis. In these patients, not only objective responses as CR/PR but although tumor growth stabilisation (MR/NC) can be regarded as an antineoplastic effect. Also, MR/NC should be regarded as a valuable result, if it is correlated with a decrease or relief of tumor related symptoms, regardless whether a survival advantage is achieved or not.
So far, there is only one published study which reports treatment results with CF/FUra in progressive colorectal cancer. In the trial of Laufman et al.(1), half of the patients had documented tumor progression prior to chemotherapy. In the two studies of our group, tumor progression was the essential eligibility criterion. In all three studies, an overall tumor growth control (CR/PR/MR/NC) of 50% - 75% could be achieved with relief of tumor related symptoms in the majority of patients. These results indicate a significant change in the natural history of patients with far advanced and progressive colorectal carcinomas.
Comparing these two sequential studies, the three-day schedule appears to be more active with regard to objective responses, overall tumor growth control, and possibly to prolongation of survival times. Toxicities of both protocols were comparable to those reported for other CF/FUra regimens except of two findings (1-7). The one-day schedule was accompanied by a high number of CNS-side effects (confusion, vertigo, ataxia) which might be due to the high single dose of FUra. With the three-day schedule, an unexpected number of cardiac side effects was observed, particularly in patients with dose escalation of FUra above 600 mg/m². The cardiac risk of patients with high dose CF/FUra is currently under investigation in a prospectively randomized trial.
The treatment results of the 3-day schedule confirm the activity of CF/FUra combinations in advanced colorectal cancer. Ac-

Table 7. Patient characteristics
(n = 33)

Male/female	22/11
Age	66 years (48 - 75)
- >65 years	22
- ≤65 years + cardiac risk	11
WHO performance status	
- 0	1
- 1	13
- 2	19
Locally advanced disease	6
metastasized disease	27

cording to these findings, future trials should include documented tumor progression prior to chemotherapy as an important eligibility criterion. Such a procedure would help define more homogeneous patient populations and contribute to a better comparibility of different studies. Moreover, an overtreatment of patients with slowly proliferating tumors can be avoided particularly with respect to subjective and objective side effects of CF/FUra combinations. Because of the therapeutic range of CF/FUra, this combination will probably become the new "standard" treatment for advanced colorectal cancer and clinicians should be encouraged to further investigate this therapeutic approach.

Gastric cancer

More than 60% of patients with advanced gastric cancer are older than 65 years and underlying diseases (cardiovascular system, lung, liver, kidney, heart) which are common in the elderly may complicate or even hinder cytostatic treatment. Except for Etoposide and FUra most drugs which are active in gastric cancer possess cumulative organ toxicities (10-15). Etoposide and FUra rarely induce severe subjective and objective side effects in conventional doses (240 - 360 mg/m² per cycle). Experimental data indicated a synergism of Etoposide and FUra in vitro (16) and in vivo (17) as well as lack of cross resistance between both drugs (16). With CF/FUra, response rates of 40% were observed in advanced gastric cancer (3). For these reasons, the combination of CF/Etoposide/FUra was of interest from the clinical point of view. After a dosage find-

Table 8. Results (n = 33)

CR	4	(12%)
CR + PR	16	(48%)
MR/NC	8	(24%)
P	9	(27%)
Locally advanced disease	5/6	
metastasized disease		
- CR	3/27	(11%)
- CR + PR	11/27	(41%)
Age		
- >65 years	10/22	(45%)
- ≤65 years + cardiac risk	6/11	(55%)

Table 9. Toxicity - WHO grade (n = 33)

	1	2	3	4
Leukocytes	9 (27%)	13 (39%)	3 (9%)	1(3%)
Thrombocytes	9 (27%)	2 (6%)	1 (3%)	Ø
Nausea/vomiting	11 (33%)	5 (15%)	Ø	Ø
Mucositis/stomat.	6 (18%)	3 (9%)	Ø	Ø
Diarrhea	4 (12%)	3 (9%)	2 (6%)	Ø
Alopezia	5 (15%)	16 (48%)	10 (30%)	Ø
Infection	1 (3%)	Ø	1 (3%)	Ø
Neurotoxicity	Ø	Ø	Ø	Ø
Cardiotoxicity	Ø	Ø	Ø	Ø

ing, a disease orientated phase II trial was initiated in June
1986.
Until October 1987, thirty-four patients (patient characteristics: table 7) with advanced gastric cancer have been entered in
this trial. Eligibility criteria included measurable +/- evaluable disease, age >65 years, age ≤65 years + cardiac disease,
WHO performance status≤ 2, no prior chemo-/radiotherapy. Most
patients had an explorative laparotomy and cytologically confirmation of metastases.
Treatment plan: CF 300 mg/m² 10 min. inf. day 1,2,3, followed
immediately by Etoposide 120 mg/m² 50 min. inf. day 1,2,3, followed immediately by FUra 500 mg/m² 10 min. inf. day 1,2,3.
Cycles were repeated day 22 (-28). If a CR was achieved, two
further cycles were given for consolidation. Patients with PR/
MR/NC recieved a maximum of 6 cycles. In case of CR/PR in patients with locally advanced and irresectable (stated by laparotomy) gastric cancer, a second look operation was planned
with resection of residual tumor.

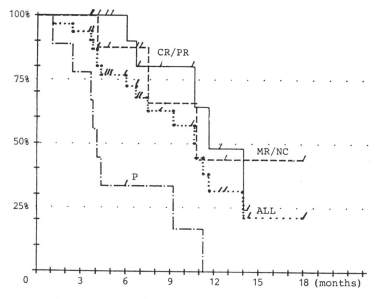

Figure 3. CF/Etoposide/FUra - Survival

Results: Thirty-three patients were evaluable for response and toxicity. One patient was lost to follow up and not included in this analysis. The overall response rate (CR/PR) was 48% (16/33; 95% confidence limit 31% - 65%) including 12% (4/33) complete remissions. Eight patients had minor remission /no change and 9 patients had progressive disease. Five of six patients with locally advanced and irresectable gastric cancer had an objective response, whereas 41% (11/27) of patients with metastases responded. In one patient a clinical CR could be confirmed pathohistologically. There was no difference between response rates of patients older or younger than 65 years (Table 8).

Median remission duration was 8 months (3 - 13+). Median time to progression in patients with MR/NC was 5,5 months. Median survival for all patients was 10,5 months (1,5 - 17,5), 11,5 months (8 - 13+) for responders, 10,5 months for MR/NC, and 4 months for progressive disease (Figure 3).

Except for one episode of WHO grade 4 leukopenia, no severe myelotoxicity was observed. Mean leukocyte nadir was $2,6 \times 10^9/1$ (0,8 - 4,2) and mean platelet nadir was $106 \times 10^9/1$ (34 - 260). Peripheral blood cell counts recovered on day 20 (17 - 24). Toxicity data are summarized in table 9.

Discussion

In this study, CF/Etoposide/FUra induced an objective response rate of 48%, a median remission duration of 8 months and a median survival time of 10,5 months in patients with risk factors (advanced age, cardiac disease, measurable disease). This regimen appears to be at least as efficient as FAM and FAM-modifications but causes less toxicity (18 - 22). CF/Etoposide/FUra is well tolerated with regard to objective and subjective side effects. It can be safely administered to older patients and to patients with cardiac risk factors and represents a valuable alternative for anthracycline-containing regimens especially in case of palliative treatment intentions. Based on these results, the addition of Cisplatin to CF/Etoposide/FUra appears to be promising in respect to the synergism between Cisplatin, Etoposide, and FUra.

References

1. Laufman, L.R., Krzeczowski, K.A., Roach, R, and Segal, M., 1987, Leucovorin plus 5-Fluorouracil: an effective treatment for metastatic colon cancer, J. Clin. Oncol., 5: 1394-1400.
2. Cunningham, J., Bukowski, R.M., Budd, T.G., Weick, J.K., and Purvis, J., 1984, 5-fluorouracil and folinic acid: a phase i-II trial in gastrointestinal malignancy, Investigational New Drugs, 2: 391 - 395.
3. Machover, D., Goldschmidt, E., Chollet, P., Metzger, G., Zittoun, J., Marquet, J., Vandenbulcke, J.M., Misset, J.L., Schwarzenberg, L., Fourtillan, J.B., Gaget, H., and Mathé, G., 1986, Treatment of advanced colorectal and gastric adenocarcinomas with 5-fluorouracil and high dose folinic acid, J. Clin. Oncol., 4: 685 - 696.
4. Zakem, M., Hines, J.D., Adelstein, D.J., and Rustum, Y.M., 1986, High-dose leukovorin and 5-fluorouracil (5-FU) in refractory and relapsed colo-rectal carcinoma, Proc. Am. Soc. Clin. Oncol., 5: 81 (abstr.).

5. Doroshow, J.H., Bertrand, M., Multhauf, P., Leong, L., Goldberg, D., Margolin, K., Carr, B., Akman, S., and Hill, R., 1987, Prospective randomized trial comparing 5-fluorouracil versus (vs) 5-FU and high dose folinic acid (HDFA) for treatment of advanced colorectal cancer. Proc. Am. Soc. Clin. Oncol., 6: 96 (abstr.).

6. Petrelli, N., Herrera, L., Stulc, J., Rustum, Y.M., and Mittelman, A., 1987, A phase III study of 5-fluorouracil (5-FU) versus 5-FU + methotrexate (MTX) versus 5-FU + high dose leucovorin (CF) in metastatic colorectal adenocarcinoma. Proc. Am. Soc. Clin. Oncol., 6: 74 (abstr.).

7. Ehrlichman, C., Fine, S., Wong, A., et al., 1988, A randomized trial of 5-fluorouracil and folinic acid in patients with metastatic colorectal carcinoma. J. Clin. Oncol., in press.

8. Carter, S.D., 1976, Large bowel cancer: the current status of treatment, JNCI, 56: 3 - 10.

9. Moertel, C.G., 1978, Chemotherapy of gastrointestinal cancer, N. Engl. J. Med., 299: 1049 - 1052.

10. Radice, P.A., Bunn, P.A., and Ihde, D.C., 1979, Therapeutic trials with VP-16-213 and VM-26: active agents in small cell lung cancer, non-hodgkin's lymphomas, and other malignancies. Cancer Treat. Rep., 63: 1231 - 1239.

11. Schmoll, H.-J., Niederle, N., and Achterrath, W., 1981, Etoposid (VP-16-213). Klin. Wochenschrift, 59: 1177 - 1188.

12. Dorr, R.T., and Fritz, W.L.,1980,5-Fluorouracil,in:"Cancer chemotherapy handbook," R.T. Dorr, and W.L. Fritz, eds., Elsevier, New York, Amsterdam, Oxford.

13. Cocconi, G., DeLisi, V., and Blasio, B., 1982, Randomized comparison of 5-FU alone or combined with mitomycin and cytarabine (MFC) in the treatment of advanced gastric cancer. Cancer Treat. Rep., 66: 1263 - 1266.

14. MacDonald, J.S., Gunderson, L.L.,and Cohn I.Jr., 1985, Cancer of the stomach, in: Cancer, principles and practise of oncology, V.T. DeVita, S. Hellman, and S.A. Rosenberg, eds., Lippincott, Philadelphia.

15. Kelsen, D.p., Magill, G., and Cheng, E., Phase II trial of Etoposide (VP-16) in the treatment of upper gastrointestinal malignancies. Proc. Am. Soc. Clin. Oncol.,123 : 96 (abstr.).

16. Hill, B.T., 1986, Potential of continous tumor cell lines for establishing patterns of cross-resistance and collateral sensitivity in vitro, Drugs Exptl. Clin. Res., 12: 685 - 696.

17. Osswaldt, H., and Kunz, W., 1987, Therapeutic synergism of Etoposide and 5-fluorouracil combined sequentially in advanced leukemia L 1210, Cancer Res. Clin. Oncol., 113 (suppl.): 53 (abstr.)

18. Beretta, G., Fraschini,P., Labianca, R., Arnoldi, E., Pancera, G., Tedeschi, L., and Luporini, G., 1986, Weekly 5-fluorouracil (F) versus combination chemotherapy for advanced gastrointestinal carcinomas, Proc. Am. Soc. Clin. Oncol., 5: 94 (abstr.).

19. Douglass, H.O.Jr., Lavin, P.T., Goudsmit, A., Klaasen, D.J., and Paul, A.R., 1984, An eastern cooperative oncology group evaluation of combinations of methyl-CCNU, mitomycin C, adriamycin, and 5-fluorouracil in advanced measurable gastric cancer (EST 2277), J. Clin. Oncol., 2: 1372- 1381.

20. MacDonald, J.S., Schein, P.S., Wooley, P.V., Smythe, T., Ueno, W., Hoth, D., Smith, F., Boiron, M., Gisselbrecht, C., Brunet, R., and Lagarde, C., 1980, 5-Fluorouracil,

doxorubicin, and mitomycin (FAM) combination-chemotherapy for advanced gastric cancer, Ann. Int. Med., 93: 533 - 536.

21. Fornasiero, A., Cartei, G., Daniele, O., Fosser, V., and Fiorentino, M. V., 1984, FAM2 regimen in disseminated gastric cancer, Tumori, 70: 77 - 80.

22. MacDonald. J.S., Gunderson, L.L., and Cohn, I.Jr., 1985, Cancer of the stomach, in: Cancer, principles and practise of oncology, V.T. DeVita, S. Hellman, and S.A. Rosenberg, eds., Lippincott, Philadelphia.

DISCUSSION OF DR. WILKE'S PRESENTATION

Audience: Are you still treating patients who are long term
   responders?

Dr. Wilke: No

Audience: When do you stop?

Dr. Wilke: We stop after 6 cycles.

EFFECTIVE SALVAGE THERAPY FOR REFRACTORY DISSEMINATED BREAST CANCER WITH 5-FLUOROURACIL AND HIGH-DOSE CONTINUOUS INFUSION FOLINIC ACID*

James H. Doroshow, Lucille Leong, Kim
Margolin, Bridget Flanagan, David Goldberg,
Marcelle Bertrand, Steven Akman,
Brian Carr, O. Odujinrin, and
Terri Litchfield

Departments of Medical Oncology
and Therapeutics Research and Biostatistics
City of Hope Cancer Research Center
Duarte, California

INTRODUCTION

Treatment options are limited for patients with dissemi-nated carcinoma of the breast whose disease has progressed after therapy with standard chemotherapeutic programs (1). In fact, the usefulness of testing investigational agents in those breast cancer patients who have been heavily pretreated, (two or more prior regimens), has been questioned recently (2). Thus, the discovery of effective therapy for this patient population is of considerable interest.

Since its introduction into clinical therapeutics, FUra has proven to be one of the most important agents for the treatment of advanced breast cancer, and remains a standard constituent of combination programs applied to the therapy of this disease (1). Because of the substantial body of experi-mental data indicating that pharmacologic concentrations of reduced folates in vitro enhance both the duration and degree of thymidylate synthase inhibition produced by FUra (3-5), a significant number of phase II and phase III trials have addressed the question of the clinical applicability of these

---

*This study was supported by Cancer Center Support Grant CA-33572 and by Lederle Laboratories. Requests for reprints should be addressed to J. Doroshow, M.D., Department of Medical Oncology and Therapeutics Research, City of Hope National Medical Center, 1500 E. Duarte Road, Duarte, CA, 91010. These results, in part, have been reported previously in Proc. Amer. Soc. Clin. Oncol. 5:65, 1986.

laboratory findings for patients with advanced gastrointestinal malignancies. To extend this area of clinical biochemical modulation, and building on our previous results using a monthly schedule of FUra and high-dose, continuous infusion folinic acid for advanced colorectal carcinoma (6), we performed a phase II trial of this regimen in women with advanced, measurable breast cancer all of whom had previously failed treatment with a FUra-containing chemotherapeutic program.

MATERIALS AND METHODS

Eligibility

Sixty patients with biopsy-proven, metastatic adenocarcinoma of the breast with bi-dimensionally measurable disease were entered on this study. All patients were required to have failed at least one prior combination chemotherapy regimen containing FUra, to have a performance status of $\geq$ 50% on the Karnofsky scale and an expected survival of at least 90 days, to have an absolute granulocyte count $\geq$ 2000/μl and platelet count $\geq$ 150,000/μl, total bilirubin $\leq$ 2.0 mg/dl, serum creatinine $\leq$ 2.0 mg/dl, no involvement of the central nervous system with breast cancer, and no history of any prior invasive malignancy. Patients having received prior radiation therapy were eligible provided that radiotherapy had been completed at least four weeks before entry on the study. Patients were required to give their written, informed consent for participation in the trial; individuals with breast cancer whose metastatic spread was limited to the axial skeleton were not entered on this study.

Pretreatment Evaluation and Follow-up Studies

Before the initiation of treatment, all patients underwent a complete history and physical examination; laboratory studies included a complete blood count with differential, platelet count, 18-function biochemical profile, chest x-ray, ECG, and abdominal CT examination. Complete blood counts with differential and platelet counts were performed weekly; serum electrolytes, BUN, creatinine and liver function tests monthly. Tumor measurements were required monthly if they could be determined by physical examination or chest x-ray; otherwise, every 2 months (or 2 cycles of therapy) if abdominal CT examinations were used for the assessment of measurable disease.

Study Design

This study was approved by the Institutional Review Board of the City of Hope National Medical Center. Patients were officially registered for the study by the Department of Biostatistics of the City of Hope Cancer Research Center after they were determined to be eligible and written, informed consent had been obtained.

Treatment

Therapy consisted of a 6-day infusion of 500 mg/m^2/day of folinic acid (calcium leucovorin; Lederle Laboratories, Pearl

River, NY) initiated 24 hours before a 5-day course of FUra given as an intravenous bolus at a dose of 370 mg/m^2/day (level 3). Treatment was repeated every 28 days. Patients with extensive bone metastases ($\geq$ 30 % total red marrow involved), extensive previous radiation therapy to the skeleton ($\geq$ 15 % total marrow), or previous treatment with mitomycin C or a nitrosourea were treated with 250 mg/m^2/day (level 1) FUra on the initial treatment cycle. Subsequent doses of FUra in these patients were increased to 300 (level 2) and then 370 mg/m^2/day where possible based on hematologic and gastrointestinal toxicity. All drug doses were calculated from surface area determinations based on ideal body weight. The folinic acid dose remained unchanged throughout the study; however, if more than moderate hematologic or gastrointestinal toxicity was observed on any course of therapy, the FUra dose was lowered one level. All patients received a minimum of 2 courses of therapy unless objective evidence of disease progression was documented after the first treatment cycle and was associated with at least a moderate level of hematologic or gastrointestinal toxicity. Therapy could only be delayed for a maximum of one week for recovery of the absolute granu-locyte and platelet counts to pre-treatment levels; patients requiring a delay of therapy of more than one week were taken off study.

Criteria for Response

Complete response was defined as complete disappearance of all objective evidence of disease on two separate measure-ments at least 4 weeks apart. Partial response was defined as a decrease of $\geq$ 50 % in the area (sum of the products of the diameters) of the measurable lesion(s), without evidence of new lesions for two consecutive evaluations separated by at least four weeks. The same criteria were used whether single or multiple lesions were evaluated. Disease progression was defined as an increase of $\geq$ 25 % in the area of the measurable lesion(s) or the appearance of new lesions. Patients with tumors not meeting these criteria for response or progression were considered stable. Response duration was measured from the onset of response until disease progression; duration of stable disease was calculated from the first day of therapy until progression. Survival was determined from the first day of treatment until death. All patient evaluations were performed by at least two of the authors.

Statistical Methods

Confidence intervals were computed as previously described (7).

RESULTS

Patient Characteristics

Sixty women with a median age of 55 years were entered on this trial (Table 1). Patients were of good performance status but were very heavily pretreated. Fifty-one of the 60 patients had previously received, and progressed on, FUra for disseminated breast cancer, and 88% had been treated with an anthracycline. A total of 21, 23, and 16 of the sixty

Table 1. Patient Characteristics

No. of Patients Entered	60
Median Age (yrs)	55
Range	27-82
Karnofsky Performance Status	
Median	80%
Range	50-100%
Patients Previously Treated	
With FUra	
Total	60
For Metastatic Disease	
Refractory to FUra	51
Patients Previously Treated	
With Anthracycline	
Total	53
For Metastatic Disease	51
No. of Prior Drug Regimens	
Total	
One	12
Two	20
Three or more	26
For Metastatic Disease	
One	21
Two	23
Three or more	16

Table 2. Therapeutic Responses

No. of Patients Entered	60
No. of Evaluable Patients	60
Complete Response, (%)	1 (2%)
Duration, Months	8.7
Partial Responses, (%)	9 (15%)
Duration, Months	1.3, 2.0, 2.0, 2.5, 3.2, 3.7, 4.1, 4.1, 12.8
Stable Disease	23 (38%)
Duration, Months	2-11+
Progressive Disease	27

patients had been treated with one, two, or three or more chemotherapeutic regimens for metastatic disease before entering this study.

Therapeutic Responses

All patients entered on the trial were evaluable for both response and toxicity. As shown in Table 2, one patient achieved a complete response lasting 8.7 months; nine patients had objective partial remissions of from 1.3 to 12.8 months for an overall response rate of 17 per cent. All of the patients experiencing an objective response had previously

Table 3. Characteristics of Objective Responders

	Complete Response	Partial Response
No. of Patients	1	9
No. of Prior Regimens for Metastatic Disease		
1		3
2	1	5
4		1
No. Patients With Prior FUra Exposure	1	9
No. Patients With Prior Progression on FUra-Containing Regimen For Metastatic Disease	1	8
Sites of Response		
Lung		2
Liver		3
Soft Tissue	1	4

Table 4. Hematologic and Other Toxicities

	Per Cent of Patients
WBC Nadir X 10^3, cells/mm^3	
1.0-1.9	12%
<1.0	10%
Granulocyte Nadir X 10^3, cells/mm^3	
0.5-0.9	23%
<0.5	22%
Platelet Nadir X 10^3, cells/mm^3	
25-49	7%
<25	3%
Stomatitis	
Ulcers, Able to Eat	18%
IV Fluids Required	5%
Diarrhea	
Well-Controlled by Therapy	18%
Poorly-Controlled by Therapy	0%
IV Fluids Required	2%

received FUra; nine of the ten responders had been treated for metastatic disease with objective evidence of disease progression on the FUra-containing program. The single complete responder had failed chemotherapy with cyclo-

phosphamide/methotrexate/FUra, FUra/vincristine/doxorubi-
cin/mitomycin C, and two prior hormonal maneuvers. Responses
were observed in visceral sites as frequently as in soft
tissues (Table 3). The median time to progression for all
sixty patients was 3.1 months. Median survival for the
entire group was 8.1 months.

Toxicity

The toxicity profile for this study is shown in Table 4.
In general, treatment was well-tolerated; no treatment-
related fatalities were observed. As expected, the major
side effects for this heavily-pretreated patient population
were hematologic, principally granulocytopenia, and gastrointestinal, including stomatitis and diarrhea. In five per
cent of patients, evidence of systemic sepsis was discovered.
Other side effects of chemotherapy, including anemia, nausea
or vomiting, alopecia, or erythematous skin changes were mild
and infrequent.

DISCUSSION

In this study, we found that the combination of a
continuous intravenous infusion of folinic acid with a daily
bolus schedule of FUra produced an objective response rate of
17% in a group of sixty women with metastatic breast cancer.
The 95% confidence limit for objective response in our study
is from 8 to 27 percent. These results are of interest
because this patient group had been heavily pre-treated for
disseminated disease with combination regimens that included
FUra, and because this response rate approaches that seen
with FUra alone in untreated patients (8). Very few, if
any, investigational agents recently tested by the Cancer
Therapy Evaluation Program of the National Cancer Institute
in patients with breast cancer refractory to standard
chemotherapy have activity that is comparable to the FUra-
folinic acid combination (2).

Two recent clinical trials have also reported preliminary results for the combination of FUra and folinic acid in
patients with advanced breast cancer; both studies support
the premise that the clinical biochemical modulation of
breast carcinomas is possible and may be explained by a
folate-related enhancement of thymidylate synthase inhibition
in vivo (9,10). The phase II study by Marini and colleagues
(9) reports a complete and partial response rate of 44% in a
group of 36 evaluable patients with metastatic breast cancer.
However, these impressive results must be interpreted in
light of the fact that fifteen patients received the bolus
folinic acid and FUra regimen as their first therapy for
metastatic disease, that only 13 patients had been treated
with doxorubicin previously, and that patients with disease
limited to the axial skeleton as the only site of metastasis
were not excluded from the assessment of the objective
response rate. In a preliminary report from the National
Cancer Institute, using a 500 mg/m^2/day folinic acid and 375
mg/m^2/day FUra schedule daily for five days every 21 days, 4
of 13 patients experienced an objective remission (10).
These patients had all failed at least one chemotherapeutic
regimen for advanced disease and 12 of 13 had progressed on

combination regimens including FUra. In two responding patients the binding of thymidylate synthase by FdUMP in tumor specimens from the chest wall was substantially enhanced after treatment with folinic acid.

Although these studies, as well as our own, suggest that the addition of reduced folates is responsible for the encouraging level of activity that was observed in such heavily pretreated women, a recent study by Mann and colleagues from the M.D. Anderson Hospital reported that FUra alone or in combination with PALA, when administered on a more dose-intensive schedule, had substantial activity in heavily pretreated patients (11). Hence, clinical progression for women with metastatic breast cancer receiving typical schedules of cyclophosphamide, methotrexate, and FUra or cyclophosphamide, doxorubicin, and FUra does not necessarily prove biochemical "resistance" to fluoropyrimidines.

Our evaluation of the toxicities associated with the use of infusional folinic acid and bolus FUra revealed, as expected, that gastrointestinal side effects, principally stomatitis, were dose-limiting. Considering the degree of prior chemotherapy received by the patients entered on our trial, hematologic toxicity was moderate and quite manageable. Differences in the folinic acid dose or schedule may explain the higher level of hematologic toxicity observed by others (9,10).

In summary, we have observed an overall objective response rate of 17 % in a group of 60 patients who received a six-day schedule of bolus FUra and high-dose, continuous infusion folinic acid as third- or fourth-line chemotherapy for metastatic breast cancer. These results and biochemical studies from other centers suggest that the efficacy of the fluoropyrimidines may be significantly enhanced in the treatment of advanced breast cancer by manipulation of the folate status of this tumor.

REFERENCES

1. I. C. Henderson, D. F. Hayes, S. Come, J. R. Harris, and G. Canellos, New agents and new medical treatments for advanced breast cancer, Sem. in Onc. 14:34 (1987).
2. E. Estey, D. Hoth, R. Simon, S. Marsoni, B. Leyland-Jones, and R. Wittes, Therapeutic response in phase I trials of antineoplastic agents, Cancer Treat. Rep. 70:1105 (1986).
3. J. A. Houghton, C. Schmidt, and P. J. Houghton, The effect of derivatives of folic acid on the fluorodeoxyuridylate-thymidylate synthetase covalent complex in human colon xenografts, Eur. J. Cancer Clin. Oncol. 18:347 (1982).
4. M. B. Yin, S. F. Zakrzewski, and M. T. Hakala, Relationship of cellular folate cofactor pools to the activity of 5-fluorouracil, Mol. Pharmacol. 23:190 (1983).
5. R. M. Evans, J. D. Laskin, and M. T. Hakala, Effects of excess folates and deoxyinosine on the activity and site of action of 5-fluorouracil, Cancer Res. 41:3288 (1981).
6. J. H. Doroshow, M. Bertrand, E. Newman, P. Multhauf, L. Leong, D. Blayney, D. Goldberg, K. Margolin, B. Carr, S. Akman, and G. Metter, Preliminary analysis of a randomized comparison of 5-fluorouracil and high-dose continuous-

infusion folinic acid in disseminated colorectal cancer, <u>NCI Monogr</u>. 5:171 (1987).

7. J. R. Anderson, L. Bernstein, and M. C. Pike, Approximate confidence intervals for probabilities of survival and quantiles in life-table analysis, <u>Biometrics</u> 38:407 (1982).

8. J. R. Harris, S. Hellman, G. P. Canellos, and B. Fisher, Cancer of the breast, <u>in</u>: "Cancer: Principles and Practice of Oncology," V. T. DeVita, Jr., S. Hellman, and S. A. Rosenberg, eds., J. B. Lippincott Co., Philadelphia (1985).

9. G. Marini, E. Simonicini, A. Zaniboni, F. Gorni, P. Marpicati, and A. Zambruni, 5-fluorouracil and high-dose folinic acid as salvage treatment of advanced breast cancer: an update, <u>Oncology</u> 44:336 (1987).

10. C. J. Allegra, B. A. Chabner, P. W. Sholar, C. Bagley, J. C. Drake, and M. E. Lippman, <u>NCI</u> <u>Monogr</u>. 5:199 (1987).

11. G. B. Mann, G. N. Hortobagyi, A. Buzdar, H-Y. Yap, and M. Valdivieso, A comparative study of PALA, PALA plus 5-FU, and 5-FU in advanced breast cancer, <u>Cancer</u> 56:1320 (1985).

DISCUSSION OF DR. DOROSHOW'S PRESENTATION

Audience: It is very difficult to determine clinical resistance but I doubt that the definition you gave is correct since
patients who have progressive disease on a regimen like CMF, who are
then put on full dose FUra single agent treatment may still respond
to this.

Dr. Doroshow: I agree with you completely. There's data from MD
Anderson to suggest that changing the schedule and dose of FUra will
produce responders.

PROGRESS REPORT ON A PHASE II TRIAL OF 5-FLUOROURACIL PLUS CITROVORUM

FACTOR IN WOMEN WITH METASTATIC BREAST CANCER

C.L. Loprinzi, J.N. Ingle, D.J. Schaid,
J.C. Buckner, and J.H. Edmonson

Divisions of Medical Oncology and
Cancer Center Statistics
Mayo Clinic
Rochester, MN

INTRODUCTION

5-fluorouracil (FUra) has definite, albeit limited, antitumor
activity against breast carcinoma (1). Inhibition of the enzyme, thymidylate
synthetase (TS) by FdUMP, an active FUra metabolite, has been postulated
as one biochemical mechanism for this antitumor activity (2). TS inhibition
is markedly augmented by the presence of increased concentrations of the
reduced folate, citrovorum factor (CF) (3). In 1985, preliminary information
suggested that FUra plus CF resulted in more substantial activity against
heavily pretreated metastatic breast cancer than would have been expected
with FUra alone (4). This current study was designed 1) to study the
antitumor activity and toxicity of FUra plus CF in metastatic breast
cancer patients who had not been "heavily pretreated" with chemotherapy,
2) to examine the impact of this regimen on tumor TS activity, and 3) to
correlate the degree of TS inhibition with clinical outcome. The protocol
continues to accrue patients and this communication provides a progress
report relating to antitumor activity and toxicity.

MATERIALS AND METHODS

Patients entering this clinical study are women with measurable
metastatic breast cancer who have received no more than one prior
combination chemotherapy regimen for metastatic disease. They must have
an ECOG performance status of ≤ 2; recovered from the acute toxicities of
previous therapy; and adequate hematologic, renal, and hepatic function
(WBC $> 4000/\mu L$, platelet $> 100,000/\mu L$, creatinine < 2 mg/dL, and total
bilirubin < 2 mg/dL).

Patients are given five consecutive days of intravenous CF, 500
mg/M^2/d in 250 cc of 5% dextrose over 30 minutes, followed, one hour
later, by FUra, 375 mg/M^2/d as an intravenous bolus. Repeat cycles are
planned at four week intervals. Dose modifications of FUra are based on
interval toxicity while CF doses are not modified.

Women with assessable tumor have had 4 mm punch biopsies obtained,
prior to, and approximately 24 hours following FUra plus CF. Samples have

255

Table 1 - Pretreatment Patient Characteristics

Age (years)
    median   56
    range   41-69

ECOG PS
    0   7
    1   8
    2   6

Previous treatment

    Chemotherapy (CFP, CMF, or CAF)*   16
        adjuvant therapy only   4
        metastatic disease only   8
        both   4

    Hormonal Therapy   17
        adjuvant therapy only   0
        metastatic disease only   13
        both   4

    Radiation therapy   13
        adjuvant therapy only   2
        metastatic disease only   10
        both   1

Disease sites
    soft tissue only   3
    osseous (+ soft tissue)   6
    visceral (+ osseous and/or soft tissue)   12

*C-cyclophosphamide, F-FUra, P-prednisone,
M-methotrexate, A-doxorubicin

been immediately frozen at -60°F and sent to the National Cancer Institute
(C. Allegra) for measurement of TS activity. These results will remain
blinded until the completion of this trial.

RESULTS

    Twenty-eight women have entered this study to date. The 21 patients
with at least cycle 1 data are the subject of this report. All 21
patients are eligible and evaluable. Pretreatment patient characteristics
are illustrated in table 1.

    Partial responses have been seen in 4/21 patients to date (19%, 95%
confidence interval, 5%-42%) with times to disease progression of 6+, 7,
8, and 9 months. Two of the 4 responding patients had received prior
FUra-based combination chemotherapy (one for metastatic disease and one as
adjuvant therapy only). Responses occurred in soft tissue (3 patients),
bone (1), and pulmonary (1) sites. Two additional patients had convincing
evidence of tumor shrinkage but did not fulfill the strict criteria for
partial response. One had flattening and healing of an ulcerated chest
wall lesion documented with serial photographs but the lateral margins of
abnormal tissue did not decrease enough to classify as a partial response.

Table II - Drug Toxicity

Toxicity	Number of patients	
Total Patients	21	
WBC		
<1000/mL	1	
1,000-2,000/mL	2	
Platelet		
<90,000/mL	0	
90,000-100,000/mL	2	
mucositis	18	
mild		5
moderate		11
severe		2
diarrhea	14	
rash	9	
phlebitis	4	
skin hyperpigmentation	3	
conjunctivitis	1	

Another had a complete disappearance of multiple chest wall nodules in the face of a markedly increased pleural effusion.

Fifteen of the 17 patients not meeting partial response criteria have been taken off study; 13 for disease progression and 2 for inordinate toxicity (hives in one patient, mucositis in another). Two of the 17 patients remain on study with stable disease at one month.

Therapy-related toxicity is summarized in table 2. The most prominent dose limiting toxicity from this regimen was mucositis, affecting 86% of the 21 patients (mild, moderate, and severe symptoms in 5, 11, and 2 patients, respectively). Fourteen patients (67%) also complained of treatment-related diarrhea which was usually mild.

Anorexia, nausea, and vomiting were seen in the majority of patients but were generally mild and well tolerated. An allergic-type rash was observed in 9/21 patients (43%). This varied from a relatively mild, transient erythema to very prominent hives requiring systemic steroids. The rash usually developed during the days of chemotherapy administration or within 3-4 days following completion of the 5 day chemotherapy course. Notably, 4 of the patients who developed an allergic-type rash during their first cycle of therapy did not develop any rash on multiple subsequent cycles of therapy. Conversely, 2 patients had recurrent rashes while 3 patients did not get further chemotherapy courses following their rash. Only one patient had therapy discontinued because of an allergic reaction (severe hives requiring systemic steroids). In addition to the above rashes, 3 patients noted generalized skin hyperpigmentation following 1-2 courses of therapy which appeared similar to that seen in some patients who have received long term FUra therapy alone. Phlebitis at the infusion site was a mild-moderate problem in 4 patients. In one of these patients, the phlebitis was alleviated in subsequent cycles of therapy by giving the FUra and CF in opposite arms.

Hematologic toxicity has not been a major problem in this study to date with median WBC and platelet nadirs of $2,600/\mu L$ and $240,000/\mu L$, respectively. A WBC nadir less than $1,000/\mu L$ was seen in only 1/65 courses while the lowest platelet nadir was $94,000/\mu L$.

DISCUSSION

Convincing results are now available demonstrating that FUra plus CF is superior to FUra alone in patients with metastatic colon cancer (5). Early phase II studies of FUra plus CF in patients with metastatic breast cancer have had encouraging results (4,6-8). Completion of protocol accrual and further data maturation are required before final conclusions can be drawn from this current study. Nonetheless, future comparative clinical trials will clearly be necessary to better define the role of FUra plus CF for patients with breast cancer.

REFERENCES

1. S. Hellman, J. Harris, GP Canellos, et al, 1982, Principals and Practice of Oncology, in: "Cancer", V. DeVita, S. Hellman, and S. Rosenberg, ed., J.B. Lippincott Col, Philadelphia, pp 183-200.
2. D. Machover, I Schwarzenberg, et al, Treatment of Advanced Colorectal and Gastric Adenocarcinoma With 5-FU Combined With High-Dose Folinic Acid: A Pilot Study, Cancer Treat Rep, 66:1803-1807.
3. S. Waxman, H. Buckner, The Enchancement of 5-Fluorouracil Anti-Metabolic Activity by Leucovorin, Menadione, and a Tocopherol, Eur J Cancer Clin Oncol, 18:685-692, 1982.
4. C. J. Allegra, B. A. Chabner, P. W. Sholar, et al, Preliminary Results of a Phase II Trial for the Treatment of Metastatic Breast Cancer With 5-Fluorouracil and Leucovorin, NCI Monogr 5:199-202, 1987.
5. M. A. Poon, M. J. O'Connell, H. S. Wieand, et al, Biochemical Modulation of Fluorouracil, Evidence of Significant Improvement of Survival and Quality of Life in Advanced Colorectal Carcinoma, (in preparation).
6. G. Marini, E. Simoncini, A. Zaniboni, et al, 5-Fluorouracil and High-Dose Folinic Acid as Salvage Treatment of Advanced Breast Cancer: An Update, Oncology, 44:336-340, 1987.
7. J. Doroshow, M. Bertrand, P. Multhauf, et al, High Dose Continuous Infusion Folinic Acid (HDFA) and IV Bolus 5-FU: An Effective Salvage Regimen for Refractory Metastatic Breast Cancer, Proc Am Soc Clin Oncol, 5:65, 1986.
8. J. L. Grem, D. F. Hoth, M. Hamilton, et al, Overview of Current Status and Future Direction of Clinical Trials With 5-Fluorouracil in Combination With Folinic Acid, Cancer Treat Rep, 71:1249-1264, 1987.

ACKNOWLEDGEMENT

Supported in part by Contract # CM 57733B from the NCI, NIH, and DHHS

DISCUSSION OF DR. LOPRINZI'S PRESENTATION

Audience: Its very difficult to assess, as you say, the response
of any regimen used as the second line. Resistance to a combination
doesn't mean a resistance to a particular drug, maybe to one on two
or some. Your patients are heavily treated with CFP and CMF and COF
but that doesn't necessarily mean that they are resistant to FUra
when you come to the second line. So in breast cancer it would be
better to go on the first line to prove the point. When you recycle
a drug used before which you show at the beginning of 70 if you use
another dosage or schedule on the top of another drug, they work.
It is not convincing all this study to me when you recycle the same
drug in different doses and different schedule and you mean that was
refractory to 5-FU and not many drugs in the prior combination.

Dr. Loprinzi: No comment.

Dr. Erlichman: I just want to add to the database of information. We
have a phase II trial in breast cancer also using the same schedule
we have used in colorectal cancer and that is in patients who have
had no prior treatment other than adjuvant at least a year before
entry on this trial. Out of 26 evaluable patients to date, 13 are
showing responses. The study continues.

ADJUVANT THERAPY FOR COLORECTAL CANCER: THE NSABP CLINICAL TRIALS

Norman Wolmark

University of Pittsburgh
Pittsburgh, Pennsylvania 15213

The current generation of the National Surgical Adjuvant Breast and
Bowel Project (NSABP) adjuvant therapy protocols assessing the utility of
5-fluouracil and leucovorin (FU-LV) in colorectal cancer was based in
large part on the data obtained from the completed Protocol C-01 for
carcinoma of the colon and R-01 for rectal cancer.

Data were derived from 1,166 patients with Dukes B and C carcinoma of
the colon who were entered into the NSABP Protocol C-01 between November
1977 and February 1983.   Patients were randomized to one of three therapeutic categories: 1) no further treatment following curative resection
(394 patients); 2) postoperative chemotherapy consisting of 5-fluorouracil
semustine, and vincristine (MOF) (379 patients); or 3) postoperative BCG
(393 patients).   The average time on study was 77.3 months.   A comparison
between patients receiving postoperative adjuvant chemotherapy and those
treated with surgery alone indicated that there was an overall improvement
in disease-free survival (P=.02) and survival (P=.05) in favor of the
chemotherapy-treated group (figure 1).   At 5 years of follow-up, patients
treated with surgery alone were at 1.29 times the risk of developing a
treatment failure and at 1.31 times the liklihood of dying as were similar
patients treated with combination adjuvant chemotherapy.   Comparison of
the BCG-treated group with the group treated with surgery alone indicated
that there was no statistically significant difference in disease-free
survival (P=.09).   There was, however, a survival advantage in favor of
the BCG-treated group (P=.03).   At 5 years of follow-up, patients randomized to the surgery-alone arm were at 1.28 times the risk of dying as
were similar patients treated with BCG.   Further investigation disclosed
that this survival advantage in favor of BCG was a result of a diminution
in deaths that were non-cancer related.   When analyses were conducted in
which events not related to cancer recurrence were eliminated, the survival difference between the BCG and control groups became nonsignificant
(P=.40); the cumulative odds at 5 years decreased from 1.28 to 1.10.   The
findings from this study are the first from a randomized prospective
clinical trial to demonstrate that a significant disease-free survival
and survival benefit can be achieved with postoperative adjuvant chemotherapy in patients with Dukes B and C carcinoma of the colon who have
undergone curative resection.

Data were also analyzed from 555 additional patients with Dukes B
and C rectal cancers treated by curative resection who were entered into

261

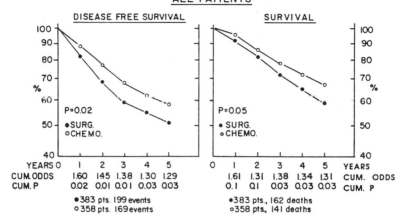

C-01
CHEMOTHERAPY vs CONTROL
ALL PATIENTS

FIGURE 1

NSABP protocol R-01 between November 1977 and October 1986. Their
average time on study was 64.1 months. The patients were randomized to
receive no further treatment (184 patients), postoperative adjuvant chemotherapy with 5-fluorouracil, semustine, and vincristine (MOF) (187
patients), or postoperative radiation therapy (184 patients). The chemotherapy-treated group, when compared with the group treated by surgery
alone, demonstrated an overall improvement in disease-free survival (P=
.006) and in survival (P=.05). Employing the proportional hazards model,
a global test was used to determine the presence of treatment interactions.
Investigation of stratification variables employed in this study indicated
that sex, and to a lesser extent age and Dukes stage, made individual
contributions to the disease-free survival and survival benefit from
chemotherapy. When evaluated according to sex, the benefit from chemotherapy at 5 years, both in disease-free survival (29% vs. 47%; P=.001;
relative odds, 2.00) and in survival (37% vs. 60%; P=.001; relative odds,
1.93), was restricted to males (figure 2). When males were tested for age
trend with the use of a logistic regression analysis, chemotherapy was
found to be more advantageous in younger patients. When the group receiving postoperative radiation (4,600-4,700 rad in 26-27 fractions;
5,100-5,300 rad maximum at the perineum) was compared to the group
treated by surgery alone, there was an overall reduction in local-regional
recurrence from 25% to 16% (P=.06). No significant benefit in overall
disease-free survival (P=.4) or survival (P=.7) from the use of radiation
has been demonstrated. The global test for interaction to identify
heterogeneity of response to radiation within subsets of patients was not
significant. In conclusion, these investigations have demonstrated a
benefit from adjuvant chemotherapy (MOF) for the management of colo-rectal
cancer. The observed advantage was present for all patients in carcinoma
of the colon and was restricted to males in patients with rectal cancer.
Postoperative radiation therapy reduced the incidence of local-regional
recurrence in carcinoma of the rectum, but it failed to affect overall
disease-free survival and survival.

Based on the findings from NSABP protocols C-01 and R-01, the NSABP initiated protocols C-03 and R-02 which were opened to patient accrual in August of 1987. Protocol C-03 is designed to compare the efficacy of postoperative FU-LV with the MOF combination that was shown to be effective in NSABP protocol C-01 in patients with Dukes B and C carcinoma of the colon. The dose and schedule of FU-LV are depicted in figure 3. To date 260 patients have been randomized into this study; the estimated sample size is 750 patients over 5 years for an 83% power to detect a 10% increase in survival probability.

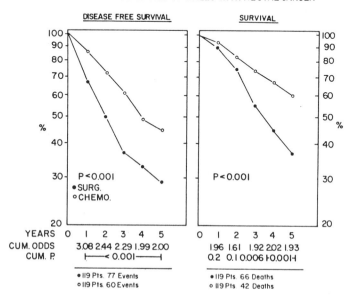

EFFECT OF ADJUVANT CHEMOTHERAPY ON DISEASE FREE
SURVIVAL AND SURVIVAL OF MALES WITH RECTAL CANCER

FIGURE 2

Protocol R-02 for patients with Dukes B and C rectal cancer is designed to address two major specific aims: 1) to determine whether the addition of radiotherapy to combination chemotherapy is more effective than combination chemotherapy alone and 2) to ascertain whether FU-LV with or without radiation is more effective than MOF with or without radiation. Because of lack of efficacy of MOF in females in protocol R-01, females are not randomized to MOF in protocol R-02. The randomization schema for protocol R-02 is shown in figure 4. Since August of 1987, 60 patients have been randomized. The main statistical goal is to be able to detect a 10% increase in 5 year survival probability for chemotherapy enhanced by radiation with 80% power using a one-sided 0.05 level log rank test. If 750 patients are accrued into the study over 5 years and are followed for an additional half year before final analysis there will be 83% power to detect a 10% increase in survival probability.

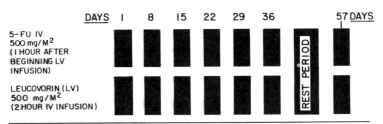

NSABP C-03, R-02
5-FU, LEUCOVORIN THERAPY

CYCLE 1

DAYS   1   8   15   22   29   36   57 DAYS

5-FU IV
500 mg/M²
(1 HOUR AFTER
BEGINNING LV
INFUSION)

LEUCOVORIN (LV)
500 mg/M²
(2 HOUR IV INFUSION)

REST PERIOD

BLOOD COUNTS WEEKLY
(PRIOR TO NEXT TREATMENT)
REPEAT x 6 CYCLES

FIGURE 3

NSABP R-02

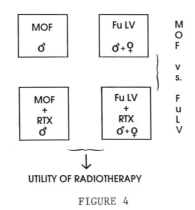

| MOF ♂ | Fu LV ♂+♀ | M O F |
| MOF + RTX ♂ | Fu LV + RTX ♂+♀ | vs. F u L V |

UTILITY OF RADIOTHERAPY

FIGURE 4

DISCUSSION OF DR. WOLMARK'S PRESENTATION

Dr. Bertino: The male/female difference is, of course, very intriguing. Have you looked at the calculated dose delivery; are females truly the weaker sex, in terms of dose tolerance?

Dr. Wolmark: There was no difference in the cumulative dose received by females relative to males. We've looked at many parameters to try to understand this sexual bias that seems to be evolving relative to chemtherapy and haven't been able to find one. The only biologic phenomenon that seems to make sense is that, from a natural history standpoint, females seem to do better than males. The untreated control female does better than the untreated control male. We are currently looking at tumor differentiation by flow cytometry to determine if there really is a difference in the tumors in males and females.

Audience: Dr. Wolmark, because of the problem that has been identified with leukemias developing in patients treated with methyl CCNU, would you please comment on how beneficial it would be to further develop a regimen which incorporates methy CCNU which may very well never be able to be marketed outside of an investigational protocol.

Dr. Wolmark: Well, out of the 480 patients who were treated with methyl CCNU we've had 3 acute nonlymphocytic leukemias in the study. Now whether this is an acceptable risk or not I think has to be weighed in light of the advantages of the therapy. As far as the marketing elements related to methyl CCNU the present generation of NSABP trials are not designed to resurrect methyl-CCNU but to bury it and we hope that FUra/CF regimen will have significant advantages over the MOF regimen. If it doesn't, I think we will all be disappointed and we'll have to reassess the value of methyl-CCNU in the adjuvant setting.

Dr. Holland: Norman, do I understand that the females are being studied with historical controls?

Dr. Wolmark: No.

Holland: What is the control for the females receiving FUra/CF?

Dr. Wolmark: The question we're simply asking in females does not assess whether FUra/CF is effective. We're simply addressing in the females whether adding radiotherapy to FUra/CF is effective.

Dr. Holland: Well if you come up with 60 months of median survival in each arm what's your conclusion going to be?

Dr. Wolmark: That radiotherapy added to FUra/CF in the female is of no value.

Dr. Holland: And that would cost you how many hundreds of thousands of dollars to do without coming up with an answer that this was a useful study for women?

Dr. Wolmark: Well I think if one assesses the cost of the number of females who are receiving radiotherapy together with chemotherapy across the country I think it would also add up to a significant cost. Probably far more than the FUra/CF.

Dr. Holland: Recognizing how hard it is and since your data are the best in not having found an adjuvant program of value for women with this disease, why don't you put an untreated control in now? Because when you finish 4 or 5 years from now and make the analysis you won't really tell us whether or not FUra/CF is useful in women.

Dr. Wolmark: Yes, I agree.

Dr. Holland: Did you run into trouble with your constituents?

Dr. Wolmark: Not so much with our constituents, perhaps our proprietors would be a more important definition of that, but I think I've said all that I know and perhaps more.

Dr. Frei: Have any of the previous studies of rectal adjuvant cancer involving FUra alone or in combination vs a control shown a sex difference?

Dr. Wolmark: No. But a good part of that data are derived from the VA which tends to cater to a male population. Looking at some of the other studies, particularly from the north central, there are really too few patients to try and address the sex issue as related to the response to chemotherapy. This is a very curious phenomenon. The global test for interaction is highly significant even accounting for multiple looks at the data. But there are no other studies that have demonstrated the same phenomenon.

266

CHEMOTHERAPY OF ADVANCED AND RELAPSED SQUAMOUS CELL CANCER OF THE HEAD
AND NECK WITH SPLIT-DOSE CISPLATINUM (DDP), 5-FLUOROURACIL (FURA) AND
LEUCOVORIN (CF)

T.M. Loeffler[1], J. Lindemann[2], H. Luckhaupt[2], K.G. Rose[2],
and T.U. Hausamen[1]

Medical Center Dortmund, Departments of Medicine[1] and
Oto-Laryngology[2], Beurhausstrasse 40
4600 Dortmund, West Germany

Abstract

58 patients with locally advanced or relapsed squamous cell head and
neck cancer were treated on 5 consecutive days with DDP 20 mg/m^2/d
IV-push, followed by CF 100 mg/m^2/d IV-bolus and Fura 400 mg/m^2/d
IV-push 60 minutes later. Treatment was recycled on day 22 (-29),
according to toxicity. CF was added to the widely used DDP/Fura
combination, because recent studies showed enhancement of Fura-activity
by CF. 45/58 patients had no prior therapy and 13/58 pts were relapsed
after chemotherapy and/or radiation therapy. All patients were
evaluable for toxicity and response. After 3 courses of induction
chemotherapy 23/45 pts in the previously untreated group had a complete
response (CR); 20/45 a partial response (PR), 2/45 were restaged as no
change (CR + PR: 95%). Induction chemotherapy was followed by radical
surgery and postoperative radiation therapy. In the pretreated group
4/13 pts had a complete response; 6/13 a partial response; no change in
3/13 pts. Median duration of remission (MDR) has not been reached in
the primarily untreated group, whereas in pretreated patients the MDR
was 3.8 months (range 2.3 - 11.7 months). Hematologic and gastrointestinal toxicity was substantial but manageable and therapy was
performed on an outpatient basis. The combination of DDP, CF and Fura
has high activity in untreated and pretreated head and neck cancer
patients. The obtained results are comparable to the widely used
DDP/Fura continuous infusion regimen.

INTRODUCTION

The combination of DDP and Fura has emerged as one of the most active
chemotherapeutic regimens for the treatment of advanced and recurrent
squamous cell head and neck cancer in recent years. In untreated
patients an overall response rate up to 90% with a 54% complete response
rate was reported, whereas a 70% response rate (27% CR) could be
achieved in recurrent and pretreated patients (1,2). Continuous infusion
of Fura in combination with DDP was found to be significant superior
when compared to bolus Fura (3). The enhancement of Fura-activity by CF
in metastatic colorectal and breast cancer has been well documented in
recent studies (9-12). Fura inhibits thymidylate synthetase (TS) and
subsequently DNA-synthesis by forming a ternary complex consisting of

the active Fura- metabolite FdUMP, TS and intracellular reduced folate. The degree of complex formation and its stability varies with the amount of available reduced folates and can be increased by the addition of exogenous folates (4-7). There is further evidence that the proposed synergism between DDP and Fura can be explained by an increase of the intracellular 5,10-methylenetetrahydrofolate pool secondary to an enhanced intracellular synthesis of methionine which is thought to be caused by DDP-mediated methionine influx inhibition (8).

Based on these findings a combination of DDP, Fura and CF for the treatment of advanced squamous cell head and neck cancer in a 5-day bolus schedule was designed. The bolus schedule was chosen because bolus Fura was found to be less active when compared to continuous infusion (3) and the proposed enhancement of Fura-activity by CF should therefore result in an increased response rate.

PATIENTS AND METHODS

58 patients, 45 untreated and 15 relapsed were enrolled into this study (See table I). All patients had biopsy proven squamous cell carcinoma. The extent of the primary lesion and involvement of regional lymph nodes were measured clinically by CT-scan and endoscopy. Further workup included a chest x-ray, abdominal ultrasound, complete blood count, blood chemistry, 24-hour creatinine clearance or isotope renal scan for GFR evaluation and an audiogram. Primary lesions were tattooed for restaging evaluation. Patients with non-compensated congestive heart failure were not eligible. Chemotherapy consisted of DDP 20 mg/m^2 IV-push x 5 days, followed by CF 100 mg/m^2 IV-bolus x 5 days. Fura 400 mg/m^2 IV-push x 5 days was administered 60 minutes after CF. Hydration and antiemetic therapy consisted of 1000 ml NS with 1 mg/kg Metoclopramide and 10 mg/m^2 Dexamethasone daily prior to DDP and was infused over 60-90 minutes. No additional hydration was administered. Chemotherapy was repeated every 3-4 weeks, depending on the actual white blood count. DDP and Fura were attenuated if hematologic and/or gastrointestinal toxicity grade III WHO and higher were observed. Response was evaluated clinically and by CT scan after 3 courses of neoadjuvant chemotherapy in the previously untreated group. All patients in this group were subsequently treated with radical surgery and postoperative radiation therapy. Relapsed patients received maximal 6 courses of chemotherapy or until disease progression was diagnosed. Complete response (CR) was defined as complete disappearance of all measurable disease; partial response (PR) was defined as 50% or the measurable lesion in the absence of new lesions; no change (NC) was defined as less response than PR or stable disease. Duration of response was calculated from the date of documented response to the date of relapse, progression of death.

Table I. Patients Characteristics

No. of Patients	: 58
Male/Female	: 49/9
Age	: 38/68
Median	: 46
Karnofsky Perf. Status	: 70-100%
Median	: 90%
Untreated/Pretreated	: 45/13

268

Table I.   Patients Characteristics (Cont'd)

Untreated Patients:

Tumor Localizations	:	Hypopharynx	16/45
	:	Oropharynx	16/45
	:	Other	13/45
Tumor Stages	:	II	6/45
	:	III	15/45
	:	IV	24/45

Pretreated Patients:

Radiation Pretreatment	:	8/13
Chemo/Radiation Pretreatment	:	5/13

Sites of Recurrence			
	:	Primary Tumor	9/13
	:	Lymphnodes	2/13
	:	Multiple Sites	2/13

RESULTS

The overall response rate in the previously untreated group after three courses of induction chemotherapy was 95% (See table 2A). A complete response was diagnosd in 24/45 patients (51%) and a partial response in 20/45 patients (44%). A no change status was noticed in 2/45 patients (5%). The percentage of pathological complete responders after induction chemotherapy needs to be determined. The inclusion of stage II disease for induction chemotherapy resulted in 5/6 complete responses (See Table 2B).

Table 2A.   Response to Chemotherapy after 3 Courses in
Untreated Patients

	N	%
Complete Response	23/45	51
Partial Response	20/40	44
Cr + PR	43/45	95
No Change	2/45	

There was no difference in response comparing stage IV hypo- and oropharynx tumors which is in contrast to the general experience that advanced hypopharynx cancer is less responsive (See table 2B).

Table 2B: Comparison of Response to Chemotherapy According
to Tumorlocalisation and Stage of Disease

Type of Remission	Complete Response			Partial Response			No Change		
Stage	II	III	IV	II	III	IV	II	III	IV
Tumor Localization									
Hypopharynx N = 16		2	4	1	8				1
Oropharynx N = 16	3	6	3	3	8				
Other N = 13	2	1	2	2	5	1			
Total	5	9	9	6	14		1		1

Response to chemotherapy of regional lymph node metastasis had a
significant impact on the overall response. 12 pts. with a complete
remission of the primary lesion had a partial remission in the
metastatic lymph nodes. Only 10 pts. with regional lymph node disease
were restaged with a complete response in both primary tumor and lymph
node metastasis.

In the pretreated group of patients 10/13 responded to chemotherapy (See
table 2C). 4/13 pts. were found to have a complete response and 6/13
pts. a partial response. No change was noticed in 3/13 pts. The median
response duration however, was short with 3.8 months (range 2.3-11.7
months).

Table 2C. Response to Chemotherapy in Recurrent and
Pretreated Patients

	N
Complete Response	4/13
Partial Response	6/13
CR + PR	10/13
No Change	3/13
Response Duration	2.3 - 11.7 Months
Median	3.8 Months

Gastrointestinal and hematologic toxicity was significant (See table 3) and required dose attenuation with grade IV toxicity. There was no toxic death. The frequency of severe gastrointestinal toxicity is probably associated with the Fura-bolus schedule, because it is not seen to that extent when giving Fura as a continuous infusion together with CF orally (13). Other toxicities included occasional lacrimation and skin hyperpigmentation without need for dose adjustment.

Table 3. Gastrointestinal and Hematologic Toxicity
- All Patients - Who-Grades III + IV

	Grade III		Grade IV	
	N	%	N	%
Diarrhea	6	10	4	7
Stomatitis	6	10	2	4
Nausea/Vomiting	0		0	
Leukocytes	17	30	4	7
Platelets	6	10	3	5
Hemoglobin	10	17	6	10

CONCLUSIONS

It was the purpose of this study to investigate if the addition of CF to a 5-day IV-bolus schedule of DDP and Fura would result in enhanced cytoxicity in pts. with advanced squamous cell head and neck cancer. Our results demonstrate that the addition of CF can achieve response rates in this disease entity which are comparable to Fura-continuous infusion schedules, although the administered dose of Fura is only 40% of the dose used in 120 hour infusion protocols. We cannot however, determine if the 5-day bolus administration of DDP has additional impact on the activity of this protocol. We also do not know if the CF-dose in our study is optimal for the modulation of Fura and it is necessary to determine if the addition of high dose continuous infusion CF to the standard DDP/Fura schedule might result in an increased number of pathological complete responders after neoadjuvant chemotherapy and/or prolonged overall survival. It is questionable if neoadjuvant chemotherapy of stage II disease, which is in a high percentage curable by surgery and radiation therapy adds any survival benefit. The observed gastrointestinal and hematologic toxicity was substantial in our study which supports a change to continuous infusion schedules for future projects because of decreased toxicity.
In summary our results suggest that the addition of CF to DDP/Fura and the treatment of advanced head and neck cancer enhances the activity of Fura.

References

1. Rooney M, Kish J, Jacobs J, et al: Improved complete response rate and survival in advanced head and neck cancer after three course induction therapy with 120 hour 5-FU infusion and Cisplatinum.
    Cancer 55:1123-1128 (1985)
2. Kish JA, Weaver A, Jacobs J, et al: Cisplatinum and 5-Fluorouracil infusion in patients with recurrent and disseminated epidermoid cancer of the head and neck.
    Cancer 53:1819-1824 (1984)
3. Kish JA, Ensley JF, Jacobs J et al: A randomized trial of Cisplatinum (CACP) + 5-Fluorouracil (5-FU) infusion and CACP + 5-FU bolus for recurrent and advanced squamous cell carcinoma of the head and neck. Cancer 56:2740-2744 (1985)
4. Evans RM, Laskin JD, Hakala MT: Effect of excess folates and deoxyinosine on the activity and site of action of 5-Fluorouracil.
    Cancer Res. 41:3288-3295 (1981)
5. Yin MB, Zakrzewski SF, Hakala MT: Relationship of cellular folate cofactor pools to activity of 5-Fluorouracil.
    Mol. Pharmacol. 23:190-197 (1984)
6. Danenberg PV, Danenberg KD: Effect of 5,10-methylenetetrahydrofolate and the dissociation of 5-fluoro-2'-deoxyuridylate from thymidylate synthetase: Evidence for an ordered mechanism.
    Biochemistry 17:4018-4024 (1978)
7. Lockshin A., Danenberg PV: Biochemical factors affecting the tightness of 5-fluorodeoxyundylate binding of human thymidylate synthetase.
    Biochem. Pharmacol. 30:247-257 (1980)
8. Scanlon KJ, Nee Dels C, Lu Y, et al: Biochemical basis for Cisplatinum and 5-Fluorouracil synergism in human tumors.
    Proc. Am. Assoc. Cancer. Res., 26:1156 (1986)
9. Machover D, Goldschmidt E, Chollet P et al: Treatment of advanced colorectal and gastric adenocarcinoma with 5-FU and high-dose Folinic Acid. J. Clin. Oncol. 4:685-696 (1986)
10. Marini G, Simoncini E, Zaniboni A, et al: 5-Fluorouracil and high-dose folinic acid as salvage treatment of advance breast cancer: An update.
    Oncology 44:336-340 (1987)
11. Bertrand M, Doroshow JH, Multhauf P, et al: High-dose continuous infusion folinic acid and 5-fluorouracil in patients with advanced colorectal cancer. A phase II study.
    J. Clin. Oncol. 4:1058-1061 (1986)
12. Allegra CJ, Chabner BA, Sholar PW et al: Preliminary results of a phase-II-trial for the treatment of metastatic breast cancer with 5-Fluorouracil and Leucovorin.
    NCI Monographs, 5:199-202 (1987)
13. Vokes EE, Choi KE, Schilsky RL, et al: Cis-Platin, Fluorouracil and high dose Leucovorin for recurrent or metastatic head and neck cancer.
    J. Clin. Oncol. 6:618-626 (1988)

DISCUSSION OF DR. LOEFFLER'S PRESENTATION

Dr. Schilsky: I thought I would make a comment in regard to the
relatively low FUra dose that you used in your study. We published
this month in the Journal of Clinical Oncology our experience with a
platinum/FUra/CF regimen that gives the FUra as a 5 day continuous
infusion following a standard platinum dose of 100mg/m^2 and uses
CF orally in divided doses on a daily dosage between 200 and
300mg/m^2/d. This is all in a group of heavily pretreated patients
with head and neck cancer. It was interesting to me that looking at
your toxicities compared to what our experience has been we've seen
virtually no diarrhea on the schedule that we've used and no significant hematologic toxicity, but have seen a considerable amount
of stomatitis as the dose limiting toxicity. We've been routinely
able to give 600mg/m^2/d of FUra as a 5 d infusion and in some
patients who have had relatively little prior therapy have been able
to up to one g/m^2/d of FUra with 300mg/m^2/d of CF. I think it
may be possible, depending upon the schedule one uses either to
deliver more chemotherapy or in some way modify the clinical
toxicities that occur.

Dr. Loeffler: I think the toxicity was caused by the push administration of FUra.

Dr. Frei: I guess a key question at this point is, is FUra/CF in this
setting with cisplatin better than FUra alone with cisplatin. There
are two ways to answer that: one way would be to do a comparative
study of the two combinations but another would be to look at
FUra/CF only, that is, without cisplatin. I would suspect that many
patients you've had who've seen cisplatin are probably not candi-
dates again for cisplatin. Have you done that or do you plan on
doing that?

Dr. Loeffler: No. I have no plans actually right now for treating
head and neck cancer patients. When I'm back in Germany I will do
that.

5-FLUOROURACIL/FOLINIC ACID/CISPLATIN-COMBINATION AND SIMULTANEOUS

ACCELERATED SPLIT-COURSE RADIOTHERAPY IN ADVANCED HEAD AND NECK CANCER

R. Hartenstein[1], T.G. Wendt[2] and E.R. Kastenbauer[3]

[1]Department of Medicine IV, Municipal Hospital
München-Harlaching, Departments of [2]Radiology and
[3]Otolaryngology, Head and Neck Surgery, University
of Munich, 8000 Munich, F.R. Germany

SUMMARY

In advanced inoperable head and neck cancer radiotherapy alone is
unsatisfying. Better results can be obtained by simultaneous 5-Fluoro-
uracil/Cisplatin-chemotherapy and irradiation. The cytotoxicity of
5-Fluorouracil can be enhanced synergistically by adding Folinic Acid
in excess.

In a clinical phase II trial 62 previously untreated patients suffering
from unresectable AJCC-stage III (4 pts.) and IV (58 pts.) squamous cell
carcinoma of the head and neck were treated with a simultaneous chemo-
radiotherapy consisting of high-dose Folinic Acid in addition to a
5-Fluorouracil/Cisplatin combination and of accelerated split-course
radiotherapy.

As results, three pts. died from tumor arrosion bleeding during
the treatment. Median follow up time of the surviving pts. is 27 +
months (range 18-44 months). 48/62 pts. (77 %) achieved complete remission, 11/62 pts. (18 %) partial remission. Presently, 32 pts. (52 %)
are without evidence of disease. Actuarial three years overall survival
rate (Kaplan-Meier method) out of 62 pts. is 53 %. Actuarial disease free
survival and local tumor control rates at three years are 58 % and 72 %.

Mucositis was severe but tolerable, bone marrow depression was
moderate to marked. In conclusion, this combined simultaneous modality
approach is highly effective in locally advanced head and neck cancer.
It seems to provide superior survival and local control rates as
compared to conventional radiotherapy or sequential chemo-radiotherapy
or as compared to simultaneous 5-Fluorouracil/Cisplatin and non-
fractionated radiotherapy. A comparative phase III study is required.

INTRODUCTION

The results of traditional treatments for patients with locally advanced unresectable stage III and IV squamous cell cancer of the upper
aerodigestive systems are poor and not acceptable. With radiotherapy
alone less than 30 % of the patients survive 5 years mainly due to of
local recurrences rather than distant metastases. Despite substantial
amount of progress in the development of effective chemotherapy in the
past decade, adjuvant chemotherapy programs preceding radiotherapy
produced high response rates but failed to alter the subsequent rate
of recurrences and long term results (1, 2, 3).

With the introduction of Cisplatin as an active agent for squamous cell cancer of the head and neck, high overall response rates were observed when Cisplatin combinations were used. In addition, Cisplatin was found to be able to potentiate the action of 5-Fluorouracil (4). In the Wayne State University Cancer Program this synergistic interaction between Cisplatin and 5-Fluorouracil is included. They reported the highest response rates of any drug combination in patients with previously untreated advanced head and neck cancer. With Cisplatin-5-Fluorouracil-chemotherapy alone an overall response rate of 93 % and a complete response rate of 54 % were achieved (5, 6).

Of greater importance is the metabolic interaction of 5-Fluorouracil and Folinic Acid. The activity of 5-Fluorouracil is enhanced by addition of Folinic Acid in excess. By using high doses of exogenous Folinic Acid in addition to 5-Fluorouracil a stabilisation and prolongation of the ternary complex consisting of thymidilate-synthetase and the substrates FdUMP and methylenetetrahydrofolate results which finally leads to a 3-to 4-fold enhanced inhibition of the DNA-de-novo-synthesis in proliferating cells (7, 8, 9. 10). These basic observations have resulted in clinical trials in which patients with a variety of cancers, especially colorectal, gastric and breast carcinoma, were treated with the Folinic Acid/5-Fluoro-uracil-combination (11,12).

Moreover, besides these drug-related interdepencies of activities on tumor cells there are radiobiologically based interactions between cyto-toxic agents and radiotherapy. The inhibition of repair of sublethal and lethal radiation damage may account for synergistic cytotoxicity when 5-Fluorouracil or Cisplatin is combined with ionizing rays (13). The description of a synergistic interaction of 5-Fluorouracil plus radiation led to the concept of a simultaneous chemo-radiotherapy resulting in an improved local control and survival rate in advanced head and neck cancer (14, 15).

An attempt to overcome radioresistence of large squamous cell carci-nomas represents accelerated fractionation and split-course procedure of radiotherapy. An increased reoxygenation and redistribution of tumor cells into the proliferation compartment of the cell cycle as well as an improved recovery of the involved normal tissue should result from this approach and improve the treatment results (16, 17).

We report of our experience in the treatment with 5-Fluorouracil enhanced by Folinic Acid and combined with Cisplatin as part of a simultaneous chemo-radiotherapy (18, 19).

PATIENTS AND METHODS

From August 1984 to October 1986 62 previously untreated patients suffering from histologically confirmed squamous cell carcinoma of the upper aerodigestive tract were selected for study. Most of the patients had poor prognosis hypopharynx carcinoma (39 %) and carcinomas of the base of the tongue (27 %). The rest suffered from carcinoma of the tonsils, the floor of the mouth, the mobile part of the tongue and the supraglottic larynx (Tab. 1). They were considered incurable with standard radiation therapy and surgical techniques because of local extension, established by inspection, palpation, endoscopy and based on radiographic findings in computerscan. Patients were considered eligible if younger than 65 years old, and a Karnofsky performance scale of at least 70 %. Patients with severe concomitant diseases such as decompensated liver cirrhosis, impairment of renal function or cardiac diseases not allowing hydration were excluded from this study. Patients were staged on the basis of the American Joint Committee on Cancer (AJCC) criteria modified by Mendenhall et al. (20). 4 patients were in stage III and 58 patients in stage IV (Fig. 1).

Table 1. Patients characteristics

n	62
age median (range)	48 (33-65)
male : female	57 : 5
histology grading	
well differentiated	0
moderately differentiated	48
undifferentiated	14
site of primary	
tonsils	10
base of tongue	17
floor of mouth /	
mobile part of tongue	8
hypopharynx	24
larynx	3

The study design provided a simultaneously over three cycles administered combined chemo-radiotherapy (Fig. 2). Chemotherapy consisted of Cisplatin 60 mg/sqm i.v., 5-Fluorouracil 350 mg/sqm i.v. and Folinic Acid 50 mg/sqm i.v. as bolus on day 1 as well as 5-Fluorouracil 350 mg/sqm and Folinic Acid 100 mg/sqm per day infused over 24 hours continuously from day 1 to day 4. Usual pre- and postchemotherapeutic hydration and antiemetic treatment was administered. Concomitant radiotherapy was given on days 2 to 4 and 7 to 10 of each course. Two fractions of 1,8 gy per day with a minimum time intervall of 4 hours were administered. Isodose distribution was calculated individually using a computertomography based treatment planning system. A combination of 60 cobalt gamma

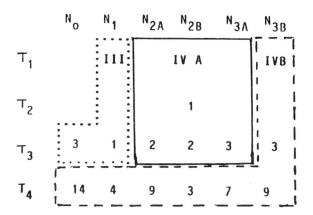

Figure 1. Distribution of patients within TN-categories and stages of modified AJCC-classification (Mendenhall et al. 1984).

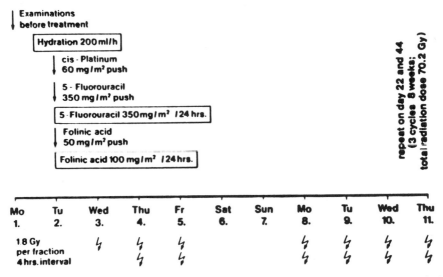

Figure 2. Treatment regimen for simultaneous chemo-radiotherapy with
5-FU/FA/Cisplatin and accelerated split-course radiation.

rays with and without wedge filters and 8 MeV photons was used. Shrinking
field technique was applied after 60 gy, when possible. For non-tumor
involved regions radiation was terminated when 50 gy were reached. This
combined treatment was repeated on days 22 and 44. The total radiation
dose amounted to 70,2 gy/8 weeks. A rest period without treatment took
place from day 11 to 21 and from day 33 to day 43.

Chemotherapy doses were reduced when one or more of the following
parameters were pathologic immediately before the second or third cycle:
White blood cell counts, platelet counts and endogenous creatinine
clearance (lower than 50 ml/min.). Radiotherapy fraction size and
rhythm were not to be altered because of acute toxicity. In case of
severe mucositis treatment-free intervals have been prolonged up to
one additional week.

Toxicity was classified according to WHO scale (21). Tumor response
was assessed 6 weeks and 3 months after the end of treatment. Complete
response was defined as the complete disappearance of all disease
clinically and in some patients on CT scans. Partial response was defined as a reduction in size of $\geq$ 50 % for both the primary and nodal
involvement.

RESULTS

Three patients (5 %) died from acute tumor arrosion bleeding early
during the treatment (Tab. 2). The median follow up time of the
surviving patients is 27 + months (range 18 - 44 months). 48 of 62
patients, corresponding to 77 %, achieved complete remmission 3 months

Table 2. Response to Treatment and Actuarial
          Survival Rates
          (Kaplan-Meier Estimate)

Pts. (treated between 8/1984 and 10/1986)	62 (100%)
Early death (arrosion bleeding during treatment)	5 (5%)
cCR (assessed clinically $\pm$ CT-scan)	48 (77%)
cPR (assessed clinically $\pm$ CT-scan)	11 (18%)
Presently NED	32 (52%)
(follow up time 18+ to 44+ months,	
median 27 months)	
Relapses loco-regional	13 (21%)
distant metastases	6 (10%)
Actuarial 3-years overall survival	53 %
(out of 62 pts.)	
Actuarial 3-years disease-free survival	58 %
Actuarial 3-years local tumor control	72 %

after the end of treatment, 11 of 62 patients, respectively 18 % had
partial tumor remission. Presently (April 1988) 32 patients, respectively
52 % are without evidence of disease. Actuarial one and three years
overall survival rate including all 62 patients, estimated by the
Kaplan-Meier method, is 74 % and 53 % (Fig. 3). The disease free survival
and local tumor control rates at one respectively three years are 71 %
and 81 %, respectively 58 % and 72 %. Until now, 27 out of 62 patients
died, including the 3 early deaths mentioned above and 7 death from
other causes than cancer. 13 patients (21 %) experienced locoregional
recurrences, 6 patients (10 %) distant metastases in the orbita, brain,
lung and bone. One patient developed a second malignancy in the lower
esophagus.

TOXICITY

    Overall acute toxicity was considered acceptable (Tab. 3). Oral
mucosa and bone marrow were the main sites of treatment toxicity.
Mucositis was considerable and most severe during the treatment free
intervall (22). Oral lesions healed rapidly within 2-3 days before
the next treatment course and were not a limiting factor. Bone marrow
depression was moderate to marked but not life-threatening in all cases.
Gastrointestinal side effects were mild. 95 % of the planned 5-Fluoro-
uracil and 98 % of the planned Cisplatin doses could be administered.

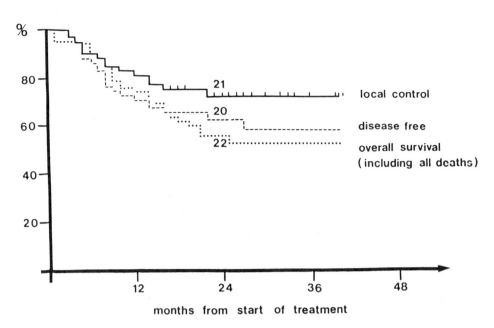

Figure 3. Kaplan-Meier survival estimate of all patients (n = 62) treated
with simultaneous chemo-radiotherapy (April 1988).

DISCUSSION

This combined simultaneous modality approach with Folinic Acid
dependent enhancement of 5-Fluorouracil, Cisplatin and accelerated
split-course radiation procedure seems to be highly effective in
locally advanced unresectable squamous cell cancer of the head and
neck (18, 19, 22).

Table 3. Acute Treatment Toxicity Graded According to
the WHO recommendations

WHO grade	0	I	II	III	IV
mucositis	0 %	66 %		34 %	0 %
leucopenia	6 %	19 %	53 %	22 %	0 %
thrombopenia	53 %	31 %	9 %	6 %	0 %
anemia	84 %	16 %	-*	- *	- *

mean weight loss start/end of treatment: 5.8 +- 3.7 %

----

*: hemoglobin < 110 g/l: Red blood cell transfusion performed

Synergistic biochemical interactions between 5-Fluorouracil, Folinic Acid and Cisplatin as well as a superadditive effect of 5-Fluorouracil and Cisplatin on radiation are supposed bo be cofactors for the improved antitumor activity (4, 13, 14, 15). The enhancement effect of Folinic Acid on 5-Fluorouracil is shown in in-vitro studies demonstrating that an excess of intracellular reduced folates is necessary for optimal and prolonged inhibition of DNA-de-novo-synthesis (7, 8, 9, 10). Several clinical trials, particularly in gastrointestinal and breast cancer confirmed the improved therapeutic activity (11, 12). Accelerated fractionation of radiation has been advocated for squamous cell carcinomas as they appear to repopulate faster than most other carcinomas and sarcomas (16). In supraglottic carcinomas the twice-a-day radiation yielded better results compared to matched historical controls (23). Comparing the results of our trial to studies with conventional simultaneous 5-Fluorouracil/Cisplatin containing chemo-radiotherapy without Folinic Acid of other institutions (24, 25), there appears to be an advantage in tumor response and in acute toxicity in favor of our simultaneous combined modality treatment program considering higher stages in our study. It also seems to provide superior survival and local control rates as compared to historical controls treated conventionally with radiotherapy alone or with sequential chemo-radiotherapy (3, 14). These promising results justify the initiation of a randomized clinical trial comparing this program with conventional simultaneous 5-Fluorouracil/Cisplatin containing chemo-radiotherapy.

REFERENCES

1. J. Tannock, B. Cummings, V. Sorrenti, and the ENT group: Combination chemotherapy used prior to radiation therapy for locally advanced squamous cell carcinoma of the head and neck. Cancer Treat. Rep. 66:1421-1424 (1982).
2. L.E. Kun, F.J. Toohill, P.Y. Holoye, J.A. Duncavage, R.W. Byhardt, T.W. Grossman, R.G. Hoffmann, J.D. Cox, and T. Malin: A randomized study of adjuvant chemotherapy for cancer of the upper aerodigestive tract. Int. J. Radiat. Oncol. Biol. Phys. 12:173-178 (1986).
3. T.G. Wendt, M. Chucholowski, R.C. Hartenstein, R. Rohloff, and N. Willich: Sequential chemo-radiotherapy in locally advanced squamous cell carcinoma of the head and neck. Int. J. Radiat. Oncol. Biol. Phys. 12:397-399 (1986).
4. J.R. Bertino, D. Cooper, J. Chang, and L. Smaldone: Overview of chemotherapeutic agents with activity in cancer of the head and neck region, in "Head and neck cancer: Scientific perspectives in management and strategies for cure", J.R. Jacobs, J.D. Crissman, F.A. Valeriote, and M. Al-Sarraf, ed., Elsevier Amsterdam, pp. 159-174 (1987).
5. A. Weaver, S. Flemming, J. Kish, H. Vandenberg, J. Jacob, J. Crissman, and M. Al-Sarraf: Cis-platinum and 5-Fluorouracil as induction therapy for advanced head and neck cancer. Am. J. Surg. 144:445-448 (1982).
6. M. Al-Sarraf, J. Kish, J. Ensley, J. Jacobs, J. Kinzie, J. Crissman, and A. Weaver: Induction Cis-platinum and 5-Fluorouracil infusion before surgery and/or radiotherapy in patients with advanced head and neck cancer. Proc. Am. Ass. Cancer Res. 25:196 (1984).

7. B. Ullman, M. Lee, D.W. Martin, jr: Increased L1210 sensitive FdUrd with LCV in-vitro. Proc. Nat. Acad. Sci. 75:980 (1978).
8. G.H. Heppner, and P. Calabresi: Increased antitumor activity with methotrexate prior to CLV 1 hr. prior to FUra in vivo-mammary tumor in C3H mice. Cancer Res. 37:4580-4585 (1977).
9. S. Waxman, H. Bruckner, and A. Wagles: Increased FUra cytotoxicity with LCV in-vitro. Proc.Am. Ass. Cancer Res. 19:149 (1978).
10. S. Waxman, and H. Bruckner: The enhancement of 5-Fluorouracil antimetabolic activity by Leucovorin, Menadione and α-Tocopherol. Eur. J. Cancer Clin. Oncol. 18:685-692 (1982).
11. D. Machover, L. Schwarzenberg, E. Goldschmidt, J.M. Towani, B. Michalski, M. Hayat, T. Dorval, J.L. Misset, C. Jasmin R. Moral, and G. Mathê: Treatment of advanced colorectal and gastric Adenocarcinomas with 5-FU combined with high-dose Folinic Acid: a piolt study. Cancer Treat. Rep. 66:1803-1807 (1982).
12. G. Marini, P. Marpicati, A. Zaniboni, G.C. Cervi, F. Gorni, and E. Simoncini: Treatment of advanced breast cancer with 5-Fluorouracil and high-dose Folinic Acid: Preliminary results. Chemioterapie 6:135-138 (1985).
13. L.A. Szumiel, H.W. Nias: The effect of combined treatment with a platinum complex an ionizing radiation on chinese hamster ovary cells in vitro. Br. J. Cancer 33:450-458 (1976).
14. T.C.M. Lo, A.L. Wily, F.J. Ansfield, J.H. Brandenburg, H.L. Davis, F.E. Gollin, R.O. Johson, G. Ramirez, and H. Vermund: Combined radiation therapy and 5-Fluorouracil for advanced squamous cell carcinoma of the oral cavity and oropharynx: a randomized study. Radiology 126:229-235 (1976).
15. J.E. Byfield, T.R. Sharp, S.S. Frankel, S.G. Tang, and F.B. Callipari: Phase I and II trial of five days infused 5-Fluorouracil and radiation in advanced cancer of the head and neck. J. Clin. Oncol. 2:406-413 (1984).
16. K.R. Trott, and J. Kummermehr: What is known about tumor proliferation rates to choose between accelerated fractionation or hyperfractionation? Radiother. Oncol. 3:1-9 (1985).
17. E. Van der Schueren, W. Van den Bogaert, and K.K. Ang: Radiotherapy with multiple fractions per day:in "The biological basis of radiotherapy", G.G. Steel, G.E. Adams, and M.J. Peckham, ed., Elsevier Amsterdam, pp. 195-210 (1983).
18. R.C. Hartenstein, T.G. Wendt, T.P.U. Wustrow, and K.R. Trott: Simultaneous twice-daily radiotherapy (RT) and Cisplatin (DDP)-5-FU-chemotherapy with Folinic Acid (FA) enhancement in advanced squamous cell cancer (SCC) of the head and neck. Proc. Am. Soc. Clinc. Oncol. 5:126 (1986).
19. T.G. Wendt, R.C. Hartenstein, T.P.U. Wustrow: Improved two years survival and local control rate in locally advanced squamous cell carcinoma (SCC) of the head and neck by simultaneous Chemo (CT)-Radiotherapy (RT): Progress report. Proc. Am. Soc. Clin. Oncol. 6:125 (1987).
20. W.M. Mendenhall, J.T. Parsons, R.R. Million, J. Cassisi, J.W. Devine, and B.D. Greene: A favorable subset of AJCC stage IV squamous cell carcinoma of the head and neck. Int. J. Radiat. Oncol. Biol. Phys. 10:1841-1843 (1984).
21. WHO Handbook for reporting results of cancer treatment. WHO Offset Publication N° 48, Geneva (1979).
22. T.G. Wendt, T.P.U. Wustrow, R.C. Hartenstein, R. Rohloff, and K.R. Trott: Accelerated split-course radiotherapy and simultaneous cis-dichlorodiammine-platinum and 5-fluorouracil chemotherapy with folinic acid enhancement for unresectable carcinoma of the head and neck. Radiother. Oncol. 10:277-284 (1987).

23. C.C. Wang, H.D. Suit, P.H. Blitzer: Twice-a-day radiation therapy for supraglottic carcinoma. Int. J. Radiat. Oncol. Biol. Phys. 12:3-7 (1986).
24. D.J. Adelstein, V.M. Sharan, A.S. Earle, A.C. Shah, C. Vlastou, D.D. Haria, C. Damm, S.G. Carter, and J.D. Hines: Combined modality therapy (CMT) with simultaneous 5-fluorouracil (5-FU), cis-platinum (DDP) and radiation therapy (RT) in the treatment of squamous cell cancer of the head and neck. Proc.Am.Soc.Clin. Oncol. 5:128 (1986).
25. S.G. Taylor, IV, A.K. Murthy, J.L. Showel, D.D. Caldarelli, J.C. Hutchinson, jr, L.D. Holinger, T. Kramer, and K. Kiel: Improved control in advanced head and neck cancer with simultaneous radiation and Cisplatin/5-FU chemotherapy. Cancer Treat. Rep. 69:933-939 (1985).

DISCUSSION OF DR. HARTENSTEIN'S PRESENTATION

<u>Dr. Hines</u>: The data that David Adelstein has presented is now matured
     after almost 5 years and is holding up. There have been no
     relapses. The interesting thing is because of the social habits of
     this kind of patient, (lots of smoking and drinking) we encountered
     almost 25% that get second primaries which are not related to the
     original tumor.

<u>Dr. Hartenstein</u>: We have one second primary in the lower esophagus.
     One point we have to reflect on too is that 7 patients died from
     causes other than cancer, some of them by cachexia not caused by the
     tumor but maybe by social habits (alcohol and smoking).

PROGRESS REPORT ON STUDIES OF FAM-CF FOR GASTRIC CANCER AND

INTRAPERITONEAL ADMINISTRATION OF FUra-CF FOLLOWED BY CISPLATIN (DDP)

S G. Arbuck, H.O. Douglass, Jr., H. R. Nava,
Y. N. Silk, M. Baroni, and Y.M. Rustum

Roswell Park Memorial Institute
666 Elm St.
Buffalo, NY 14263

INTRODUCTION

Randomized controlled trials have demonstrated that the response rate to 5-fluorouracil (FUra) in combination with leucovorin (CF) is approximately two-fold higher than the response rate to single agent FUra in patients with colorectal carcinoma (1-5). Since FUra alone has activity in other gastrointestinal cancers, our work has been directed toward evaluating the role of this combination for the treatment of other gastrointestinal cancers, using both the intravenous (IV) and intraperitoneal (IP) routes.

Previous studies have demonstrated that FUra in combination with CF has activity in gastric carcinoma (6,7). To date, there have been no randomized controlled trials comparing FUra and CF with single agent FUra. Although we and others recognize the need for Phase II trials of new agents in previously untreated patients with gastric cancer, many patients are treated first in the community with FAM (8) chemotherapy. Therefore, another approach to assess the contribution of CF to FUra activity in gastric cancer is to compare standard FAM chemotherapy, (FUra, Adriamycin and Mitomycin-C) to standard FAM chemotherapy given with CF, in a randomized controlled trial. A pilot study was initiated at Roswell Park Memorial Institute to assess the toxicity of FAM-CF and to make preliminary observations about the efficacy of the drug combination.

Intraperitoneal chemotherapy is being investigated in an effort to develop effective adjuvant chemotherapy for gastrointestinal cancer. Using the IP route, IP FUra concentrations 2-3 logs higher than peak plasma concentrations are achieved (9, 10). Since therapeutic plasma levels are also obtained, drug delivery occurs via both local diffusion and the standard veno-capillary route. Further, it has been demonstrated that IP FUra administration achieves portal vein FUra concentrations similar to those obtained in the hepatic artery following hepatic artery perfusions (11). Since liver metastases from GI cancers occur initially via the portal vein and since there are preliminary reports of effectiveness of adjuvant portal vein FUra infusions in colorectal carcinoma (12), the intraperitoneal route of administration warrants further investigation.

In a previous study we demonstrated that FUra and CF can be administered via the intraperitoneal route (10). FUra, in escalating concentrations, was administered in combination with CF (25 mg or 125 mg) for eight consecutive four hour exchanges. The maximally tolerated dose of 4 mM FUra (1040 mg), for 8 consecutive four-hour dwells, and the toxicity observed, were the same as those reported when FUra was administered as a single agent using the IP route and the same schedule (9). At the 25 mg CF dose, plasma CF and 5-methyltetrahydrofolate (5-CH_3-H_4PteGlu) were undetectable (<0.5uM) and t1/2 of CF in the peritoneal cavity was 127+49 minutes (10).

Rustum and colleagues have demonstrated that DDP administered 24 hours after FUra and CF results in prolonged thymidylate synthase inhibition and increased cytotoxicity in model systems (13,14). On the basis of this and other reports, a pilot study of sequential intraperitoneal administration of FUra/CF followed by DDP was initiated.

This report summarizes the current status of 2 ongoing trials evaluating FUra and CF:
1. in combination with standard FAM chemotherapy for gastric cancer.
2. in combination with sequential DDP with all three drugs administered via the intraperitoneal route.

METHODS

Pilot Study of FAM-CF in Gastric Carcinoma

Patients with advanced gastric cancer that was incurable by surgery were eligible. Previous chemotherapy was permitted if it did not include Adriamycin or Mitomycin-C. WBC >3500/mm^3, platelets >100,000/mm^3 were required as was bilirubin <2 mg%. Higher bilirubin values were permitted if they were due to liver involvement by tumor. Adriamycin doses were decreased in these patients. No active heart disease was permitted.

Since responses to FAM have been reported in patients with poor performance status, any patient who was judged to be a candidate for FAM chemotherapy was enrolled. Informed consent meeting institutional and federal regulations was required. Measurable disease was not a requirement for study entry since the primary objective was to assess toxicity of the drug regimen. Those patients who had an area of known malignant disease that was measurable by palpation, chest x-ray or computerized axial tomography, were assessed for response to treatment.

Patients received CF 500 mg/m^2 by 2-hour infusion with FUra 600 mg/m^2 IV push mid-infusion on Days 1, 8, 29, and 36 of an 8 week cycle. Adriamycin 30 mg/m^2 was given on Days 1 and 29. Mitomcyin-C 10 mg/m^2 was administered on Day 1.

Disease status was re-evaluated in all patients at the end of each 8 week cycle. Re-evaluation was undertaken sooner if there was clinical evidence of progression. A complete response was defined as absence of all clinically detectable tumor. A partial response was defined as a reduction of at least 50% of the sums of the products of the longest perpendicular diameters of all clearly measurable tumor masses. No increase in the size of any lesion and no new areas of malignant disease could appear. There could be no significant deterioration in weight and no deterioration in performance status in patients who were responders. Objective progression was defined as a 25% increase in any measurable lesion, the appearance of new areas of malignant disease, or symptomatic deterioration of the performance status by more than one level.

National Cancer Institute Toxicity Criteria were used.

Intraperitoneal FUra and CF Followed by DDP

Patients with histologic evidence of advanced inoperable tumor, primarily involving the peritoneal cavity were eligible if they had WBC >4000/mm^3, platelets >100,000/mm^3, and creatinine clearance >50 cc/min. or serum creatinine <1.5 mg%. Patients were entered with 1) measurable disease, 2) evaluable disease with cytologically documented malignant ascites or 3) following an exploratory laparotomy where residual but clinically non-measurable disease was found. Previous IV chemotherapy with FUra, DDP or other agents was permitted if the last dose was 3 or more weeks prior to entry and if recovery from toxicity was complete. An estimated life expectancy of at least 2 months and informed consent meeting institutional and federal guide-lines were required.

Treatment consisted of 8 sequential 4-hour exchanges that were administered into the peritoneal cavity using a Tenckhoff catheter or a Tenckhoff catheter connected to an implanted port (Port-a-Cath, Pharmacia, St. Paul, Minn.). The first four exchanges consisted of FUra 1 gram and CF 125 mg in 2 liters of 1.5% Dianeal containing 8 mEq KCl, 50 mEq NaHCO$_3$ and 1000 units heparin. These were followed by 4 consecutive exhanges of DDP 25 mg/m^2 in 2 liters of 0.9% NaCl with electrolytes. Patients were hydrated and given diuretics in order to maintain a urine output of >100 cc/hour during and for at least 12 hours after DDP administration. Patients who did not have systemic toxicity received additional FUra by the IV route in subsequent courses. Antiemetics were administered to all patients during DDP treatment.

Treatment was repeated monthly. Patients were evaluated following two courses of treatment or sooner if there was clinical suspicion of progression. Re-evaluation consisted of physical examination, abdominal fluid cytology (when possible), and computerized axial tomography of the abdomen and pelvis (usually with 2 liters of dialysis fluid that contained Hypaque (15)).

RESULTS

FAM-CF in Gastric Carcinoma

To date, fourteen patients (12 males and 2 females) have been entered. The median age is 63.5 years (range 44-76) and median ECOG Performance Status is 1 (range 0-4). Seven patients had previous chemotherapy and two had prior radiotherapy.

Ten patients have completed one 8 week course and are evaluable for toxicity. Ten patients had leucopenia (5 Grade 3, 1 Grade 4). Only 1 patient required hospitalization for fever. Three patients had thrombocytopenia (2 Grade 1, 1 Grade 2). Grade 1 diarrhea, nausea, and mucositis each occurred in 1 patient.

Eleven patients had measurable disease. Two patients are too early to evaluate for response. In the remaining patients, responses,

Table 1

Clinical Characteristics of Patients Treated with
Intraperitoneal 5-FU and CF, Followed by DDP

No. of Patients	12
Males/Females	6/6
Median Age in Years (range)	58 (27-65)
Median ECOG Performance Status (range)	2 (0-3)

Tumor Type	
Adenocarcinoma, unknown primary	3
Pancreas	2
Stomach	2
Small Bowel	1
Pseudomyxoma peritonei	1
Colon	1
Cholangiocarcinoma	1
Appendix	1
Previous Treatment	6
Malignant Ascites	7

including 1 complete response have been seen. To date, too few patients with measurable disease have been treated to report a response rate with acceptable confidence limits. Of the responding patients, three had been treated previously with chemotherapy and one with radiotherapy.

Intraperitoneal FUra and CF Followed by DDP

To date, 12 patients have been treated (Table 1). The median age is 58 years and median ECOG performance status is 2. Diagnoses are recorded in Table 1.

Toxicity in all 12 patients has been acceptable and has included nausea and vomiting in 6 (Grade 1 in 2 patients, and Grade 2 in 4 patients), Grade 2 leucopenia in 1 patient and Grade 3 leucopenia in 2 patients, and Grade 1 thrombocytopenia in 1 patient. Abdominal and/or chest pain occurred in 5 patients. DDP was discontinued in 1 patient who developed Grade 1 renal toxicity after 11 courses of treatment. Renal impairment was mild and is resolving. There have been 2 episodes of infectious peritonitis: one was the result of a surgical infection and unrelated to the Tenckhoff catheter.

Only two patients had measurable disease. Of 7 patients with massive malignant ascites, 4 had a clinically significant reduction in ascites for 49+ to 337+ days. One had a minor, clinically insignificant reduction in ascites, one is too early to evaluate, and one died early of tumor-related causes.

DISCUSSION

FAM-CF in Gastric Carcinoma

Evaluation of toxicity in 10 patients who have received at least 1 course of treatment demonstrated that CF can be combined safely with other active drugs used for the treatment of gastric cancer. When FUra and CF are administered during 4 weeks of an 8 week cycle, diarrhea is not dose-limiting as it is when the same doses are administered weekly for 6 weeks of an 8-week schedule.

Patients with measurable gastric cancer, including those who were previously treated, have responded to the combination of FAM-CF. Forty-two percent of 62 previously untreated gastric cancer patients achieved partial responses with standard FAM chemotherapy (8). Others have reported similar results (16). It is possible, therefore, that the responses seen in our study could have been achieved with standard FAM chemotherapy. Until a randomized controlled trial comparing FAM to FAM-CF is performed, no conclusions about the contribution of CF to the FAM regimen for the treatment of gastric cancer can be made.

In this study, chemotherapy is administered only if WBC $>3000/mm^3$ and platelet count $>100,000/mm^3$. If a delay of more than one week is necessary for day 8 or 36 FUra, that treatment is omitted. FUra doses are also decreased for nadir WBC <2000 or nadir platelet counts $<60,000$. The dose intensity of FUra administered on this schedule is being monitored carefully. If FUra doses are frequently omitted or decreased because of myelotoxicity due to Mitomycin C and Adriamycin, a randomized Phase III trial comparing standard FAM to FAM-CF may not be the optimal test of the usefulness of FUra and CF in gastric cancer.

In view of the Phase II results that are currently available, and the improved response rates observed when CF is added to FUra for the treatment of advanced colon carcinoma, a well designed definitive trial is warranted to determine the usefulness of CF combined with FUra in the treatment of gastric cancer.

Intraperitoneal FUra and CF Followed by DDP

Evaluation of the efficacy of intraperitoneal chemotherapy presents several difficulties. Available data suggest that drug penetration via local diffusion is limited to the outer cell layers (17). It is not expected, therefore, that IP chemotherapy will be more effective than IV therapy for bulky measurable disease. Patients who have small volume metastases documented at surgery are not evaluable for response using currently available imaging procedures. These patients can, however, be followed for sites of progression and time to progression. Patients with malignant ascites can be followed for subjective response to therapy, but are not considered measurable by standard objective criteria. There are, therefore, no objective response criteria to apply to those patients who might be expected to respond to an effective IP regimen.

Although malignant ascites cannot be monitored using objective response criteria, a substantial decrease in ascites can provide effective palliation. In this study, significant palliation was achieved in four of six evaluable patients with massive malignant ascites. In our experience, such palliation has been infrequent when systemic chemotherapy, peritoneal-venous shunting or repeated paracentesis has been used.

Pharmacokinetics of CF (dl and l) are being evaluated in plasma and peritoneal fluid samples from these patients. Preliminary results suggest that additional IV CF may be required to ensure that plasma l-CF concentrations reach 10 uM. A precise recommendation will be made when the pharmacokinetic studies are completed.

This regimen administered via the intraperitoneal route is well tolerated and can be evaluated in the adjuvant setting. Modifications will be made based on our clinical experience and on the pharmacokinetic studies. Patients who undergo curative resections for gastric cancer, but who are at high risk of disease recurrence (those with serosal invasion or regional lymph node metastasis) will receive intraperitoneal chemotherapy with treatment begining in the operating room. In addition, studies will continue in patients with malignant ascites.

Acknowledgements: The assistance of research nurses Suzanne Milliron and Pat Goodwin, and of Juliann Eddy, who prepared this manuscript, is gratefully acknowledged.

This work was supported in part by CA 21071 and CA 24538 from the National Cancer Institute, Bethesda, Maryland.

References

1. Doroshow JH, Bertrand M, Multhauf P, et al: Prospective Randomized Trial of 5-FU versus 5-FU and High-Dose Folinic Acid (HDFA) for Treatment of Advanced Colorectal Cancer. Proc Am Soc Clin Oncol 6:96, 1987

2. Petrelli N, Herrera L, Rustum YM, et al: A Prospective Randomized Trial of 5-Fluorouracil versus 5-Fluorouracil and High-Dose Leucovorin versus 5-Fluorouracil and Methotrexate in Previously Untreated Patients with Advanced Colorectal Carcinoma. J Clin Oncol 5:1559-1565, 1987

3. Erlichman C, Fine S, Wong A, et al: A Randomized Trial of Fluorouracil and Folinic Acid in Patients with Metastatic Colorectal Cancer. J Clin Oncol 6:469-475, 1988

4. Petrelli N, Stablein D, Bruckner H, et al: Phase III Evaluation of 5-Fluorouracil (5-FU) vs 5-FU and High-Dose Leucovorin (HDCF) vs 5-FU and Low-Dose Leucovorin (LDCF) in Patients with Metastatic Colorectal Adenocarcinoma. A Report of the Gastrointestinal Tumor Study Group. Proc Am Soc Clin Oncol, In Press, 1988

5. O'Connell MJ and Wieand HS: A Controlled Clinical Trial Including Folinic Acid at Two Distinct Dose Levels in Combination with 5-Fluorouracil (5FU) for the Treatment of Advanced Colorectal Cancer: Experience of the Mayo Clinic and North Central Cancer Treatment Group, Proceedings of the International Symposium on "The Expanding Role of Folates and Fluoropyrimidines in Cancer Chemotherapy". Buffalo, NY, April 1988

6. Arbuck SG, Douglass HO Jr, Trave F, et al: A Phase II Trial of 5-Fluorouracil and High-Dose Intravenous Leucovorin in Gastric Carcinoma. J Clin Oncol 5:1150-1156, 1987

7. Machover D, Goldschmidt E, Chollet P, et al: Treatment of Advanced Colorectal and Gastric Adenocarcinomas with 5-Fluorouracil and High Dose Folinic Acid. J Clin Oncol 4:685-696, 1986

8. MacDonald JS, Schein PS, Wooley PV: 5-Fluorouracil, Doxorubicin and Mitomycin (FAM) Combination Chemotherapy for Advanced Gastric Cancer. Ann Intern Med 93:533-536, 1980

9. Speyer, JL, Collins JM, Dedrick, R L, et al: Phase I and Pharmacological Studies of 5-Fluorouracil Administered Intraperitoneally. Cancer Res 40:567-572, 1980

10. Arbuck SG, Trave F, Douglass HO, Jr, et al: Phase I and Pharmacologic Studies of Intraperitoneal Leucovorin and 5-Fluorouracil in Patients with Advanced Cancer. J Clin Oncol 4:1510-1517, 1986

11. Speyer, JL, Sugarbaker PH, Collins, JM, et al: Portal Levels and Hepatic Clearance of 5-Fluorouracil After Intraperitoneal Administration in Humans. Cancer Res 41:1916-1922, 1981

12. Taylor I, Machin D, Mullee M: A Randomized Controlled Trial of Adjuvant Portal Vein Cytotoxic Perfusion in Colorectal Cancer. Br J Surg 72:359-363, 1985

13. Trave F, Rustum YM, Goranson J: Synergistic Antitumor Activity of Cisplatin (DDP) and 5-Fluorouracil in Mice Bearing Leukemia L1210 Cells. Proc Am Assoc Cancer Res 26:322, 1985

14. Rustum YM, Trave F: Personal Communication

15. Dunnick, NR, Jones RB, Doppman JL, et al: Intraperitoneal Contrast Infusion for Assessment of Intraperitoneal Fluid Dynamics. Am J Rad 133:221-223, 1979

16. Douglass, HO Jr, Lavin PT, Goudsmit A, et al: An Eastern Cooperative Oncology Group Evaluation of Combinations of Methyl-CCNU, Mitomycin C, Adriamycin, and 5-Fluorouracil in Advanced Measurable Gastric Cancer (EST 2277). J Clin Onc 2:1372-1381, 1984

17. Ozols RF, Locker GY, Doroshow JH, et al: Pharmacokinetics of Adriamycin and Tissue Penetration in Murine Ovarian Cancer. Cancer Res 39:3209-3214, 1979

DISCUSSION OF DR. ARBUCK'S PRESENTATION

Dr. Pandya: Susan, you probably mentioned it but how often do you repeat this i.p.?

Dr. Arbuck: We repeat it monthly. Every 28 days.

Dr. Schilsky: Platinum and FUra together intraperitoneally is highly effective in management of patients with malignant ascites. You have a unique opportunity here in these patients with malignant ascites to collect the tumor cells and look at the pharmacodynamics of FUra/CF and platinum intracellularly. I'm just curious to know if you're going to be doing that

Dr. Arbuck: We tried 3 or 4 years ago when we first starting doing the FUra/CF i.p. We did collect cells and try to measure enzyme levels, but there are several difficulties. One, if you look under the microscope you see that there are a number of cells besides the tumor cells and sometimes they're in fairly large proportion. The other thing is that, as Dr. Rustum pointed out, it's important to freeze these cells quickly and as you know draining the abdominal cavity takes some time so we were also faced with not having an optimal specimen. Of course we also have nothing to control it with. I think you're right it's a wonderful opportunity, but we haven't figured out how to do it yet.

Audience: Susan, as a follow-up on the cytology, I was wondering if you have any information with respect to the openness of the peritoneal cavity. Is the palliation that you're achieving as far as reduction in ascites related directly to tumor kill (i.e. by cytology or by whatever other methodology) or it is just related to sclerosis and sort of sealing down of the peritoneal cavity?

Dr. Arbuck: Well, again it's small numbers of patients so it's hard to draw conclusions. I can tell you several things. One is that some of these patients who have been palliated still have positive cytology so we're clearly not curing tumor. We do have a couple of patients with measurable disease. We haven't seen anything particularly in them in terms of shrinkage of the bulk tumor. We do follow these patients by hypaque CAT scans and we even have palliation in a patient where we don't get complete distribution throughout the abdominal cavity. The one patient that I mentioned who we've treated for almost a year we've recently noted thickening of her peritoneal surfaces on the CAT scan which we didn't see when we started treatment. Certainly I can't tell without a microscope whether it's tumor or something we did, but it's a strong possiblility that it's something we did.

Audience: Having had experience with intraperitoneal chemotherapy for G.I. malignancies we have found that measuring intraperitoneal or ascitic levels of CEA has been a very good indicator of response in the absence of any better indicator. Have you tried to measure CEA levels? Usually there is a very great gradient of at least 2-3 logs between the serum levels and the ascitic fluid level.

Dr. Arbuck: What kinds of patient numbers are you talking about and what did you Ca actually correlate with?

Audience: You have a decrease in the ascites you don't see tumor masses but you have patients that have serum CEA levels of say 10 - 30 and ascitic fluid levels of 3,000, so it's a few log differences. I'd recommend using that if you want to try.

CLINICAL EXPERIENCE WITH 5-FU/DDP ± OHDW COMBINATION CHEMOTHERAPY

IN PATIENTS WITH ADVANCED COLORECTAL CARCINOMA

Stefan Madajewicz, John J. Fiore, and Mohammad H. Zarrabi

State University of New York at Stony Brook
Division of Oncology, Health Sciences Center, T-17, 080
Stony Brook, NY 11794-8174

INTRODUCTION

Many avenues are being explored in an effort to develop more effective and selective treatment of patients with advanced colorectal carcinoma. One approach termed biochemical modulation is based on "immortal", although minimal, 5-fluorouracil (5-FU) activity. At least six types of modulation have been attempted based on the current understating of 5-FU metabolism: 1) Methotrexate, 2) Thymidine, 3) PALA, 4) Allopurinol, 5) Folinic acid (FA), and 6) cisPlatin (DDP).

We shall focus our attention on the last two mechanisms. Folinic acid, upon its conversion to 5,10 methylene tetrahydrofolate (CH_2FH_4), would increase the binding of 5-fluorodeoxyuridine monophosphate (FdUMP) to thymidylate synthetase (TS) with consequent inhibition of DNA synthesis (1).

CisPlatin can act on several levels. It blocks sodium-dependent methionine transport in tumor cells generating increased levels of folate cofactors, therefore acting as a substitute for FA (2,3,4). CisPlatin may also interact with the sulfhydryl groups of the enzyme TS resulting in its irreversible inhibition (5).

Based on this information, we designed a clinical randomized study of 5-FU/DDP continuous infusion (CI) versus 5-FU/DDP CI with oral high dose Wellcovorin (OHDW) in patients with advanced colorectal cancer.

PATIENTS AND METHODS

Thirty patients (pts) entered this study. All had metastatic, progressive disease and expected survival of at least two months. Fifteen patients had prior therapy. All patients had normal hematologic, renal, hepatic and cardiac function unless abnormalities resulted from tumor invasion. All the patients had at least evaluable disease. Patients' characteristics are presented in Table 1.

TABLE 1

PATIENT CHARACTERISTICS

Total		28 (15)*
Male/Female		15/13
Age median range		62 (36-81)
	0.2	23
PS	3-4	5
Metastases:		
Liver		20
Lung		4
Bones		3
Lymph Nodes		3
Previous Therapy:		
5-FU	7]	
FUDR Pump	3]	
Immunotherapy	4]	– total of 15 (7)*
RT	7]	
None	13]	

*Wellcovorin group

Treatment Protocol

5-FU 600mg/M^2 in 1000cc dextrose in 0.45% normal saline was administered CI intravenously over 24 hours for five consecutive days; the dose was lowered to 450mg/M^2 in the last 10 patients. DDP 20mg/M^2 in 1000cc normal saline + 25gm mannitol was given CI concomitantly with 5-FU over 24 hours for five days. Hydration as 1000cc D_5 0.45% NS + 20mEq KC1 + 1000mg $MgSO_4$ was given IV over 24 hours for five days. Wellcovorin (25mg tablets, Burroughs-Wellcome) 500mg/M^2 was given orally in four equally divided hourly doses (125mg/M^2 X 4) at the beginning of each daily treatment over a five day period. Treatment was provided every four weeks.

Evaluation Criteria

Prior to each course of therapy, every patient had a complete blood count, electrolytes, liver function tests, creatinine, BUN and chest x-ray. Liver scan, abdominal and pelvic CT scans or ultrasound were performed prior to the first course, after the second, fourth and at the end of treatment (after the sixth course). The tests were repeated every 2-3 months as a part of the follow-up examination until progression. Complete disappearance of all recognizable masses constituted a complete response (CR). A 50% reduction in the product of the largest perpendicular diameter of the most clearly measurable area (or 75% reduction of the evaluable mass) constituted a partial response (PR). Individual patients were removed from the study when toxic effects were unacceptable or when objective tumor progression occurred.

RESULTS

Twenty eight of 30 patients are currently evaluable for response and toxicity and two patients are too early into the course of treatment to be evaluated. Fifteen of 28 patients received OHDW.

TABLE 2

THERAPEUTIC EFFECT

PR   3 (1)*

CR   1

Total   4 (1)* - 14% (7%)*

Remission duration - weeks 52, 15+, 11, 10

*Wellcovorin group

Response Rate (RR) - Table 2

A median dose of 5-FU was 9,600mg (range 4,150-24,036mg) and DDP was 380mg (range 150-1,110mg). The last 10 patients received a reduced dose of 5-FU consisting of 450mg/M^2 daily for five days. Complete response was seen in one patient and partial responses were seen in an additional two patients for a total response rate of 23% in the 5-FU/DDP group. The complete responder was a 60 year old male status post abdominoperineal resection for rectal adenocarcinoma who presented with recurrent lung metastases. He was originally treated with 5-FU. One partial responder was a 62 year old female who developed peritoneal and liver metastases post surgery and radiation therapy for rectal adenocarcinoma. The third patient was a 67 year old male who developed liver and lung metastases after surgery and tumor specific antigen immunotherapy for colon carcinoma.

One PR was seen in the group of patients who received OHDW for a RR of 7%. This patient was a 39 year old female with liver and lung metastases as the result of a familial type of colon carcinoma. Five other patients demonstrated significant reduction or normalization of the previously elevated "liver enzymes" or CEA levels. A median survival time for the entire group from treatment to death was 26 weeks (range 4-52) and a median survival time from the diagnosis to death was 60 weeks (range 12-260 weeks).

TABLE 3

TOXICITY

	5-FU/DDP	5-FU/DDP/OHDW
Nausea and Vomiting	13	15
Mucositis	13	15 (5 severe)
Diarrhea	13	15 (5 severe)
Leukopenia <4,000	8	11
<2,000	5	0
<1,000	0	4
Thrombocytopenia <50,000		4
Hypomagnesemia <1.8mg%	19	
<1.5mg%	9	
Weakness - "washed out"	19	
Peripheral Neuropathy	9	

All patients experienced nausea, vomiting, mucositis and diarrhea. Five patients in the OHDW group and two in the 5-FU/DDP group had to be hospitalized for dehydration and/or sepsis. One of these patients developed an intestinal obstruction complicated by severe neutropenia and thrombocytopenia; he died 2 days post-operatively. Another patient reported mild chest pain following the second course of chemotherapy. She expired at home before being able to come to the hospital. This patient experienced severe mucositis, diarrhea and dehydration after the first course of 5-FU/DDP with OHDW. The subsequent 10 patients received a reduced dose, $450mg/M^2$ of 5-FU. They have experienced only mild gastrointestinal toxicity. All patients experienced weakness and fatigue, increasingly bothersome after the third course of therapy. Nine patients complained of hand/foot syndrome as early as soon after the first and as late as six months after the last course of treatment.

DISCUSSION

For the last 27 years 5-FU has been the mainstay of colorectal carcinoma chemotherapy, despite its being effective in fewer than 20% of patients and the responses being short-lived. Its acceptance as "standard" therapy can be attributed only to the relative lack of efficacy of any other therapies, including single agents and 5-FU-containing combination regimens. Several 5-FU/DDP studies in advanced colorectal carcinoma generated considerable enthusiasm and interest (6,7). It has also been shown that the 5-FU cytotoxic activity can be greatly enhanced by the availability of reduced folates (8). The clinical value of this hypothesis was confirmed by several researchers, including ourselves (9,10). However, this randomized study fails to confirm any therapeutic significance of 5-FU/DDP combination or the same plus folinic acid. Some potential explanations exist for these observations. First, the cells resistant to 5-FU require high concentrations of reduced folates to form and maintain a complex between FUdMP, CH_2FH_4 and TS (11,12). The mean peak plasma concentration of the two diastereoisomers of FA were approximately $80\mu M$ at 80 minutes and $10\mu M$ at 24 hours and L-FA above $8\mu M$ at 80 minutes after $500mg/M^2$ intravenous infusion of FA (1). In our present trial, we have been using oral FA. This mode of administration results in a saturation of gastrointestinal absorption lasting up to 2 hours at doses exceeding 50mg of FA (13). Vokes and colleagues reported mean plasma concentration of FA between $2-3\mu M$ after the oral dose of $200-300mg/M^2$ (13). They also found relatively high mean plasma concentration of 5-methyl FH_4, namely $1.54-2.35\mu$ (13). Perhaps the plasma FA concentration achieved with oral administration is not adequate to sustain TS inhibition. Also, $5-CH_3FH_4$ may have an inhibitory effect on CH_2FH_4 (9).

Secondly, the dose and mode of administration of DDP resulting in optimal modulation of reduced folates and thus of 5-FU, has not been established. It is conceivable that the five days CI of DDP inhibition of methionine synthesis might result in profound deficiency of this amino-acid. That, in turn, would "trap" most of the total tetrahydrofolate as CH_3FH_4 (Fig. 1). A consequence of the trapping of folates as CH_3FH_4 is the decrease in the concentration of free tetrahydrofolate (14). Thus, the potential action of DDP in increasing the pool of reduced folates has been lost or even reversed in our protocol.

MECHANISM OF 5-FU/DDP INTERACTION

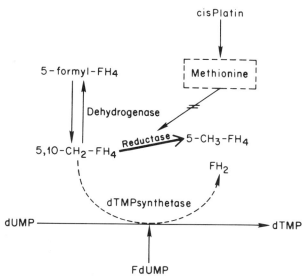

dUMP = deoxyuridylate FH_4 = tetrahydrofolate

FdUMP = fluorodeoxyuridylate $5,10-CH_2-FH_4$ = methylenetetrahydrofolate

dTMP = thymidylate $5-CH_3-FH_4$ = methyltetrahydrofolate

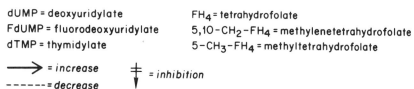

Figure 1

CONCLUSION

Neither protocol arm has shown significiant therapeutic benefit as a result of this specific combination. The response rate can, perhaps, be attributed only to the 5-FU activity. Despite this, it is apparent that the combination of 5-FU/DDP ± OHDW as administered in this study, was associated with a greater degree of toxicity than historically observed with 5-FU alone. This suggests at least some synergistic "toxic" effect. Further, modification of dose and schedule will be required in order to take advantage of the observed biochemical modulation of DDP on folate metabolism.

REFERENCES

1. Y.M. Rustum, S. Madajewicz, J. Campbell, S. Zakrzewski, N. Petrelli, L.O. Herrera, A. Mittelman, P.J. Creaven. Clinical biochemical pharmacology 5-formyltetrahydrofolate in combination with 5-fluorouracil in patients with advanced colorectal carcinoma: correlation with clinical response. In: Advances in Cancer Chemotherapy. The Current Status of 5-Fluorouracil-Leucovorin Calcium Combination. H.W. Bruckner and Y.M. Rustum, eds., Div. of Park Row Publishers (1984).
2. K.J. Scanlon, R.L. Safirstein, H. Thies, R.B. Gross, S. Waxman, J.B. Guttenplan. Inhibition of amino acid transport by cis-diamminedichloro-platinum(II) derivatives in L1210 murine leukemia cells. Cancer Res. 43:4211 (1983).
3. H.A. Krebs, R. Hems, B. Tyler. The regulation of folate and methionine metabolism. Biochem. J. 158:341 (1976).
4. K.J. Scanlon, E.M. Newman, Y. Lu, D.G. Priest. Biochemical basis for cisplatin and 5-fluorouracil synergism in human ovarian carcinoma cells. Proc. Natl. Acad. Sci. 83:8923 (1986).
5. J.L.Aull, A.C.Rice, L.A. Tebbetts. Interactions of platinum complexes with the essential and non-essential sulfhydryl groups of thymidylate synthetase. Biochem. 16:672 (1977).
6. S. Madajewicz, F. Trave, N. Petrelli, Y. Rustum, L. Herrera, A. Mittelman, P. Creaven. Preclinical and clinical studies with 5-fluorouracil and cisplatin. Proc. Am. Soc. Clin. Oncol. 4:47 (1985).
7. J. Cantrell, R. Hart, R. Taylor, J. Harvey. A phase II trial of continuous infusion 5-FU and weekly low dose cisplatin in colorectal carcinoma. Proc. Am. Soc. Clin. Oncol. 5:84 (1986).
8. A. Lockshin, P.V. Danenberg. Biochemical factors affecting the tightness of 5-fluorodeoxyuridylate binding of human thymidylate synthetase. Biochem. Pharmacol. 30:247 (1980).
9. S. Madajewicz, N. Petrelli, Y.M. Rustum, J. Campbell, L. Herrera, A. Mittelman, A. Perry, P.J. Creaven. Phase I-II trial of high dose calcium leucovorin and 5-fluorouracil in advanced colorectal cancer. Cancer Res. 44:4667 (1984).
10. D. Machover, E. Goldschmidt, P. Chollet, G. Metzger, J. Zittoun, J. Marquet, J.M. Vandenbulcke, J.L. Misset, L. Schwarzenberg, J.B. Fourtillan, H. Gaget, G. Mathe. Treatment of advanced colorectal and gastric adenocarcinomas with 5-fluorouracil and high-dose folinic acid. J. Clin. Onc. 4:685 (1986).
11. J.A. Houghton, S.J. Maroda, J.O. Phillips, P.J. Houghton. Biochemical determinants of responsiveness to 5-fluorouracil and its derivatives in xenographs of human colorectal adenocarcinoms in mice. Cancer Res. 41:144 (1981).
12. K. Keyomarsi, R.G. Moran. Folinic acid augmentation of the effects of fluoropyrimidines on murine and human leukemic cells. Cancer Res. 46:5229 (1986).
13. E.E. Vokes, K.E. Choi, R.L. Schilsky, W. Moran, C.M. Guarnieri, R.R. Weichselbaum, W.R. Panje. Cisplatin, fluorouracil, and high-dose leucovorin

for recurrent or metastatic head and neck cancer. J. Clin. Oncol. 6:618 (1988).

14. H.S. Krebs, R. Hems, B. Tyler. The regulation of folate and methionine metabolism. Biochem. J. 158:341 (1976).

ACKNOWLEDGEMENT

I gratefully acknowledge the Burroughs Wellcome Company for supplying the free drug used in these studies.

DISCUSSION OF DR. MADAJEWICZ'S PRESENTATION

Dr. Peters: Do you see more responses in lung metastases because lung metastases are more easily measured? Secondly, is your better response rate in rectal cancer due to the fact that rectal cancers are more likely to have lung metastases?

Dr. Madajewicz: One of our partial responders with rectal carcinoma had extensive lung metastases and huge local pelvic disease. She responded in both places. Patients do respond in both liver and lung metastases, it is not a question that you can better measure responses in lung metastases than in liver; however, if the patient did not have measurable disease, our criteria for PR was a 75% decrease of those not measurable markers. I would like to mention the very first patient that we started to treat at Roswell Park, a remarkable lady with rectal carcinoma and massive lung metastases and huge pelvic tumor which extended to the bladder, her vagina was outside. The patient was in, forgive me for the words, in delivery position; she couldn't walk. She was one of our first if not first patient on cis-platin/FUra. She is now into her fifth year in complete response, pathologically confirmed, perhaps cured. Another patient from University Hospital in Jackson who failed FUra and radiation therapy received cis-platin and FUra. Again, the patient had an enormous pelvic mass; she is now 2 years in complete response.

Dr. Scanlon: I've always found it a little bit easier to explain how results work rather than how they don't work. I can pose several possibilities of why you weren't able to achieve the response with platinum and FUra. The obvious one would be the pharmacology of the platinum as well as the FUra at the doses used. Perhaps at the higher doses of the platinum you are not seeing the subtle effects that we tried to explain yesterday or the activation of the FUra in your patients to achieve high enough levels of FdUMP and the other optimizing conditions of the ternary complex that was discussed yesterday. There may be some possibility that the folates stay in the form of 5-methyltetrahydrofolate and a possible lack of methionine synthetase in some of these patient cells may limit the conversion to increase the 5,10-methylene pool. There are obviously several possibilities to explain why the patients don't respond.

5-FLUOROURACIL AND FOLINIC ACID: SUMMARY OF CLINICAL EXPERIENCE

Patrick J. Creaven

Department of Clinical Pharmacology and Therapeutics
Roswell Park Memorial Institute
Buffalo, New York, 14263

INTRODUCTION

   In summarizing the clinical experience with 5-fluorouracil (FU) and
folinic acid (FA) I shall approach it in the context of some critical
questions which may be used to determine where we currently stand and
where information still needs to be sought with respect to the clinical
activity of this modulation.   These questions are listed in Table 1.

Table 1.   CLINICAL EVALUATION OF FU/FA:
                   MAJOR QUESTIONS

---

1.   Does FA significantly increase the response rate (RR) of colon
     carcinoma to FU?
2.   If so, is this an increase in therapeutic index or merely an
     increase in intensity of therapy?
3.   Does this increase in RR result in increased survival?
4.   Is it seen in other FU responsive tumors?
5.   Is the combination active against tumors with natural or
     acquired resistance to FU?
6.   Is the dose of FA critical to response?
7.   Can modulation of FU by FA be increased by addition of:
       a) cisplatin
       b) other compounds

COLORECTAL CARCINOMA

   The early data on FU as a single agent in colorectal carcinoma have
been assembled by Livingston and Carter (1).   These are compared in Table
2 with published data on studies of FU/FA in patients with no prior
therapy (2-20).

Table 2. RESPONSE IN COLORECTAL CARCINOMA:
FU VS FU/FA

	No. of Studies	No. of Patients	Response Rate Median	Overall
FU	32	1255	20	24
FU/FA[a]	20	999	27	27

a - No prior chemotherapy

Such a comparison is very crude and lacks statistical validity, and can
serve only as a point of departure in considering whether the addition of
FA to FU represents a therapeutic advance. For an accurate comparison
one must select out those studies in which a randomized comparison has
been made between the two treatments. Two types of such comparisons will
be considered: those in which the control and the experimental group
both receive the same dose and schedule of FU and the experimental group
also receives FA, and those in which the FU dose and schedule in the
control arm are adjusted to give a regimen which is equitoxic to the
FU/FA combination. The first design attempts to answer such questions as
"does the addition of FA to FU increase the response rate and/or toxicity
of FU". It does not answer the question "is FU/FA a more effective
therapy than FU alone?" This question is best answered by the second
design. A mixed design has also been used in which the two groups start
out receiving the same dose of FU but in subsequent courses the dose is
adjusted to make the two arms equitoxic. The data on comparative studies
where essentially the same starting dose of FU in both arms was used, are
shown in Table 3.

Table 3. FU VS FU/FA COLORECTAL CARCINOMA
RANDOMIZED COMPARISONS.
I. FU DOSE A = B

AUTHOR (Ref)	DOSE[a] FU	FA	R/T[b]	RR (%)[b]	
Erlichman et al (19)	A) 1850[c] B) 1850	1000	4/61 21/65	7 33	p < 0.005
Doroshow et al (6)	A) 1850 B) 1850	3000	5/34 13/29	15 45	
Canobbio et al (17)	A) 2400 B) 2400	2000	2/39 7/43	5 16	NS
Petrelli et al (18)	A) 2500 B) 2400	2000	13/107 31/109	12 28	p < 0.01

a - Doses are mg/m^2/4 weeks of treatment
b - R/T Responders/treated, RR Response rate (CR+PR)
c - Escalated to make the regimens equitoxic in subsequent courses

For the purposes of comparison in this and in subsequent tables the total dose of FU and of FA planned for the first four weeks of treatment are used as a basis for comparison, even in cases where the initial treatment course extended beyond a 4 week period. Toxicity was, in general, more severe in the FU/FA groups than in the FU alone groups and more directed towards the GI tract. In the study by Erlichman et al (19), patients receiving FU/FA had significantly more mucositis and diarrhea from course 1, than those receiving FU alone (p <0.0005); median nadirs of neutrophil counts were respectively 1.9 and 3.2 x 10^9/L in the two groups after course 1. Stomatitis was more severe in the combination group (p <0.02) in the study by Doroshow et al (6); both stomatitis and severe diarrhea were more frequent in the FU/FA group than in the FU alone group in the study by Cannobio et al (17).

The tendency for FU/FA to change the pattern of toxicity of FU complicates the attempt to design studies in which FU and FU/FA are given at equitoxic doses. The result of three attempts to achieve this are given in Table 4.

Table 4. FU VS FU/FA COLORECTAL CARCINOMA[a]
         RANDOMIZED COMPARISONS.
         II. FU DOSE A > B

AUTHOR (Ref)		DOSE FU	FA	R/T	RR (%)	
Petrelli	A)	3450		2/19	11	p = 0.009
et al (21)	B)	2400	2000	12/30	40	
O'Connell	A)	2000		4/39	10	p = 0.001
et al (20)	B)	1700	100	16/37	43	
Valone	A)	3885		9/49	18	NS
et al (15)	B)	2000	1000	15/96	16	

a – See footnotes Table 3

The two treated arms were roughly equitoxic in the study by Petrelli et al.(21), with more hematologic toxicity in the FU alone group and more GI toxicity in patients treated with the combination. The FU/FA arm was somewhat more toxic in the study by O'Connell et al (20). Both hematologic and non-hematologic toxicity were significantly greater in the FU alone arm in the study by Valone et al (15)

A summary of the overall results of the randomized trials is shown in Table 5.

Table 5. FU VS FU/FA COLORECTAL CARCINOMA[a]
         RANDOMIZED COMPARISONS:
         OVERALL RESULTS

	R/T	RR (%)
FU	39/348	11
FU + FA	115/409	29

a – See footnote Table 3

305

The data on the effect on survival of FU/FA as compared with FU are more preliminary. The data from the randomized trials are shown in Table 6.

Table 6. FU VS FU/FA COLORECTAL CARCINOMA:
EFFECT ON SURVIVAL

| AUTHOR (Ref) | MEDIAN SURVIVAL (MONTHS) | | p |
	FU	FU/FA	
Petrelli et al (RPMI) (8)	11[a]	12[a]	N.S.
Petrelli et al (GITSG) (18)	Too early		
Erlichman et al (19)	9.6	12.6	0.05
Doroshow et al (6)	13.2	14.6	N.S.
O'Connell et al (20)	7.5	13.75[b]	0.004[b]
		12.25[c]	0.01[c]
Cannobio et al (17)	12.7	8.6	N.S.
Valone et al (22)[d]	Too early		

a - Estimated
b - Low dose CF (See Table 8)
c - High dose CF (see Table 8)
d - Preliminary evidence suggests survival is equal

BREAST CARCINOMA

The effect of modulating FU action with FA in FU responsive tumors other than colorectal carcinoma is only now being examined. Data on breast carcinoma from 4 trials in which most patients had received extensive pretreatment are summarized in Table 7.

Table 7. FU/FA IN BREAST CARCINOMA[a]

AUTHOR (Ref)	R/T	RR (%)
Allegra et al (23)	12/50	24
Doroshow et al (24)	10/60	17
Loprinzi et al (25)	4/21	19
Marini et al (26)	16/36	44
Overall	42/167[b]	25

a - See footnote Table 3
b - Prior FU in 90%

Recently, Fine et al (27) have published a phase II study of FU/FA as first line treatment for breast carcinoma (10/25 prior adjuvant therapy, 15/25 no prior chemotherapy). The response rate was 48% (12/25). Zaniboni et al (28) have incorporated FU/FA into a combination with cyclophosphamide and epirubicin. The responses were CR 7/30 and PR 15/30 (overall 22/30, 73%).

OTHER TUMORS

In previously untreated patients with gastric carcinoma, Machover et al (29) have reported a response rate of 50% (13/26) and Arbuck et al, 8% (1/13) (30). Encouraging preliminary results in pancreatic carcinoma have been reported by Bruckner (31).

The data on activity of the FU/FA combination in tumors with natural or acquired resistance to FU are incomplete. Early results indicating that the combination was highly active in patients with colorectal carcinoma who had failed FU (7) have not been confirmed by later studies. A phase II trial in non-small cell lung cancer showed no activity in this disease (32).

OPTIMUM MODULATING DOSE OF FA

The question of the appropriate dose of FA for modulation of FU activity is complicated by the fact that the response rate and toxicity will be a function of the dose of both agents and that the requirement for exogenous reduced folate for maximum activity of FU probably varies from patient to patient. High doses of FA which attempt to reproduce clinically the extracellular concentration of FA shown by Hakala and co-workers to be optimal in an in vitro system (33) were used in the original studies by Machover (29) while much lower doses were used in the early studies reported by Bruckner (2). A review of the literature shows no immediately obvious dose response relationship in colorectal carcinoma for the FA used in the FU/FA combinations. Two prospective randomized studies have addressed the question of high vs low dose of FA and the results are presented in Table 8. The question of whether there is a subgroup of patients who would benefit from even higher doses of FA than conventional 'high dose' is only now being addressed and no data are available.

Table 8. FU vs FU/FA COLORECTAL CARCINOMA
HIGH DOSE VS LOW DOSE FA[a]

STUDY (Ref)	FA Dose	R/T	RR (%)
GITSG	0	13/107	12
(Petrelli et al, 18)	100	21/112	19
	2000	31/109	28
Mayo Clinic	0	4/39	10
and NCCTG	100	16/37	43
(O'Connell et al,	1000	10/35	29
20)			

a – See footnote to Table 3

MODULATION OF FU WITH FA + CISPLATIN

Attempts further to modulate the activity of FU by addition of cisplatin to FU/FA are underway. Data are fragmentary and widely variable. Responses that have been reported in colorectal carcinoma include 1/15 by Madajewicz et al (34), 2/12 by Scheithauer et al (35) and 7/15 by Chiarion Sileni et al (36). Very high response rates to the three drug combinations in previously untreated squamous cell carcinoma of the head and neck are reported in the present proceedings by Loeffler et al (37) (43/45, 95%).

DISCUSSION

In discussing the clinical data presented at this Symposium and some data recently reported in the literature, I shall do so in the context of the questions presented in Table 1. A comparison of the response rate to FU/FA and the response rate to FU reported in the older literature (Table 2), is not suggestive of a marked therapeutic benefit for the combination. However, it is clear from the overall summary of the prospective randomized clinical trials comparing FU with FU/FA (Table 5), that the older literature markedly overestimates the true response rate to FU alone and that the response rate of the combination is approximately three times that of FU used alone. Three of the four studies in which FA was added to a dose of FU showed a significant improvement in response rate for the combination with an overall increase from 10% to 30% (Table 3). Of the 3 studies in which a greater dose of FU was used in the control arm (Table 4), one failed to show an advantage for the combination, but in this study the FU alone arm was significantly more toxic than the combination arm. Thus, it seems reasonable to conclude from the data now available that FU/FA not only increases the response rate of FU in colorectal carcinoma, but also represents a therapeutic advantage over FU used alone.

The data on survival benefit are much more mixed. Only 2/5 studies show a survival advantage for the combination and in one of these the advantage is quite small. A definitive conclusion on this question must await the maturation of the present studies and perhaps further more extensive investigations.

Investigations in other tumor types have been much more limited. Initial studies in breast cancer have shown significant activity in heavily pretreated patients. At least two groups have felt this activity to be sufficiently encouraging to warrant moving the combination into front line therapy. The paucity of data in gastric carcinoma is disappointing in the light of the high response rate reported by Machover et al (29), and further studies are clearly needed in this area. The data on activity against tumors resistant to FU are too preliminary to warrant comment at this stage.

The available data on the effect of the dose of FA is surprising in the light of the original data of Hakala and co-workers indicating that 10 μM 1-CF was necessary for full activity in their in vitro system. The marked difference in the results of the GITSG study and the Mayo Clinic study is difficult to interpret and suggests that possibly patients may fall into several groups; those who will respond to FU alone, those who will respond to FU plus low dose CF, those who require high doses of CF, and those who will be resistant to the combination at any dose. If this is so, the development of predictive biochemical assays to distinguish prospectively between members of these subtypes constitutes an important area for current and future investigation.

The data currently available are insufficient to draw any conclusion on the effect of attempting to modulate FU activity further by the addition of cisplatin to the combination. The very high response rate reported for the 3 drug combination in untreated squamous cell carcinoma of the head and neck (37) must be seen in the context of the already high response rates achievable with FU and cisplatin without addition of FA.

In the above discussion I have attempted to summarize very briefly the major conclusions to be drawn from the clinical data presented at this Symposium and to delineate the present status of clinical knowledge of the FU/FA combination. Studies currently ongoing should, in the next several years, clarify many of the questions still open.

REFERENCES

1. R.B. Livingston and S.K. Carter, "Single Agents in Cancer
    Chemotherapy", IFI/Plenum, New York, 1970, pp. 202-206.
2. H. Bruckner, J. Roboz, M. Spiegelman, et al. An efficient leucovorin
    and 5-fluorouracil sequence: dosage escalation and pharmacological
    monitoring. Proc Am Assoc Cancer Res 24:547 (1983).
3. D. Machover, E. Goldschimidt, P. Chollet, et al. Treatment of
    advanced colorectal and gastric adenocarcinoma with 5-fluorouracil
    and high-dose folinic acid. J Clin Oncol 4:685 (1986).
4. P. Byrne, J. Treat, M. McFadden, et al. Therapeutic efficacy of the
    combination of 5-fluorouracil and high-dose leucovorin in patients
    with advanced colorectal carcinoma: single daily intravenous dose
    for five days, in: "The Current Status of 5-Fluorouracil-Leucovorin
    Combination," H.W. Brucker and Y.M. Rustum, eds., Park Row
    Publishers, Inc., New York, 1984.
5. G.T. Budd, T. Fleming, J.D. Bukowski, et al. 5-Fluorouracil and
    folinic acid in the treatment of metastatic colorectal cancer: a
    randomized comparison. A Southwest Oncology Group Study. J Clin
    Oncol 5:272 (1987).
6. J.H. Doroshow, M. Bertrand, P. Multhauf, et al. Prospective
    randomized trial comparing 5-FU versus (vs) 5-FU and high dose
    folinic acid (HDFA) for treatment of advanced colorectal cancer.
    Proc Am Soc Clin Oncol 6:96 (1987)
7. S. Madajewicz, N.J. Petrelli, Y. Rustum, et al. A phase I trial of
    high dose calcium leucovorin and 5-fluorouracil in advanced
    colorectal cancer. Cancer Res 44:4667 (1984).
8. N.J. Petrelli, Y.M. Rustum, H. Bruckner, et al. The Roswell Park
    Memorial Institute and Gastrointestinal Tumor Study Group phase III
    experience with the modulation of 5-fluorouracil by leucovorin in
    metastatic colorectal adenocarcinoma. in: "International Symposium
    on the Expanding Role of Folates and Fluoropyrimidines in Cancer
    Chemotherapy," Y. Rustum and J. McGuire, eds., Plenum Press, New
    York, 1988, pp.
9. J.D. Hines, D.J. Adelstein, J.L. Spiess, et al. High-dose weekly
    oral leucovorin and 5-fluorouracil in previously untreated patients
    with advanced colorectal carcinoma: a phase I study. in:
    "International Symposium on the Expanding Role of Folates and
    Fluoropyrimidines in Cancer Chemotherapy," Y. Rustum and J.
    McGuire, eds., Plenum Press, New York, 1988, pp.
10. J. Cunningham, R.M. Bukowski, G.T. Budd, et al. 5-Fluorouracil and
    folinic acid: a phase I-II trial in gastrointestinal malignancy.
    Invest New Drugs 2:391 (1984).
11. J. Mortimer and C. Higano. Continuous infusion 5-fluorouracil (FU)
    and folinic acid (FA) in disseminated colorectal cancer: a phase
    I-II study. Proc. Am. A. Cancer Res. 26:171 (1985).
12. H. Greene, A. Desai, S. Levick, et al. Combined 5-fluorouracil
    infusion and high dose folinic acid in the treatment of metastatic
    gastrointestinal cancer. Proc Am Soc Clin Oncol 5:89 (1986).
13. H.-J. Schmoll and S. Le Blanc. Sequential high dose folinic acid
    (FA) and 5-fluorouracil (5-FU) in advanced colorectal cancer with
    measurable, progressive disease. Proc Am Soc Clin Oncol 4:94
    (1985).
14. H. Wilke, H.-J. Schmoll, P. Preusser, et al. Folinic acid
    (CF)/5-fluorouracil (FUra) combinations in advanced gastrointestinal
    carcinomas. in: "International Symposium on the Expanding Role of
    Folates and Fluoropyrimidines in Cancer Chemotherapy," Y. Rustum
    and J. McGuire, eds., Plenum Press, New York, 1988, pp.

15. F.H. Valone, T. Drakes, M. Flam, et al. A Northern California Oncology Group randomized trial of single agent 5-FU vs high-dose folinic acid + 5-FU vs methotrexate + 5-FU + folinic acid in patients with disseminated measurable large bowel cancer. Abst. of The Expanding Role of Folates and Fluoropyrimidines in Cancer Chemotherapy. April 1988, Buffalo, New York.

16. L.R. Laufman, W.D. Breckman, Jr., K.A. Stydnicki, et al. Clinical experience with CF-FUra. in: "International Symposium on the Expanding Role of Folates and Fluoropyrimidines in Cancer Chemotherapy," Y. Rustum and J. McGuire, eds., Plenum Press, New York, 1988, pp.

17. L. Canobbio, M.T. Nobile, A. Sobrero, et al. A randomized trial of 5-fluorouracil alone versus 5-fluorouracil and high dose leucovorin (LV) in untreated advanced colorectal cancer patients. in: "International Symposium on the Expanding Role of Folates and Fluoropyrimidines in Cancer Chemotherapy," Y. Rustum and J. McGuire, eds., Plenum Press, New York, 1988, pp.

18. N. Petrelli, D. Stablein, H. Bruckner, et al. A prospective randomized phase III trial of 5-fluorouracil (5FU) versus 5FU + high dose leucovorin (HDCF) versus 5FU + low dose leucovorin (LDCF) in patients (pts) with metastatic colorectal adenocarcinoma. A report of the Gastrointestinal Tumor Study Group. Proc Am Soc Clin Oncol 7:94 (1988).

19. C. Erlichman. 5-Fluorouracil (FUra) and folinic acid (FA) therapy in patients with colorectal cancer. in: "International Symposium on the Expanding Role of Folates and Fluoropyrimidines in Cancer Chemotherapy," Y. Rustum and J. McGuire, eds., Plenum Press, New York, 1988, pp.

20. M.J. O'Connell. A controlled clinical trial including folinic acid at two distinct dose levels in combination with 5-fluorouracil (5FU) for the treatment of advanced colorectal cancer: experience of the Mayo Clinic and North Central Cancer Treatment Group. in: "International Symposium on the Expanding Role of Folates and Fluoropyrimidines in Cancer Chemotherapy," Y. Rustum and J. McGuire, eds., Plenum Press, New York, 1988, pp.

21. N. Petrelli, L. Herrera, Y. Rustum, et al. A prospective randomized trial of 5-fluorouracil versus 5-fluorouracil and high-dose leucovorin versus 5-fluorouracil and methotrexate in previously untreated patients with advanced colorectal carcinoma. J Clin Oncol 5:1559 (1987).

22. F.H. Valone, P.S. Wittlinger, M.S. Flam, et al. A Northern California Oncology Group randomized trial of single agent 5-FU vs. high-dose folinic acid + 5-FU vs. methotrexate + 5-FU + folinic acid in patients with disseminated measurable large bowel cancer. in: "International Symposium on the Expanding Role of Folates and Fluoropyrimidines in Cancer Chemotherapy," Y. Rustum and J. McGuire, eds., Plenum Press, New York, 1988, pp.

23. C. J. Allegra, G.F. Egan, J.C. Drake, et al. The treatment of metastatic breast cancer with 5-fluorouracil and leucovorin. in: "International Symposium on the Expanding Role of Folates and Fluoropyrimidines in Cancer Chemotherapy," Y. Rustum and J. McGuire, eds., Plenum Press, New York, 1988, pp.

24. J.H. Doroshow, L. Leong, K. Margolin, et al. Effective salvage therapy for refractory disseminated breast cancr with 5-fluorouracil and high-dose continuous infusion folinic acid. in: "International Symposium on the Expanding Role of Folates and Fluoropyrimidines in Cancer Chemotherapy," Y. Rustum and J. McGuire, eds., Plenum Press, New York, 1988, pp.

25. C.L. Loprinzi, J.N. Ingle, D.J. Schaid, et al. Progress report on a phase II trial of 5-fluorouracil plus citrovorum factor in women with metastatic breast cancer. in: "International Symposium on the Expanding Role of Folates and Fluoropyrimidines in Cancer Chemotherapy," Y. Rustum and J. McGuire, eds., Plenum Press, New York, 1988, pp.

26. G. Marini, E. Simoncini, A. Zaniboni, et al. 5-Fluorouracil and high-dose folinic acid as salvage treatment of advanced breast cancer: an update. Oncology 44:336 (1987).

27. S. Fine, C. Erlichman, L. Kaizer, et al. Phase II trial of 5FU + folinic acid (FA) as first line treatment for metastatic breast cancer. Proc Am Soc Clin Oncol 7:41 (1988).

28. A. Zaniboni, E. Simoncini, P. Marpicati, et al. Cyclophosphamide (C), epirubicin (E), high-dose folinic acid (HDFA) and 5-fluorouracil (5-FU) as first line chemotherapy in metastatic breast cancer (MBC). Preliminary results. Proc Am Soc Clin Oncol 7:18 (1988).

29. D. Machover, E. Goldschmidt, P. Chollet, et al. Treatment of advanced colorectal and gastric adenocarcinomas with 5-fluorouracil and high-dose folinic acid. J Clin Oncol 4:685 (1986).

30. S.G. Arbuck, H.O. Douglass, Jr., F. Trave, et al. A phase II trial of 5-fluorouracil and high-dose intravenous leucovorin in gastric carcinoma. J Clin Oncol 5:1150 (1987).

31. H. W. Bruckner. Mount Sinai clinical experience with leucovorin and fluorouracil. in: "International Symposium on the Expanding Role of Folates and Fluoropyrimidines in Cancer Chemotherapy," Y. Rustum and J. McGuire, eds., Plenum Press, New York, 1988, pp.

32. P.J. Creaven, H. Takita, Y. Rustum, et al. Unpublished data.

33. R.M. Evans, J.D. Laskin, M.T. Hakala. Effect of excess folates and deoxyinosine on the activity and site of action of 5-fluorouracil. Cancer Res 41:3288 (1981).

34. S. Madajewicz, J.J. Fiore, M.H. Zarrabi. Clinical experience with 5-FU/DDP + OHDW combination chemotherapy in patients with advanced colorectal carcinoma. in: "International Symposium on the Expanding Role of Folates and Fluoropyrimidines in Cancer Chemotherapy," Y. Rustum and J. McGuire, eds., Plenum Press, New York, 1988, pp.

35. W. Scheithauer, D. Depisch, R. Schiessel, et al. High dose leucovorin (CF), 5-fluorouracil (5-FU) and cisplatin (DDP) for treatment of metastatic colorectal cancer. Proc Am Soc Clin Oncol 7:108 (1988).

36. V. Chiarion Sileni, F. Figoli, M. Gulisano, et al. 120 Hours 5-fluorouracil (5-FU) continuous infusion (c.i.) plus cisplatinum (P) and folinic acid (F) in metastatic colon cancer (M.C.C.). Proc Am Soc Clin Oncol 7:109 (1988).

37. T.M. Loeffler, J. Lindemann, H. Luckhaupt, et al. Chemotherapy of advanced and relapsed squamous cell cancer of the head and neck with split-dose cisplatinum (DDP), 5-fluorouracil (Fura) and leucovorin (CF). in: "International Symposium on the Expanding Role of Folates and Fluoropyrimidines in Cancer Chemotherapy," Y. Rustum and J. McGuire, eds., Plenum Press, New York, 1988, pp.

PANEL DISCUSSION OF FUTURE DIRECTIONS

Dr. **Wittes:** I'd like to begin the panel discussion. We have a group
of people who are very experienced in clinical oncology and in
experimental oncology. I thought the best way of dealing with the
question of future directions would be to let each panel member have
a few minutes to react to whatever portion of the material presented
in the last 2 days particularly interested them by way of making
suggestions for the important priorities that ought to occupy the
FUra/CF story over the next couple of years. First, it seems to me
that some discussion ought to center around the issues of optimization of dose and schedule; what sorts of issues need to be addressed
in order to do this in less than a completely empirical way?
Second, there is the issue of predictive tests and mechanistic
studies as they relate to clinical trials results. We've heard a
fair amount about the potential uses of biochemical pharmacology in
helping either to optimize therapy or helping to select patients,
much in the manner that the estrogen receptor helps to select breast
cancer patients who are likely to respond to endocrine manipulation. Third, what is the propriety of moving FUra/CF based regimens
into the adjuvant setting now, knowing what we do about their
activity in advanced disease? Is this a reasonable thing to do or
should we fine tune the situation further and await more data as to
what would constitute a more nearly optimal regimen before doing
this? Fourth, what is the propriety of incorporating FUra/CF into
other regimens that are FUra sensitive? One thinks of breast cancer
particularly, not only because data have been presented here in
partial support of the notion that CF may increase the therapeutic
index of FUra in certain situations in breast cancer, but also
because although breast cancer has plenty of other individual agents
that are active, it still remains true that most of the responses
that one sees in metastatic breast cancer are partial. We badly
need regimens in advanced disease that can increase the complete
response rate. With that introduction, let me ask Dr. Mihich to
begin by saying a few words.

Dr. **Mihich:** It was very interesting to hear all this progress in these
2 days. I think that in this case of metabolic modulation the issue
that is really important is to increase selectivity. Potency is
useful but if we increase potency without an advantage in selectivity we really have not gained as much as we would like to. In
this respect, there are indications, and we can speak only about
indications at this moment, that there is a change in pattern of
limiting toxicity to normal tissues as a result of the addition of
CF. Even though we are dealing here with a change in limiting
toxicity between normal tissues (hematopoietic versus gastrointestinal), this is, in a sense, encouraging because it indicates
the addition of the normal cofactor is selectively modifying one

tissue versus the other. We would of course like to exploit this maximally by increasing selectivity for the antitumor activity, which brings us to the next question. Can we do this with that combination by modifying doses, schedules, routes, pharmacological parameter, i.e., the devices that are often used in attempts to increase selectivity? Here there is confusion, at least for me, because we saw what I would define as contradictory results in terms of effects of low versus medium versus high. The issue is that at the same dose level of 20-25 mg/m^2 of CF there were differences in effectiveness and response. The question is how to define the optimal dose and schedule. We should try to avoid the classical chemotherapy "rational-empirical" approach to dose and scheduling which is to try various combinations with various schedules and then look at the results in a chemotherapeutic sense. That's fine but it's going to be, it seems to me, given the complexity of the problem, very time consuming. It may be disappointing because of contradictory results. I wonder whether, now that many centers in the country are involved in biochemical pharmacological measurements in humans, we could use such measurements to speed the process. The question is, how can we do this? Which parameter of a biochemical nature could be selected such that it would monitor the effectiveness of CF administration in a particular patient? This is a problem that we have in BRMs, too, in terms of identifying a biological response modification that is relevant in a particular patient. So the issue is, which parameter? Inhibition and duration of inhibition of TS would be the obvious endpoint; however, that may be very difficult to do in every case, almost impossible in many cases. Another possibility would be to develop a correlation between that parameter and a more accessible parameter; which one, would have to be determined. One might try blood levels, but those are modified by so many factors that they may not be appropriate. Once TS inhibition can be correlated with a more readily accessible parameter, that parameter might be used to identify in each case whether that particular CF regimen is the optimal one for selectivity.

Dr. Bertino: I was struck by a couple things that I would like to make comments on. One is the fact, mentioned by Howard Bruckner, that the dose schedule for CF may depend upon the dose schedule of FUra used. I think that is brought out by the Mayo Clinic and the North Central Group data; that, if one gives FUra daily for 5 days, maybe we don't need massive doses of CF each day. You have to ask, why is that? It may be that with the low-doses we essentially are giving a low-dose, continuous type of infusion because we are generating 5-methyltetrahydrofolate. Although we're measuring accumulation in tumor tissue 1 hr or so after the first dose, what is probably important is what happens after, say, the fifth dose; are we seeing accumulation of CF levels or, more importantly, methylenetetrahydrofolate levels in tissues as a consequence of those repeated doses. In support of that, we've been doing a trial of intrahepatic infusion therapy with FUdR together with CF in a pump. Even at doses of 30 mg/m^2 of CF, but given continuously over the 14 day period with FUdR, we have seen increased local toxicity of the combination over what we would have expected with FUdR alone (Nancy Kemeny will report on those studies at the ASCO Meeting), but the response rates and the degree of responses have been very impressive. The other point to be made is that if, in human tumors, CF utilizes the same kind of transport system we know about in terms of MTX uptake, then we are dealing with a carrier-mediated limiting transport system. Thus, even though we increase the dose 10-fold we're not going to get much more than perhaps 2-fold more folate transported across the membrane because of that limitation and the need for some passive diffusion as well.

The other point I thought might be worth making is that one of the arms of the Mayo Clinic-North Central Trial which was not discussed today was sequential MTX and FUra, and they did it right. They gave a high dose of MTX, they waited 7 hr before they gave FUra, and they gave a high dose of FUra. It was encouraging to see that the response rate in that trial was as good as the FUra/CF arm, and I think we should not abandon MTX/FUra as another alternative in terms of future exploration. Finally, I think the biochemical tests on human tumor tissue are, of course, very important. It's loaded with problems and we didn't really go into many of the problems that one has to deal with. I'm not sure that measuring inhibition of TS activity 30 or 60 min post-treatment is going to be all that predictive, although the data look reasonably good, because we know from many of the studies from yesterday and Joe Rustum's studies in particular that duration of inhibition of TS seems to be important rather than the transient early inhibition. I certainly would encourage those types of studies and we are also beginning that kind of research.

Dr. Wittes: Joe, how would you deal with the question of sorting out the relation between CF scheduling and FUra scheduling?

Dr. Bertino: - I think the key thing is trying to get more tumor measurements of methylenetetrahydrofolate and not just once but after different time points and after the 2nd, 3rd or 4th day dose as well.

Dr. Wittes: The point is that you would approach it initially biochemically and not with randomized comparative trials at this point

Dr. Bertino: Well, that's a harder way.

Dr. DeLap: It was nice to be a part of this conference and get a unique perspective as to how the field developed. It called to mind again that progress can be made in this area beginning with good science. I was struck by Dr. Santi's comment to the effect that the enzymologists had shown the way here, and it has led to good, important clinical work. The other thing that I'm struck by is that we're talking about treatment of colorectal cancer which, in its metastatic form, has been one of the toughest nuts to crack in the clinical oncology area and so any progress in this area, even if it is fairly modest, is symbolically very important and I think gives everyone encouragement to continue. Specifically, in terms of things that might be done, I certainly agree with what Dr. Bertino was saying regarding the importance of the biochemical measure-ments. The randomized clinical trial is certainly one of the most powerful tools we have, but it makes little sense to go into randomized clinical trials if you can first make sure biochemically that you are doing what you want to do. I think we can see a way to do that now; we've certainly seen fine examples of it here. One can find patients with accessible tumors, one can determine if TS inhibition is adequate, the technology is emerging to determine if adequate folate levels are achieved and if they are the kind of folates one wants with the proper polyglutamylation status, etc. These kinds of things can be settled before one moves into a very long term and very resource intensive randomized clinical trial. I would encourage more of that research before jumping in and trying to compare all of the permutations and combinations of CF and FUra. I think one of the things that I'm hopeful about in the future is that we will develop even better surrogate endpoints. What I mean by surrogate endpoint is, for example, measuring TS inhibition in a tumor sample. That is still a somewhat invasive technique and has some limitations technically. I would hope that we will develop some more non-invasive measurements to tell us what is going on inside the tumor after treatment with drugs. Then we can take the same patient and treat them a couple of different times with different drug combinations, for example, different ratios of FUra to CF, and see if a better effect on the tumor is observed with treatment A or treatment B within the same patient. I think that is a very powerful technique for moving the field more quickly than just relying on the underlying trials. This is exactly what Dr. Allegra was doing with FUra and FUra/CF at different times in the same patient by looking at biochemical parameters in tumor samples. Finally, I think we don't want to overlook optimizing safety in these clinical regimens as well as efficacy. I think that there are some real safety differences between the different regimens that have been discussed. One of the things that we might do fairly promptly without so much investment in patient resources is to look at the comparative safety of some of these regimens which we think are at least globally of comparable efficacy. I think we have to recognize the fact that these regimens already are going into widespread clincal use and at least we should do what we can to optimize the safety as promptly as we can.

Dr. **Wittes:** I was interested yesterday in Rick Moran's suggestion that one of the things we might do with this whole area is get off the fluoropyrimidine wagon entirely and, if we really want to inhibit TS, do it with an antifol. Rick, have you heard anything in the last day or so, that changes your opinion of that?

Dr. **Moran:** No. I actually have a few things I want to say. I wanted to echo what Dr. Mihich said and go back to what I think is a major question facing us at the moment. When you have a situation where you are seeing complete responses in colorectal carcinoma, you're knocking the hell out this tumor. This is a surprise for me to see and it's a very pleasant surprise. You clearly have increased the activity of the drug against the tumor. In spite of the difference in types of toxicities we're seeing, it's not an overwhelmingly greater increase in toxicity. So we've done something here. This is the first time I've ever seen a combination which seems to be selectively cytotoxic and I think we all ought to be cognizant of the fact that none of us has addressed the selectivity question experimentally. It is amazing that none of us have and I think that is certainly something that has to be done very quickly. One gets the feeling that what we're dealing with in terms of selectivity of this combination has to do with metabolism of the CF or, by the time it hits the plasma, of 5-methyltetrahydrofolate, into other folate forms that are useful to stimulate binding to enzyme. One jumps to the conclusion that there's a difference in polyglutamation between the tumors that are responding and either the tumors that are not responding or normal tissues. That may well be the case, but here we have a problem. We've used CF in 2 different circumstances. In high dose CF with FU we're saying that normal tissues don't polyglutamate the folates all that well, and the tumor does. The other case is MTX with CF. The mechanism of MTX/CF is really, I think, fairly dark and darkly understood and there are only 2 papers that bear on it, one by Frank Sirotnak in

Cancer Research about 15 years ago and one slightly before that by
Dr. Frei in the New England Journal of Medicine. They clearly
showed that there was a difference in response between the tumors
and the normal tissues to CF. This seems like a contradiction. In
one case we're saying that the normal tissues don't convert CF into
polyglutamates, etc., as fast as tumors and in the other case we're
saying that they convert it better than the tumor. I don't understand what's going on here, but I think this is certainly a place
that needs some pretty hardcore work. I suggested the other day,
that compounds of the nature of CB3717 be thought of seriously. I
also suggested that hydroxyurea be added to some of these combinations. I was very pleased to get some positive feedback on that
from some of the members of this audience and panel. I guess I'd
like to put a pitch in here at this point and that is that I've seen
a number of clinical studies today that are squeezing the very last
drop out of a combination which you have to look at hard and very
carefully to make sure you get the proper effect. I have to wonder
what you people would do with a really good new drug. I would like
to find out, and one of the reasons that that's going to be
difficult is that over the past 15 years we've selectively weeded
out the synthetic chemists in this country by not funding them and
by giving them a hard time and I think we have to reverse that
process.

Dr. Clendenin: I do feel there is quite a bit of work that we need
to do in a situation where clinically we're already beginning to use
this combination and, since these drugs are already available, any
physician may begin to use them. We've heard today many clinical
schedules and differing results. We're going to have a lot of
patients being treated with FUra/CF whether or not they are going to
be receiving an appropriate schedule. I agree with Joe Bertino's
comment that the schedule used with FUra may be predictive of the
dose of CF. However, I also think I'm going to hear out in the
general community that, no matter what the evidence, maybe we should
be using less CF and what's going to happen is that less CF will be
used, and maybe not appropriately. We don't know the answer to the
question of whether less CF is necessary or appropriate. In this
area we do need really a lot more work from the biochemist to understand folates and folate pools, the importance of the different
folate cofactors and how the pools are changing. I'm still somewhat
confused about if when we measure 5-methyl in the serum and total
folates we are really measuring what we should be measuring; just
because a patient has a high 5-methyltetrahydrofolate level, are we
really delivering the right amount of CF to that patient. I think
we need to do a lot more work in that area. In addition, we need a
really good animal model that we could do some of the work in.
Animals are not men, so that is always a difficulty, but if we could
find an animal tumor where we could do some of the scheduling and
modeling I think that would be very helpful to speed some of the
correct clinical trials in their development. I am a little worried
about the use of this combination in the adjuvant setting in
clinical trials. Although I think it probably was the next logical
step, I'm not sure we're really going to be using the right
schedules. Hopefully there will be enough of them that will use
enough different schedules that we'll be able to say at least one of
them was potentially right and repeat it again. My fear is we're
just going to have the situation we have now with a lot of conflict-
ing results and not really being able to tell what was the correct
way to do the dosing.

Dr. Frei: I think this is a very important conference which brings together what I think is clearly the first evidence that one can modulate an important antitumor agent in the direction of an improved therapeutic index in the clinic. I think historically maybe that's very important; when you have a positive study all kinds of building becomes possible. In terms of what the emphasis should be on comparative studies versus phase I-II studies, versus biochemical studies applied to the clinic, I think all three fronts are important and the important thing to do is to make sure that the study is rigorous, that there are endpoints and that answers are obtained. There are many things that could be discussed. I would agree with Rick Moran but put a little different slant on it. I don't think we're using the right fluoropyrimidine and I don't think we're using the right leucovorin. It would make much more sense to me to use FUdR since FUdR by continuous infusion, at least biologically, is probably much closer to inhibiting DNA synthesis than FUra. That's always been an argument with respect with FUra. So using that fluoropyrimidine may make a big difference and I would suspect that that's going to come into the clinic with respect to CF fast and relatively furious and may replace FUra. The same is true of CF. When we give CF, we give a lot of 6R isomer and we've heard over the last 2 days that that may complicate life very considerably. I think very major emphasis should be given at this point by whatever resources (including the National Cancer Institute, the pharmaceutical industry, and those of us who can influence policy) to getting sufficient quantities of the 6S isomer to do the necessary studies. All the considerations with respect to dosing and schedule of CF are going to have to be reconsidered in the light of the purified 6S isomer material when that becomes available and I think that it should be sooner rather than later. We have tried many times in the past to use pharmacologicbiochemical approaches to modulate phase I and phase II clinical studies. The technology wasn't ready; it worked with steroid receptors, it worked perhaps with asparaginase but with the more complex material, it hasn't worked. But I think times have changed and the biochemical pharmacology is highly sophisticated and should be applied in parallel with many phase I, phase II clinical trials.

I can understand, on a biochemical basis, why CF increases the activity of FUra. What I don't understand is why there should be selection against tumors as compared to the host? I think that is a critical question. Until we have some leads with respect to that critical question, it's going to be somewhat empirical and somewhat difficult to apply the biochemical factors to the clinic. We know enough about the biochemistry from beginning to end to actually look at the differential with respect to the biochemistry and perhaps find the basis for selectivity. For example, polyglutamation is quantitatively different with respect to the gut as compared to many other tissues on the basis of Sirotnak's studies. Let us assume that polyglutamation is excessive in the gut. To this extent CF might be expected to modulate FUra more with respect to the gut than other sites. This would be consistent with the fact that the one thing that seems to be more prominent when you modulate is diarrhea. Tumors of the gut may also be expected to have that difference and maybe that's the basis for selectivity. Another possible basis of selectivity is that solid tumors have vascular problems. Access into solid tumors can be diminished, perhaps for CF. Tumors are metabolically and cytokinetically active which means they consume folates; so one can consider solid tumors potentially as folate deficient and it may be that the basis for selectivity is simply that large ambient concentrations of CF selectively upgrade in solid tumors as compared to normal tissues. There're many other postulates that can be made and these are the simplest ones, but it does mean that we can address them with biochemistry.

I think two things in terms of our clinical trials. For breast cancer its very important to do the studies up front in patients with metastatic disease where its possible. There are clinical trials now to the effect that this can be done with safety. Finally, most of the emphasis has been on how we can make FUra sensitive tumors more responsive by modulation. But I think it opens the door to the possibility that FUra insensitive tumors, and there are many clinically such, might be rendered sensitive by virtue of these kinds of modulations and that's another very big opportunity.

Dr. Holland: I wanted to talk about polyglutamation but Peter Houghton said he was going to and since they're his data I just would like to second whatever he is going to say. It does appear to me that Norman Wolmark didn't pay too much attention to my commentary, but I think for the NCI to be funding a multi-institutional, several hundred person trial of a phenomenon as important as this, in women with breast cancer, not to have either a FUra arm alone or a no treatment arm could be improved upon. I think that there are thousands, probably tens of thousands, of women in this country who will be getting CMF sometime in the next calendar year and although I don't personally believe that's the best adjuvant treatment they can get for their breast cancer, they will get it nonetheless. I think that the Cancer Institute could and should establish a trial, which could be conducted in the CCOP, to test adding CF to the FUra in that regimen since it could potentially give just a little bit more and that may be all it takes to change the cure rate considerably. Folic acid may be the dietary constituent that leads to some of the alleged benefits of macro-biotic diets. It seems to me rather than talk about pharmacologic treatment 1/2 hr before the administration of FUra one might be talking about a daily dietary treatment, and folic acid is sub-stantially cheaper than CF, and that needs studying.

As Howard Bruckner pointed out, this regimen is indeed active in many other neoplasms of the GI tract and the same schedule of FUra and of CF will not necessarily be applicable to each tumor in each site but be determined perhaps by the inherit characteristics of the tumor, let alone by the specific cytokinetics for each one. So I agree with Dr. Frei, this is a major step forward in chemotherapy and as such deserves a great deal of attention and effort. I don't disagree with Rick Moran that in fact we have identified, it seems to me in the GI tract particularly, TS as the target enzyme that makes most sense. That may not be true in sarcomas. In the GI tract, that is the target and it seems to me you could legitimately and profitably begin by studying the enzyme in vitro biochemically as a screen for other inhibitors and then back off so that you have to take it through a cell membrane and back off so that you have to take it through an animal and its liver, etc. to demonstrate a compound that is worthy to put in man, but knowing what the target is makes a huge difference in how much energy and emphasis you can place on it.

Dr. Mittelman: What we've being hearing for the past 2 days, is the natural history of a new therapy. I don't know whether we will find an optimal schedule, but for the short run I'm sure that given the multiplicity of interest and people, we'll probably find a useful

one. One of the things that seems to me to stand out as we listen
to our friends in the laboratory, is the repeated observation that
the epithelial tumors (ovarian, colon) have, as a rule, low levels
of folate and folate metabolites. We were totally unaware of this
as a general phenomenon. It was seen by Maire Hakala and others in
tissue culture and forms the basis of their experimentation. We
never until recently appreciated this, it would be wrong to call it
a deficiency, observation within a variety of human epithelial
tumors. We don't understand why the levels are low. Obviously it's
not true in every tumor or in every cell but it's a generality. We
don't understand why this occurs and we certainly are not clear as
to whether we can modulate this phenomena. Some of the evidence for
our ability to do so we heard today. There are obviously some
tumors in which we can give 20 mg, 50 mg, 500 mg, or perhaps a gram
and increase the levels of intracellular folates. It is unlikely
that we will find a schedule that will do so for every tumor. Is
there a way in which we can determine how to do it for classes of
tumor? Is there anything in our technical or scientific knowledge
which will enable us to make such a judgment? I think some of the
work from Gustavsson's laboratory gives us a hint in that direction
and some of the work that the Bergers presented yesterday offers us
a way of looking at these tumors. In other words, can we with
relative ease look at a tumor and identify certain of its biochemical and genetic features that will tell us something about what
we ought to give it. I would like to end on a more practical note.
I would like to propose at least for us to consider, that those
laboratories and groups that have the technical and scientific
capability to look at gene expression, to look at folate levels, to
look at the other things we are interested in, could perhaps come
together. Reliable human tissue is not easily come by. It isn't
the same as the leukemias but even among our colleagues who treat
the leukemias there is a shared resource of materials. What I would
like to suggest is that we do something comparable with FUra/CF and
some of the tumors that we have discussed today.

Dr. Schacter: I was struck yesterday while listening to some very
elegant biochemistry and pharmacology by the rather unpleasant and
nagging doubt that sometimes we're a little bit like the drunk who
looks for his keys under the lamp post because that's where the
light is. Often we do biochemistry on enzymes which we know how to
assay and we may not be looking at the only or even the primary
event in the cell. With that large caveat one is still stuck with
the observation that there appears to be a synergy with FUra and
CF. I think that it is critical that be rigorously explored in a
clinical setting at the earliest practical time and I think it gives
the opportunity to test in man some of the hypotheses which are
current at the moment. I would agree with the comment made earlier
that we don't have a very long time before FUra/CF becomes the
regime du jour as so many other combinations have before. I think
we owe it to ourselves at an early time to try to look at some of
the critical issues in a clinical setting to see whether current
biochemical concepts have much bearing on the clinical situation.
If you simply look at a multi-factoral situation there at least 24
combinations and permutations that one can look at. Fortunately, we
have a lot of patient material and it is possible with the help of
the people who have developed the theoretical basis to attempt to
answer some questions critically now rather than waiting. I think
there is a window of opportunity now, because of the growing
interest in this regimen, to set up clinical trials which will test
some of the biochemical hypotheses and see whether the keys are
indeed under the lamp post or someplace else.

Dr. Budd: I think we've made one of those small incremental steps that was referred to in the first talk yesterday, although we are at the bottom of the staircase looking up. In looking over the large number of clinical studies, particularly those big phase III trials in colon cancer, I'm struck both by the anomalies and consistencies. I think the consistency is that we can conclude that in the setting of a multi-institutional group such as the Southwest Oncology Group, when we studied this combination a few years ago finding a response rate of about 22%, or in the NCOG of the North Central Group, the response rate is about 20%. This is one small incremental step better than this same group of institutions would see with a dose of FUra producing equal toxicity. The one apparent anomaly would be the NCOG trial which showed that this was not superior to FUra but in looking at it I think that this supports the argument that an equally toxic dose of FUra/CF is more active in as much as an equiactive dose was twice as toxic. So that I think we do have evidence that an equally toxic dose of FUra/CF is more active than FUra alone. In looking at the anomalies in the North Central group, I am very intrigued by the finding that the low dose CF arm seemed to be superior to the high dose CF arm. I think that this is encouraging in a way for it shifts our focus away from the pharmacokinetics in the plasma to that in the tissue and I'm glad to see that the studies have been extended to the tumors and I would await the extension of these studies to the normal tissues which are manifesting the toxicity or are in fact spared the toxicity.

Dr. Houghton: I would like to take 3 pieces of data that were presented which struck me as really exciting and to say how they will influence short term the sort of experiments that we would be involved in at the preclincal level. Then I want to deal with what I think this meeting has achieved not just from the people presenting but from people in the audience who are involved in folate metabolism. Some of the ideas that have been generated may lead to long term approaches to devising somewhat better therapy than FUra/CF is currently achieving.

Three things struck me as being of real interest: one is the data of Dr. Duch who showed that you could get a lot of folate within a tumor and it didn't get anywhere. That data is so similar to the data that Janet Houghton has produced in her human xenograft systems that I think it is telling us something. It's telling us that by using high levels of precursors such as CF, we may in fact be working against ourselves. From our data we know that we have to produce a minimum of triglutamate of 5,10-methylenetetrahydrofolate to have a significant impact upon stabilization of the covalent ternary complex. The data that Dave Duch presented and analysis of Janet Houghton's data suggest that when we maintain a high level of a monoglutamate, such as CF or mainly 10-Formyltetrahydrofolate monoglutamate, within the cells this may in fact be preventing the formation of higher polyglutamates. So we're working against ourselves. The data of Dr. O'Connell, from the Mayo Clinic, gives further impetus at the preclinical level to re-exploring what would happen if we gave continuous but low levels of the precursor; to see whether we would in fact generate higher levels of the polyglutamates that we think are essential to modulate this interaction. So in the short term we're going to be looking at the role of low doses by continuous infusion. Dr. O'connell's data is very, very interesting.

The third piece of data that to me was exciting was that of Dr.
Gustavsson showing the difference in survival between patients with
tumors that have low levels of TS and those that have high levels.
I think if that data can be shown to exist in untreated tumors such
that it is a measure of some facet of the natural history of the
disease, I think that is really very remarkable. Certainly I look
forward to seeing more data from that same group.

Gratifying was the fact that, now that one is using human material
and measuring pools of 5,10-methylenetetrahydrofolate and tetrahydrofolate, the levels are very low and they are almost identical
to the levels that we predicted for human colon cancers back in
1981. I think the whole field has grown and now the methods for
looking at these pools, the polyglutamates, and the activities of
the enzymes involved in folate metabolism are now available to more
laboratories. One word of caution, however, these assays are not
trivial assays. To do them correctly, to do them precisely, takes a
fair degree of skill. So in some respects one looks at the data and
one has to perhaps weigh the data with the experience of the people
who are doing it. Perhaps Dr. Mittelman's idea of making some sort
of collaborative agreement with the laboratories involved in some of
these sophisticated methods may be a very good one.

I think what has come out of this whole area of FUra/CF and the fact
that the methylenetetrahydrofolate pools seem to be very low, is
that I talked with at least 3 chemists in the audience over the last
2 days who are suddenly thinking about how we can target this area
of folate metabolism. Suddenly, we're realizing that methylenetetrahydrofolate may be a major restriction within colorectal adenocarcinoma cells. Changing or ordering the fluxes through the
methylenetetrahydrofolate pool by inhibiting some of the other
enzymes that utilize 5,10-methylenetetrahydrofolate suddenly becomes
a realistic possibility. A second possibility is that we can design
analogs of CF that may either spontaneously within the cell generate
tetrahydrofolate, which is a lot closer to methylenetetrahydrofolate, or possibly act as slow release forms of CF that would after
bolus administration remain in the plasma for very considerable
amounts of time but constantly generate low levels of CF. These
ideas have been generated by getting a lot of people together who
have become interested in the idea of modulating FUra with CF. From
this are emerging new concepts of where we should be going.

Dr. Wittes: Let me just clarify what I think the sense of the panel
is, and that is that despite the very considerable unknowns that
remain and all the work left to be done, you feel that the modulation of FUra by CF in the clinical setting results in, among other
things, better therapy than with FUra alone; although the nature of
the improvements still leaves a lot to be desired. Is that correct?

PANEL ASSENTS

OPEN DISCUSSION WITH MEMBERS OF THE AUDIENCE

Dr. Santi: I still have a question. Do you people feel confident now
that if one had a truly selective inhibitor of TS, that it would be
a good anti-cancer agent; that is, do you really know or believe
that the selectivity you're seeing is due to differences in inhibition of that enzyme or due to transport or metabolism or polyglutamation or something else? The reason I think that is still an

important question to ask is that I think that, especially with the technologies that are available today, if you could point to that enzyme and be confident that a new, good inhibitor would work, I think that it could be done. I don't know how much energies are worth investing in that particular direction until that question is answered.

Dr. Mihich: In that connection, I think that perhaps when we are more sophisticated in relation to tumor sampling and analysis in the tumor, in addition to what I indicated initially in terms of individual sensitivity to some parameters, other avenues might be explored. In particular, the presence of iscenzymes of TS, originally described by Heidelberger and later confirmed by others, should be explored to see whether in those cases where there is not a response whether that is due to pharmacological factors like those which you alluded to or whether to the presence of a TS which in that particular tumor is not the target enzyme because of reduced affinity. It is part of the mosaic of biochemical parameters that one should try to identify in the individual tumor in attempting to correlate the response to modification of the biochemistry of the cell.

Dr. Houghton: The question is whether TS in human cells is a relevant target. I think that may well depend upon the tumor type. Our experience, so far with colorectal adenocarcinomas, suggests that if you delete TS, that is a major detriment to this cell. We have selected now 17 independent clones and all of them have great difficulty in surviving even under high levels of thymidine, whereas in mouse cells that doesn't seem to be the case. Perhaps in the colorectal adenocarcinomas their ability to salvage pre-formed thymidine is not going to be that great, so TS becomes a valid target.

Dr. Santi: So the answer is?

Dr. Houghton: So the answer is for at least some human cancers, TS is an important target.

Dr. Santi: If that's true, I think that you could seriously think about entering the inhibitor game again. If you're now at the level where you have identified a target that you feel confident is going to be successful then you can start playing games with deazafolates, for example, which are totally different, in terms of their behavior, than CF. The TS FdUMP-methylenetetrahydrofolate complex, at least in vitro, has a half-life, under conditions we use, of several hours. The off rate of the CB3717-dUMP-TS complex is about 24 hours and the FdUMP-CB3717-TS complex off rate has a half-life of 38 hours. So you can start answering questions about duration. If it is truly worth doing, I think that the technologies could be used to develop new targeted inhibitors of this enzyme. I'm not sure it's truly worth it at this point. That is why I asked the question.

Dr. Rustum: Since there are tumors in which TS is the target, it would be very worth while, to develop drugs toward that target. There are 2 points I want to make about Dr. Houghton's comment about low doses for continuous infusion. The reality of the clinical situation is the following: in patients with no prior chemotherapy, Dr. Doroshow has demonstrated in his trials a 50-55% response rate by continuous infusion of 500 mg/m^2 CF. In relapsed patients with advanced colorectal cancer, infusion of the same dose gives a response rate anywhere between 10-15%. This is continuous infusion for 5 days achieving a plasma concentration of 1-5 ?M 6S-CF. That tells us something; that it is the nature of the disease. In one type of disease you have 50% response rate by continuous infusion versus zero response rate using the same schedule in the same disease type. So if we're dealing with just the fact of the polyglutamation, which is a very important determinant, then continuous infusion in both cases should be comparable, yet the response rates in patients were very different. We have to deal with the issue of drug delivery to the tumor before we deal with drug metabolism. You may be delivering a small amount especially when you're dealing with solid tumors in patients or in the mouse for that fact. When you're dealing with a large solid tumor in the animal or the human, by infusing low doses you're delivering very little drug to that tumor. So we have to balance between drug delivery and drug metabolism in that tumor and I think we have to learn from the clinical realities in order to better design our pre-clinical experiments.

Dr. Houghton: I think your argument is not necessarily correct because both you and I could give at least 17 mechanisms of resistance to FUra without trying. It's very clear that you can have changes in just about every single enzyme involved in the metabolism. What I was proposing was that we look at the effect of low-dose continuous infusion of CF in pre-clinical models and determine what is happening to polyglutamate formation. If you look at the concentration of the monoglutamate that gives you a dissociation time of 100 min, it is 385 ?M, but with tetraglutamate it is less than 1 ?M. One is dealing with enormous differences in the concentration that are actually going to be useful. What I'm saying is that in the model systems we should go back and look at it. We can look at solid tumors in model systems, where we can very accurately look at the polyglutamates formed. I don't think that technology has been applied to clinical samples yet to look at the polyglutamates of 5,10-methylenetetrahydrofolate, maybe it will be more difficult to do that, and explore it. I think we should not have a closed mind. Whether we have entered the medical folklore that one has to use high doses of CF in the same way that we have entered medical folklore in terms of high-dose MTX, I don't know, but what I'm saying is we should go back and, with human tumors under defined conditions, look again.

Dr. Rustum: I don't think there is disagreement on the point of going back to the model system. I think the data during the last day clearly have demonstrated that we need to do studies in the model system based on what we know clinically to date. There is no question about this and the question of looking at polyglutamate formation at low doses, at different doses, different modes of administration is clearly an important area. All I'm saying is that the clinical findings are telling us something that should help us to re-think the designing of studies in the pre-clinical model systems. Certainly there are major differences between relapsed and newly diagnosed patients, and the mechanisms of resistance could be a hundred different things. If we for the moment concentrate on TS and if the folate pools play a role in this process there is something different here. In the 8 patients that we presented yesterday looking at the ability to modulate at the 2 hr infusion with 500 mg in previously untreated and previously treated patients, the difference in 5,10-methylenetetrahydrofolate is somewhere around 3-4 fold. You may say this is not a significant difference. We don't know what the polyglutamates are, but if you look at TS inhibition you find 80-90% inhibition when modulation increases pools by 3-4 fold versus 30% inhibition when you have only changed these folate pools 2-fold. That is the difference between newly diagnosed and relapsed patients so there is something there that we should try to learn from, I think.

Dr. Hakala: I just want to agree with Joe that the basis of the selectivity certainly can be thousands of different reasons. Even though this combination of FUra/CF is based on rational knowledge from enzyme and cell systems, we still do not know how many different variations we would find; let us say, metabolism of FUra can differ even from patient to patient in one type of tumor and then metabolism of CF, uptake and metabolism, etc. I was thinking when I listened to the talk from the Mayo Clinic where they said the low doses of CF are statistically better. In a cellular system we have observed that the higher the intracellular content of FdUMP the less CF you need for potentiation, thus we need to know how much FdUMP is formed from FUra. Not every cell is the same in this regard. It becomes an enormous project if one wants to do good and thorough work. I feel that the clinical testing is still very empirical and that it would be impossible to do everything that one should do. I agree with Dr. Houghton when he said that whatever we are going to test, it should be done using identical, absolutely reliable testing methods, otherwise we can't compare from one place to another. Is there is anybody who is ambitious to be a service laborabory?

Dr. Spears: I'm not going to volunteer to do all of those specimens Dr. Hakala, but I wanted to make just a couple of comments. It is unfortunate that Dr. Heidelberger can no longer share some of this success. FUra was the first successful rationally synthesized anti-metabolite. Now today I think we're hearing that this is the first rational biochemical modulation that seems to have come of age. What we usually hear in medical oncology is an attempt to find out why patients respond by listening to patient characteristics for 80% of most clinical presentations. We try to find out why the tumors are different by finding out why the patients are different. Now we have a chance to really do things rationally by looking at the tumors. I disagree with the comments that I keep hearing repeatedly that these methods are difficult. They are all simple, direct binding assays or tritium release assays. The tritium release assay proposed by you Peter, for example, can be done in 1 mg size tissue needle aspirates. Your suggestion for a neutral charcoal clean up at the end of the TS incubation is readily applicable. What I would like to do in my manuscript is put down a little bit of cook book approach to what we have had experience in doing in applying David Priest's folate binding assay, your tritium release assay from Memphis, Rick Moran's FdUMP and [C^{14}] dUMP assays and some of our FdUMP binding experiences that would make it easy for other laboratories to follow.

Dr. Rustum: About a year ago I sent a letter to NCI proposing a "Task Force" to get together on the methodology (which is extremely difficult, in my opinion, and variable among different laboratories) and to decide which things need to be done and how they need to be done. I must say that I have not heard a response to my letter. I still think a Task Force for getting people together to plan, discuss, and have a common methodological approach to the measurement of TS, or of the polyglutamates or the tissue handling, etc. would be very worthwhile and I think it is timely.

When we talk about the difficulty in using tumors from human tissues, let me tell you what we did 5 years ago. We took a tumor from pathology with the pathologist present and cut it into 2 pieces. One piece was frozen very quickly right in surgery, the other was left on ice. Within 1 hr after removal of the tissue on ice, there was no assayable TS in that tissue. When we talk about level of TS activity in human tumors, low versus high, this is an extremely variable parameter and we have to be extremely careful about processing of these tumors from surgery before one can do reliable assays. Quality control is extremely important when you are dealing with clinical material and when you are dealing with solid tumor in general, either from the mouse or rat or human. Dr. Allegra said he could measure TS in only 60% of his tumors. In 60% of pieces coming from our clinic, I could not measure TS although under the most rigorous means of getting the tumor into the laboratory. Is it really low? I think the biochemical assay for TS which requires maybe 200 - 300 mg is not going to be very feasible when we try to apply it to clinical material. There are cDNAs for TS available to certain groups but not to the other and some of us are frustrated to try to get these things. There are laboratory needs to develop some new approaches toward accurate measurement and quantitation of thymidylate synthase in clinical material and/or pre-clinical tumors. I think there is a lot that needs to be done in the laboratory and the model systems. I fully agree with Peter on this. We should not lose sight of that.

Dr. **Mihich**:   I think that in summing up the conversation that occurred in the last 15-20 min it is as important to understand why a treatment acts on a particular tumor as it is why it does not act on a particular tumor. When you are talking about these different results with infusion versus high dose, etc., I think that it becomes very important to correlate the non-activity as well as the activity with a parameter of response. The question then can be summarized in 2 aspects: (1) the quality control of the technology, whatever the technology is; and (2) the establishment of the priorities. One cannot do everything. One has to identify on the basis of biochemical acumen which priorities are more cost effective in terms of effort to measure, in trying to correlate response or non-response.

Dr. **Wittes**   Let me just add in closing that I'm really in complete sympathy with these goals as well. I might even have been a year ago if you had let me know that they were on your mind. I think we will give reasonable priority to convening a small group of people who can perhaps set forth some ideas about how things ought to proceed from here. One last comment and I think we'll go to Dr. Rustum's closing remarks.

Dr. **Santi**:   I would like to say that in terms of the assays, it seems to me that measuring mRNA levels is obviously one approach that hasn't been used. Because we could not get the extant clones made available to us, we have isolated all the cDNA probes from human DNA that you would want and I would be very happy to give them to you if there was some central place to put them. Also, for the enzyme assay systems we have an expression system of the L.casei enzyme that is producing an order of magnitude more enzyme than the natural resistant mutant that I would also be quite willing to give to anybody who wants. I think if there is some central source I could put them in, I would do that next week.

Dr. Wittes: We thank the members of the panel and the speakers of the day Joe.

Dr. Rustum: I think the hour is getting late and scientifically I have very little to add to what has been said and talked about during the last couple days. I think the panel discussions and the various discussants summarized it very nicely. I just want to take this opportunity to thank everyone for coming to Buffalo and certainly from my point of view it has been very educational, very useful, and I am glad we did it. Lastly but not least I again want to take this opportunity to thank very much the people who helped us to organize this meeting. Without them there it certainly would not have been a meeting. The RPMI personnel in the Medical Illustration and Medical Photography Departments and the projectionist Mr. Fred Haller certainly did an absolutely superb job and I thank them very much for their time and effort. Gayle Bersani, of the Education Department, and my secretary Geri Wagner, have done a superb job. I want to thank the companies who have contributed significant monies to this namely, Lederle, Burroughs Wellcome, Kyowa Hakko Kogyo of Japan; without their generosity and support certainly this meeting would not have come about.

ADJOURNMENT

ABBREVIATIONS

CH$_2$-H$_4$PteGlu   5,10-methylenetetrahydrofolate
5-CHO-H$_4$PteGlu*   5-formyltetrahydrofolate
5-CH$_3$-H$_4$PteGlu   5-methyltetrahydrofolate
CNS   central nervous system
CF*   citrovorum factor
                              (folinic acid, leucovorin)
CR   complete response
dTMP   thymidylate
dUMP   2'-deoxyuridylate
dUrd   2'-deoxyuridine
ECOG   Eastern Cooperative Oncology Group
FA*   folinic acid
FdUMP   5-fluoro-2'-deoxyuridylate
FdUrd   5-fluoro-2'-deoxyuridine
5-formyl-H$_4$PteGlu*   5-formyltetrahydrofolic acid
FPGS   folylpolyglutamate synthetase
FUra   5-fluorouracil
GI   gastrointestinal
GITSG   Gastrointestinal Tumor Study Group
H$_2$PteGlu   dihydrofolate
H$_4$PteGlu   tetrahydrofolate
HPLC   high performance liquid chromatography
IC$_{50}$ concentration of drug to inhibit
                              growth by 50%
IMP   inosinic acid
IV   intravenous
k$_{off}$ rate constant for dissociation
k$_{on}$ rate constant for association
LV*   leucovorin
MTX   methotrexate
NR   no response
PD   progressive disease
PR   partial response
Pts   patients
PteGlu   folic acid
TS   thymidylate synthase

* Folinic acid, citrovorum factor, and leucovorin are all used to
  describe racemic (6R,S) 5-formyltetrahydrofolate (5-HCO-H$_4$PteGlu).
  CF is the preferred abbreviation for this volume.

  Poly-gamma-glutamyl metabolites of all derivatives of folic acid
  (PteGlu), including all reduced and one-carbon substituted forms, are
  indicated by a subscript number following Glu, e.g., PteGlu$_2$. The
  subscript indicates the total number of glutamate residues in the
  molecule, thus PteGlu$_2$ is pteroylglutamyl-gamma-glutamate.

AUTHOR INDEX

SUBJECT INDEX

Since this symposium dealt with the topic of chemotherapy using the
combination of 5-fluorouracil and citrovorum factor (called by one or
another of its synonyms), the index does not include citations to every
contribution under each of these headings. Citations were included only
in the cases where the editors decided that they were warranted.
Similarly, since citrovorum factor is called by many different names
(5-formyltetrahydrofolate, leucovorin, folinic acid) each reference does
not appear under all the titles. Abbreviations used are those defined
on p. 329.

333